AF572642

Cardiac Drug Therapy

Cardiovascular Clinics Series

Brest	1/1	Hypertensive Cardiovascular Disease
Brest	1/2	Coronary Heart Disease
Brest	1/3	Cardiovascular Therapy
Downing	2/1	Congenital Heart Disease
Dreifus	*2/2	Arrhythmias
White	2/3	International Cardiology
Gifford	3/1	Peripheral Vascular Disease
Harken	*3/2	Cardiac Surgery 1
Harken	*3/3	Cardiac Surgery 2
Burch	*4/1	Cardiomyopathy
Edwards	*4/2	Clinical-Pathological Correlations 1
Engle	4/3	Pediatric Cardiology
Edwards	*5/1	Clinical-Pathological Correlations 2
Likoff	*5/2	Valvular Heart Disease
Fisch	*5/3	Complex Electrocardiography 1
Fisch	*6/1	Complex Electrocardiography 2
Melmon	*6/2	Cardiovascular Drug Therapy
Fowler	6/3	Diagnostic Methods in Cardiology
Vidt	7/1	Cleveland Clinic Cardiovascular Consultations
Brest et al.	7/2	Innovations in the Diagnosis and Management of Acute Myocardial Infarction
Spodick	7/3	Pericardial Diseases
Corday	8/1	Controversies in Cardiology
Rahimtoola	8/2	Coronary Bypass Surgery
Rios	8/3	Clinical Electrocardiographic Correlations
Onesti, Brest	9/1	Hypertension
Kotler, Segal	9/2	Clinical Echocardiography
Wenger	*9/3	Exercise and the Heart
Roberts	*10/1	Congenital Heart Disease in Adults
Willerson	*10/2	Nuclear Cardiology
Brandenburg	10/3	Office Cardiology
Castellanos	11/1	Cardiac Arrhythmias: Mechanisms and Management
Engle	11/2	Pediatric Cardiovascular Disease
Rackley	11/3	Critical Care Cardiology
Noble, Rothbaum	12/1	Geriatric Cardiology
Vidt	12/2	Cardiovascular Therapy
McGoon	12/3	Cardiac Surgery
Rahimtoola	13/1	Controversies in Coronary Artery Disease
Spittell	13/2	Clinical Vascular Disease
Fowler	13/3	Noninvasive Diagnostic Methods in Cardiology
Goldberg	14/1	Coronary Artery Spasm and Thrombosis
Dreifus	14/2	Pacemaker Therapy

*Not Available

Cardiac Drug Therapy

C. Richard Conti, M.D. | Editor

Professor of Medicine
Chief, Division of Cardiology
University of Florida
Gainesville, Florida

CARDIOVASCULAR CLINICS

Albert N. Brest, M.D. | Editor-in-Chief

James C. Wilson Professor of Medicine
Director, Division of Cardiology
Jefferson Medical College
Philadelphia, Pennsylvania

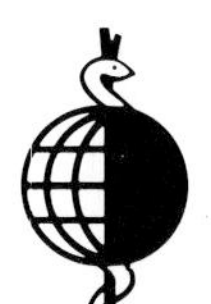

F. A. DAVIS COMPANY, PHILADELPHIA

Cardiovascular Clinics, 14/3, Cardiac Drug Therapy

Printed in the United States of America

NOTE: As new scientific information becomes available through basic and clinical research, recommended treatments and drug therapies undergo changes. The authors and publisher have done everything possible to make this book accurate, up-to-date, and in accord with accepted standards at the time of publication. However, the reader is advised always to check product information (package inserts) for changes and new information regarding dose and contraindications before administering any drug. Caution is especially urged when using new or infrequently ordered drugs.

Library of Congress Cataloging in Publication Data
Main entry under title:

Cardiac drug therapy.

(Cardiovascular clinics ; 14/3)
Includes bibliographical references and index.
1. Cardiovascular agents. 2. Heart—Diseases—Chemotherapy.
I. Conti, C. Richard. II. Series.
RM345.C33 1984 616.1′061 83-15440
ISBN 0-8036-1975-8

Preface

Twenty-five years ago, drug therapy for cardiovascular problems was relatively simple. Heart failure was treated with digitalis and mercurial diuretics, hypertension with reserpine, arrhythmias with quinidine and procainamide, angina with sublingual nitroglycerin, myocardial infarction with morphine and oxygen, and hyperlipidemia with diet. Bacterial endocarditis was treated with penicillin, streptomycin, vancomycin, and a few other antibiotics. Beta blockers and calcium-channel blockers were unknown to the physician taking care of patients.

Since that time, an enormous number of new drugs have become available. The clinician is now armed with a variety of drugs that can be used alone or in combination with other agents for the management of conditions that were inadequately treated in the past.

The purpose of this book is to consolidate current thinking about the management of common cardiac conditions with currently available drugs. By design, there is some overlap of the chapters because some deal with clinical pharmacology of specific drugs whereas others discuss specific conditions such as myocardial infarction treated with a variety of drugs. Some of the drugs that are mentioned in this text are not available for clinical use in the United States at this time, but either they or their congeners probably will be introduced here in the future.

This text is authored by experts in their field and should be of use to the student as well as the experienced, demanding clinician. It can be a reference source for all those interested in understanding some basic concepts of cardiac drug therapy, for example, basic pharmacology of beta blockers, calcium-channel blockers, antiarrhythmic agents, and inotropic drugs. In addition, I believe that it will serve a useful function as a quick reference for physicians who manage acutely ill patients in the coronary care unit.

We have included a chapter dealing with platelet-suppressive therapy in cardiovascular disease. This is an area considered to be of great importance but relatively new to most physicians caring for patients with cardiac disease.

As mentioned before, in the past 25 years, enormous strides have been made in the development of cardiac drugs and the use of these drugs for treating common cardiac conditions. I suspect that many of the currently available drugs will still be used 25 years from now, but the editor of a textbook on cardiac drug therapy at that time will have a book twice the size of this one.

C. Richard Conti, M.D.
Guest Editor

Editor's Commentary

During the past decade, no aspect of cardiology has flourished more than the advances in cardiac drug therapy. Better understanding of the adrenergic nervous system has permitted important developments and expanded uses for beta and alpha blockade. Attention to afterload reduction has enhanced our ability to manage low cardiac output syndromes and congestive failure. The advent of calcium-channel blockers has expanded our understanding and treatment of anginal syndromes. Thrombolytic therapy has provided an entirely new dimension to the handling of acute myocardial infarction. Antiplatelet therapy has proved to be increasingly important, as the role of platelets in cardiovascular disease has unfolded. There have been many other significant advances in the management of hypertension, hyperlipidemia, cardiac arrhythmias, myocardial ischemia, and valvular disease. These various developments are reviewed and put into perspective by the outstanding group of investigators who have contributed to this issue of CARDIOVASCULAR CLINICS. I am extremely grateful to C. Richard Conti for his guidance in the formulation of this book, and both of us are indebted to the contributors for their scholarly contributions.

Albert N. Brest, M.D.
Editor-in-Chief

Contributors

P. C. Adams, B.A., M.R.C.P.
British Heart Foundation Junior Research Fellow; Registrar, Department of Cardiology, Freeman Hospital, Newcastle upon Tyne, England

Andrew G. Bodnar, M.D.
Instructor in Medicine, Harvard Medical School; Assistant in Medicine, Cardiac Unit, Massachusetts General Hospital, Boston, Massachusetts

Eugene Braunwald, M.D.
Hersey Professor of the Theory and Practice of Physic and Herman Ludwig Blumgart Professor of Medicine, Harvard Medical School; Chairman, Department of Medicine, Brigham and Women's Hospital and Beth Israel Hospital, Boston, Massachusetts

Albert N. Brest, M.D.
James C. Wilson Professor of Medicine; Director, Division of Cardiology, Jefferson Medical College, Philadelphia, Pennsylvania

R. W. F. Campbell, F.R.C.P.
Senior Lecturer, Department of Cardiology, University of Newcastle upon Tyne, Freeman Hospital, Newcastle upon Tyne, England

Wilson S. Colucci, M.D.
Assistant Professor of Medicine, Harvard Medical School; Associate Physician, Cardiovascular Division, Brigham and Women's Hospital, Boston, Massachusetts

C. Richard Conti, M.D.
Professor of Medicine; Chief, Division of Cardiology, University of Florida, Gainesville, Florida

Michael J. Cowley, M.D.
Associate Professor of Medicine, Medical College of Virginia, Richmond, Virginia

Debra S. Echt, M.D.
Clinical Assistant Professor of Medicine; Director of the Cardiac Pacemaker Service, Stanford University Medical Center, Stanford, California

Robert L. Feldman, M.D.
Associate Professor of Medicine, Division of Cardiology, University of Florida, Shands Teaching Hospital and Gainesville Veterans Administration Hospital, Gainesville, Florida

John T. Flaherty, M.D.
Associate Professor of Medicine, Division of Cardiology, The Johns Hopkins Hospital, Baltimore, Maryland

Frank A. Franklin, Jr., M.D., Ph.D.
Assistant Professor, Department of Pediatrics; Division of Lipid Research—Atherosclerosis, Johns Hopkins University School of Medicine, Baltimore, Maryland

Sidney Goldstein, M.D.
Clinical Professor of Medicine, University of Michigan School of Medicine; Head, Division of Cardiovascular Medicine, Henry Ford Hospital, Detroit, Michigan

Andrea Hastillo, M.D.
Director, Coronary Intensive Care Unit; Associate Professor of Medicine and Cardiology, Medical College of Virginia, Richmond, Virginia

Philip D. Henry, M.D.
Professor of Medicine, Baylor College of Medicine, Texas Medical Center, Houston, Texas

J. O'Neal Humphries, M.D.
O. B. Mayer Sr. and Jr. Professor of Medicine; Chairman, Department of Internal Medicine, University of South Carolina School of Medicine, Richland Memorial Hospital, Columbia, South Carolina

Adolph M. Hutter, Jr., M.D.
Associate Professor of Medicine, Harvard Medical School; Director, Coronary Care Unit, Massachusetts General Hospital, Boston, Massachusetts

D. G. Julian, M.D., F.R.C.P.
British Heart Foundation Professor of Cardiology, Department of Cardiology, Freeman Hospital, Newcastle upon Tyne, England

T. H. Le Jemtel, M.D.
Assistant Professor of Medicine, Albert Einstein College of Medicine, Bronx, New York

David T. Lowenthal, M.D.
Professor of Medicine and Pharmacology; Director, Clinical Pharmacology and Cardiac Fitness Center, Likoff Cardiovascular Institute, Hahnemann University, Philadelphia, Pennsylvania

Simeon Margolis, M.D., Ph.D.
Professor of Medicine and Physiological Chemistry, Division of Endocrinology and Metabolism, Department of Medicine, The Johns Hopkins University School of Medicine, Baltimore, Maryland

Carol S. Maskin, M.D.
Assistant Professor of Medicine, Albert Einstein College of Medicine, Bronx, New York

Jay W. Mason, M.D.
Professor of Medicine; Chief, Division of Cardiology, University of Utah Medical Center, Salt Lake City, Utah

Jawahar Mehta, M.D.
Associate Professor of Medicine, Division of Cardiology, University of Florida College of Medicine; Director, Coronary Care Unit, Veterans Administration Medical Center, Gainesville, Florida

Suzanne Oparil, M.D.
Professor of Medicine; Associate Professor of Physiology and Biophysics, The University of Alabama in Birmingham, School of Medicine, Birmingham, Alabama

Carl J. Pepine, M.D.
Professor of Medicine/Cardiology; Associate Director of Cardiology, University of Florida; Chief, Cardiology, Veterans Administration Medical Center, Gainesville, Florida

Julio E. Pérez, M.D.
Assistant Professor of Medicine, Department of Medicine (Cardiovascular Division), Washington University School of Medicine, St. Louis, Missouri

Reuben Ramphal, M.D.
Assistant Professor of Medicine, University of Florida College of Medicine, Gainesville, Florida

Howard S. Rosman, M.D.
Clinical Assistant Professor of Medicine, University of Michigan School of Medicine; Senior Staff Physician, Cardiovascular Medicine, Henry Ford Hospital, Detroit, Michigan

Louis Roy, M.D.
Research Fellow, Division of Cardiology, University of Florida College of Medicine, Gainesville, Florida

Stanley A. Rubin, M.D.
Assistant Professor of Medicine, UCLA School of Medicine; Associate Cardiologist, Cedars-Sinai Medical Center, Los Angeles, California

Joseph W. Shands, Jr., M.D.
Professor of Medicine and Chief, Infectious Disease, University of Florida College of Medicine, Gainesville, Florida

Edmund H. Sonnenblick, M.D.
Professor of Medicine; Chief, Division of Cardiology, Albert Einstein College of Medicine, Bronx, New York

H. J. C. Swan, M.D., Ph.D.
Professor of Medicine, UCLA School of Medicine; Director, Division of Cardiology, Cedars-Sinai Medical Center, Los Angeles, California

Sherry Winternitz, M.D.
Assistant Professor of Medicine, Cardiovascular Research and Training Center, University of Alabama in Birmingham, School of Medicine, Birmingham, Alabama

Contents

Inotropic Drugs for Treatment of the Failing Heart

Carol S. Maskin, M.D., T.H. Le Jemtel, M.D., and Edmund H. Sonnenblick, M.D.

Congestive heart failure is a systemic disease manifested variously by abnormalities in neuroendocrine, renal, hepatic, peripheral vascular, and respiratory function caused by an intrinsic depression of myocardial contractility and a failure of compensatory mechanisms to maintain an adequate cardiac output. Clinically, patients with heart failure are limited by symptoms of dyspnea related to elevated pulmonary venous pressures, and of fatigue related to a markedly reduced ability to augment cardiac output as required by metabolically active organs, for instance, during exercise.[1–5] Worsening symptoms and deterioration of functional capacity in these patients are generally due to progression of the underlying cardiac disease, as well as to the effects of enhanced activity of compensatory mechanisms, such as increased activity of the sympathetic[6,7] and renin-angiotensin-aldosterone systems[8–10] on peripheral vascular resistance and hence impedance to left ventricular ejection, and on regional distribution of blood flow.

Optimally, a therapeutic intervention should directly or indirectly alter the progression of the underlying myocardial disease responsible for depressed contractility, as manifested in the intact heart by reduced maximum developed tension at any given ventricular end-diastolic volume.[11,12] Failure of the heart as a pump generally occurs in the presence of a hemodynamic overload, with myocardial cell loss, segmental (coronary artery disease) or diffuse (cardiomyopathies),[13] and subsequent fibrosis and hypertrophy of remaining myocardial cells. As the compensatory hypertrophy fails, ventricular dilatation ensues as well.[14–16] Unfortunately, the structural and/or biochemical derangements responsible for depressed contractility remain unclear[17] and may indeed differ with respect to the etiology of heart failure (i.e., ischemic heart disease; pressure/volume overload; diffuse cardiomyopathy) and with the stage of the disease. Whether a primary process such as microvascular spasm and cell loss contributes to the development of progressive myocardial failure[17] is yet to be fully explored. Thus, specific therapeutic modalities are yet to be developed, and congestive heart failure remains largely an enigmatic and progressive disease.

Thus, currently, the overall aim of therapy in heart failure is to improve symptoms of congestion, exercise tolerance, and hence quality of life, and is focused on optimizing cardiac output via pharmacologic manipulation of the four determinants of left ventricular performance: ventricular filling pressure (preload), arterial pressure and the resistance to ventricular emptying (afterload), myocardial contractility, and cardiac rate and rhythm.

The use of inotropic agents to stimulate the depressed myocardium is predicated on the existence of residual myocardial function,[18] or a "contractile reserve," as suggested in animal models of heart failure,[19–21] and in the failing human heart by postextrasystolic beat potentiation, demonstrated with paired electrical stimulation.[22] To be clinically meaningful, however, the increase in myocardial contractility thereby induced must be of sufficient magnitude to significantly augment global cardiac performance and systemic perfusion. Relative to this condition, the effectiveness of any given inotropic agent may be limited by the relative potency and toxic/therapeutic ratio of the drug; its mechanism of action; and the quantity of "contractile reserve" available, which may indeed vary greatly depending on the severity, chronicity, and etiology of heart failure. Furthermore, it is important to recognize that the ability of an inotropic agent to acutely improve maximum aerobic exercise capacity in patients with chronic heart failure may be limited, despite substantial augmentation of pump function, by a diminished and fixed capacity to acutely increase maximum blood flow in exercising muscles related to factors such as salt and water retention in the vessel walls and interstitial edema with consequent increased tissue pressure.[23–25]

Regardless of the magnitude of acute hemodynamic improvement achieved with any cardioactive agent, the substantive issue remains whether the patient will continue to feel and function better with chronic therapy and without adverse effects. Indeed, it has been observed that the magnitude of acute hemodynamic response to an agent does not predict the patient's long-term outcome with continued therapy.[26–28] Other important considerations include the ability of the drug to induce long-term improvement of cardiac performance without development of tachyphylaxis; the drug's ability to eliminate excess sodium and water and to attenuate the heightened activity of the sympathetic and renin-angiotensin-aldosterone systems, with consequent reduction of impedance to left ventricular ejection, and improvement of regional distribution of blood flow and organ function in general; and the drug's effect on the progression of the underlying myocardial disease. Indeed, to understand the clinical response during long-term therapy, it may be most helpful to repeat hemodynamic evaluation on maintenance therapy and after withdrawal and reinstitution of the drug, using the patient as his or her own control.[27,29]

Table 1. Inotropic agents

1. CALCIUM		
2. DIGITALIS GLYCOSIDES		Na-K ATPase inhibition
3. CATECHOLAMINES		
	Norepinephrine	
I.V.	Epinephrine	β_1 stimulation → ↑ Cyclic AMP
	Isoproterenol	
	Dopamine	
	Dobutamine	
	Prenalterol (Astra)	
	Butopamine (Lilly)	β_1 stimulation
Oral	H 80/63 (Ciba-Geigy)	
	Pirbuterol (Pfizer)	β_1 and (?) β_2 stimulation
	Salbutamol	Dopaminergic receptor stimulation
	Ibopamine (Smith, Kline, French)	β_1 stimulation and partial β_1 inhibition
	ICI 118,587	
4. XANTHINES		
	Theophylline	Phosphodiesterase inhibition → ↑ cyclic AMP
	Caffeine	↑ Ca^{++} movement
5. GLUCAGON		Cyclic AMP
6. New Agents		
	Amrinone (Sterline)	↑ Ca^{++} movement (?)
	WIN 47203 (Sterling)	Phosphodiesterase inhibition
	ARL-115 BS (Vardex)	
	MDL 17043 (Merrell)	

A further consideration relative to the use of inotropic agents is their potential contribution to the progression of the cardiac disease. For example, stimulation of the inotropic state can directly augment myocardial oxygen demand or it may reduce metabolic demands via a reduction of heart size and hence wall tension.[30–32] Furthermore, these metabolic effects may differ with respect to the etiology of heart failure and the stage of the disease. Although several investigators have described the acute effects of various inotropic agents on cardiac metabolism and function in humans,[30,33–37] these responses may not predict the effects of chronic therapy on the myocardium. Indeed, to address these issues, long-term controlled studies are needed.

Inotropic stimulation of the failing heart appears to work ultimately by increasing the amount of activating calcium available for the contractile system. There is no evidence that inotropic agents "cure" the specific contractile abnormalities of the failing myocardium; thus, it is important to recognize that to maintain the desired effects, these agents must be administered on a long-term basis. As illustrated in Table 1, the list of inotropic agents currently available is not very long, and their mechanisms of action are few. Indeed, the net hemodynamic effect observed with several of these agents is related to their concomitant effects on peripheral vascular tone and cardiac rate and rhythm, as well as on inotropic state.

CATECHOLAMINES

Catecholamines exert an inotropic effect by stimulation of myocardial $beta_1$-adrenergic receptors. Stimulation of $beta_1$ receptors in the sarcoplasmic reticulum activates adenyl cyclase, which in turn catalyzes the conversion of ATP to 3′5′-cyclic AMP. Protein kinases are then activated, which allow phosphorylation of multiple membrane systems, resulting in enhanced transfer of ionized calcium. The positive inotropic effect results from increased calcium availability to the contractile proteins and/or enhanced removal of ionized calcium from the myoplasm and thus more rapid relaxation.[38] Activation of $beta_1$ receptors, however, also enhances sinoatrial discharge and atrioventricular conduction. The resulting tachycardia and/or arrhythmia may indeed limit the tolerable dose and thus the maximum inotropic effect achieved clinically by various sympathomimetic agents.

In addition to the desired $beta_1$ effects, most available sympathomimetic agents also stimulate vascular $beta_2$-adrenergic receptors, which in turn mediate peripheral vasodilation and/or alpha-adrenergic receptors that stimulate vasoconstriction. Clinically, the hemodynamic effects produced by a given sympathomimetic agent reflect the absolute and relative activation of these receptors (Fig. 1).

Several catecholamines are available for parenteral use.

Norepinephrine may substantially augment contractility and cardiac performance via stimulation of myocardial $beta_1$ receptors. Concomitant alpha-adrenergic effects, however, may cause considerable elevation of arterial pressure that may be desirable only when heart failure is accompanied by severe hypotension. Similarly, isoproterenol greatly enhances contractility; however, concomitant $beta_2$ stimulation may lower systemic vascular resistance and arterial pressure. The clinical benefits of both agents are further complicated by their marked positive chronotropic effect at doses required to produce the desired inotropic response, and by a significant incidence of malignant ventricular arrhythmias.

Dopamine is a biologic precursor in the endogenous synthesis of norepinephrine. Its inotropic effect is mediated in part by direct $beta_1$-receptor stimulation and partly via release of myocardial stores of norepinephrine,[39] thereby potentially limiting its activity in advanced heart failure when such stores may be largely depleted.[6] In addition to its inotropic properties, dopamine has the unique ability to stimulate vasodilatory dopaminergic receptors in the kidney and thereby facilitate diuresis. Intravenous administration in doses ranging from 2 to 5 $\mu g/kg/min$ has been shown to augment cardiac output with little change in left ventricular filling pressure. Doses greater than 6 $\mu g/kg/min$ are associated with increased heart rates and with a predominant alpha-adrenergic effect, similar to that of norepinephrine.

Adrenergic-Receptor Activity of Sympathomimetic Amines.

	α	β_1	β_2
	PERIPHERAL	CARDIAC	PERIPHERAL
Norepinephrine	++++	++++	0
Epinephrine	++++	++++	++
Dopamine*	++++	++++	+
Isoproterenol	0	++++	++++
Dobutamine	+	++++	++
Methoxamine	++++	0	0

*Causes renal & mesenteric dilatation by stimulating dopaminergic receptors.

Figure 1. Relative effects of various catecholamines on receptors.

Dobutamine is a synthetic catecholamine that is available for parenteral use. Its predominant action is direct stimulation of myocardial $beta_1$ receptors, with lesser effects on $beta_2$ and alpha receptors.[40,41] Furthermore, it appears to exert a lesser effect on the sinoatrial node than on ventricular contractile tissue. Thus, dobutamine increases contractility with little effect on blood pressure or heart rate when administered in doses ranging between 5 and 10 μg/kg/min and thereby constitutes a very useful catecholamine for acute stimulation of the failing heart when severe hypotension is not present. It is important to be aware, however, that an attenuation of the hemodynamic effects of dobutamine may occur, even within 8 hours of administration,[42,43] requiring upward dose titration to maintain the desired response. Indeed, this observation is suggestive of a rapid induction of a "down-regulation" of myocardial $beta_1$ receptors.

Of special interest is the description of ultrastructural myocardial changes observed in association with prolonged (72 hours) dobutamine infusion[44] and sustained hemodynamic improvement. These changes included reduction of the number of electron-dense particles per 100 mitochondria, an increased cristae-to-matrix ratio within the mitochondria, and a decrease in mitochondria size. Although the mechanisms by which dobutamine may induce morphologic improvements are not understood, the possibility that an inotropic intervention could trigger certain reparative myocellular processes is certainly exciting. Interesting as well is the recent description of improvement of functional capacity following repeated brief infusions of dobutamine, in a form of "pulse therapy."[45] The physiologic changes responsible for this observation remain speculative.

A small number of orally active synthetic catecholamines have been developed and are presently under investigation. Unfortunately, use of the parenteral compounds has been associated with several problems including lack of myocardial $beta_1$-receptor selectivity, tachycardia, arrhythmias, and tachyphylaxis. Furthermore, the use of catecholamines with significant $beta_2$-agonist activity may be complicated by noncardiovascular side effects including tremulousness and anxiety.

Pirbuterol is an oral catecholamine with hemodynamic effects that appear to be mediated predominantly via stimulation of vascular $beta_2$-adrenergic receptors. Therefore it appears to act largely as a vasodilating agent rather than as an inotropic agent.[34,35,46–48] Similarly, *salbutamol* acts predominantly via stimulation of $beta_2$ receptors.[35,49] It is of interest that both agents have been shown to augment left ventricular dp/dt in patients with heart failure.[34,35,49] It is unclear, however, whether the latter effect reflects direct drug actions or results from reflex release of catecholamines in response to the reduced systemic vascular resistance. Regardless of the mechanism responsible for increased dp/dt, pirbuterol has been variously reported to have both a beneficial effect[35–37] and a detrimental effect[37] on myocardial oxygen consumption in patients with severe heart failure. Indeed, such disparity may reflect differences in the study populations and a variability of drug effect on peripheral vascular resistance and hence impedance to left ventricular ejection relative to the severity of the underlying disease.

Preliminary clinical studies have demonstrated acute and short-term improvements in cardiac performance following oral administration of pirbuterol to patients with severe heart failure. These hemodynamic benefits have not been accompanied by acute improvements in exercise capacity and maximum oxygen uptake. Furthermore, the long-term clinical experience with pirbuterol in uncontrolled studies has been variable.[50–54] Indeed, whereas some investigators have observed significant improvements in indices of cardiac performance and in treadmill exercise tolerance during 6 weeks of continued therapy, others have reported attenuation of both symptomatic and clinical benefits following only 1 month. Of special interest, attenuation of drug effect has been associated with a reduction of lymphocyte beta-adrenergic receptor density.[54] Whether a similar "down-regulation" of beta-adrenergic receptors occurs in myocardial and vascular tissues, thereby effectively limiting responsiveness to pirbuterol, is unknown. Recently, however, using a controlled double-blind protocol, Weber and associates[28] could not demonstrate significant improvements in functional status or in exercise capacity and maximum oxygen uptake during chronic pirbuterol therapy in patients with severe heart failure, despite initial hemodynamic benefits. Furthermore, in this study, adverse effects attributable to beta$_2$-agonist activity, including tremulousness and nervousness, limited the tolerable dosage in 37 percent of patients to less than the optimal daily dose of 60 mg. These data suggest that the role of pirbuterol in the chronic management of heart failure is very limited. The poor correlation observed between the acute hemodynamic response to pirbuterol and the subsequent clinical improvements derived during chronic therapy is consistent with previous experience with vasodilating agents such as hydralazine[26] and with inotropic agents such as amrinone.[27] Indeed, as mentioned previously, this observation suggests that the long-term clinical response to any given pharmacologic intervention reflects a variety of variables, including sustained hemodynamic efficacy, the severity and/or rate of progression of the underlying disease, and secondary abnormalities in neuroendocrine function and peripheral circulation.

An oral catecholamine that is predominantly a dopaminergic agent, *ibopamine,* is currently under investigation.[55] Its potential clinical importance, however, appears to be largely related to its activity as a renal vasodilator and its ability to improve renal function in severe heart failure, rather than to its direct effect on myocardial contractility. Indeed, this drug may prove to be an important adjunct to therapy with a specific inotropic agent.

Prenalterol appears to be largely a selective beta$_1$ agonist, with only minimal beta$_2$-agonist effect, and has been demonstrated to augment myocardial contractility and cardiac performance when administered either parenterally or orally.[56–58] In some patients, this improvement may be stimulated at the expense of increased myocardial oxygen requirements, as suggested by the recent observations of Wahr and associates.[37] In a preliminary report, Sharfe and Coxon[59] observed functional improvements for as long as 1 month in patients treated with oral prenalterol. However, the long-term clinical usefulness of oral beta$_1$-specific agonists is yet to be determined and, at least in part, may be related to whether hemodynamic tolerance caused by "down-regulation" of myocardial beta receptors develops during chronic therapy.

Recent interest has been focused on a new class of catecholamines that have both intrinsic beta$_1$-agonist and antagonist activity. The concept supporting their use derives from data suggesting that chronic stimulation of the heart by excessively elevated levels of catecholamines is ultimately detrimental to myocardial function,[60,61] that is, resulting in depletion of cardiac norepinephrine and associated with decreased density of myocardial $beta_1$ receptors as well as reduced myocardial responsiveness to catecholamines.[62] Indeed, some studies have suggested that treatment with beta-receptor blockade improves myocardial function and prolongs survival in patients with congestive cardiomyopathy.[63] Other studies, however, suggest that adequate cardiac performance in patients with severe heart failure is dependent on the inotropic support provided by increased sympathetic tone,[64] making beta-adrenergic blockade fairly hazardous. Thus, theoretically, to be of clinical benefit, such an agent must provide inotropic support to the failing myocardium via its beta-agonist effect, while via its antagonist effect narrowing the range over which sympathetic nerves can modulate cardiac function to a level equal to the agonist activity of the drug. Clinically, the relative agonist or antagonist effect of the agent would further depend on the individual's level of sympathetic tone at rest and during exercise. Thus, whereas these agents may ultimately prove to offer unique long-term benefits in patients with milder stages of congestive heart failure by both improving cardiac function and altering the progression of the myocardial disease, their use in advanced heart failure may be inappropriate. *ICI 118,587* is a prototype of this group and is currently undergoing clinical investigation.[64,65] Although conceptually intriguing, the ultimate role and safety of these sympathomimetics in the management of heart failure remain to be established.

Though most of the aforementioned sympathomimetic agents can induce acute hemodynamic improvements in patients with chronic heart failure, their ability to effect an appropriate distribution of increased blood flow to actively metabolizing organs will largely determine their clinical usefulness during long-term therapy. Indeed, as already described, the increased cardiac output induced by pirbuterol did not afford increased maximum oxygen uptake and hence failed to improve exercise capacity acutely or during chronic therapy. Therefore, we recently evaluated the acute hemodynamic and metabolic effects of dobutamine,[66] a catecholamine with both $beta_1$- and $beta_2$-agonist effects, and of dopamine,[67] a $beta_1$ agonist largely devoid of $beta_2$ activity, during maximal upright graded exercise in patients with severe heart failure. Interestingly, as illustrated in Figure 2, dobutamine administration induced substantial improvements in cardiac performance both at rest and during maximal exercise; however, there was no improvement in exercise capacity and only minimal change in maximum oxygen uptake. Indeed, the increased cardiac output induced during exercise was accompanied by a narrowing of the arteriovenous oxygen difference reached at exhaustion when compared with a control period of exercise, suggesting an increased blood flow to non–metabolically active tissues rather than to the exercising muscles. These observations suggest that although the $beta_1$-agonist effect of dobutamine may augment inotropy and cardiac performance during exercise, concomitant $beta_2$-receptor stimulation may produce effects similar to those of vasodilating agents[66–71] and result in a "shunting" of the increased blood flow to nonexercising circulations. However, it is also possible that the failure of dobutamine to acutely improve aerobic exercise capacity, despite the significantly increased cardiac output, may have been more a function of a markedly reduced and fixed vasodilating capacity in the exercising limbs, as suggested by the recent study of LeJemtel and coworkers[72] in patients with chronic congestive heart failure. Furthermore, the improvements in cardiac performance observed during maximal exercise on dobutamine may have been largely due to the lowering of left ventricular afterload afforded by $beta_2$-receptor stimulation rather than to its direct $beta_1$-agonist effect. Indeed, during administration of dopamine to patients with severe heart failure, although cardiac performance was substantially improved at rest, this beneficial effect was not maintained during maximal exercise, and maximum oxygen uptake and exercise capacity were not improved. This apparent loss of the inotropic effect of dopamine during exercise was somewhat surprising. These findings, however, imply that during maximal exercise in patients with severe heart failure, myocardial $beta_1$ receptors may already be almost fully saturated by elevated levels of circulating endogenous catechol-

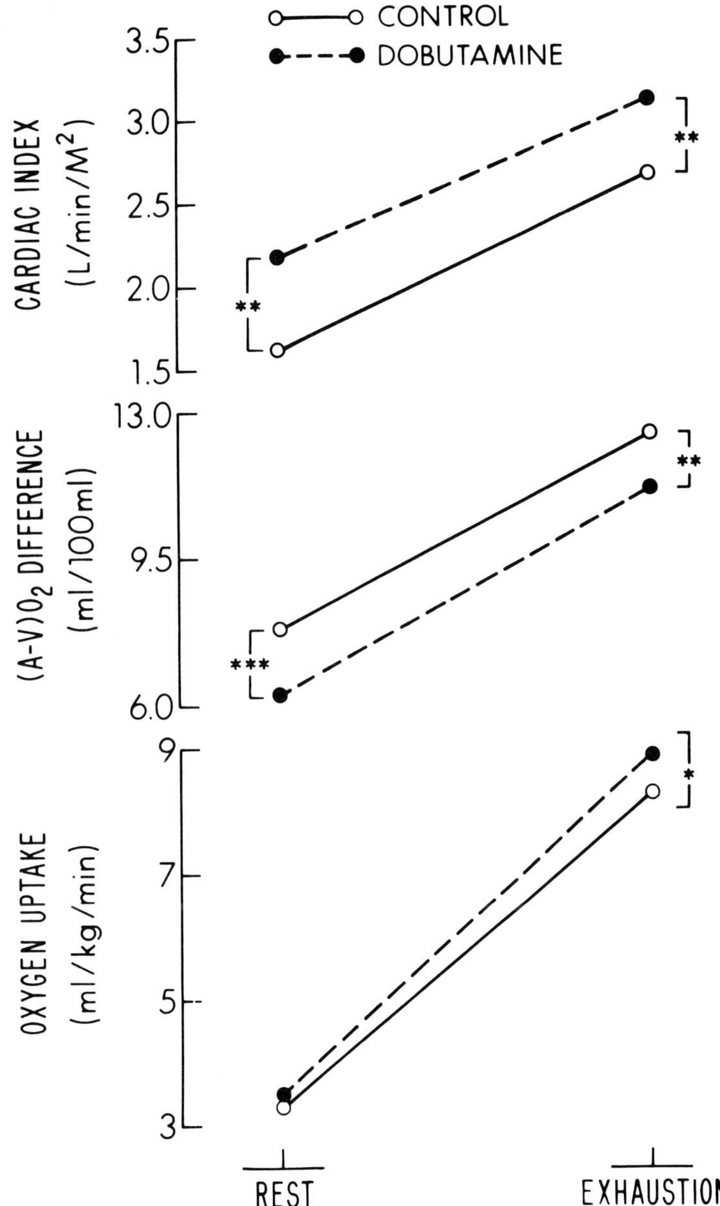

Figure 2. Hemodynamic and metabolic effects of dobutamine administration during maximal exercise. *Top,* Cardiac index at rest and at exhaustion, during control period and during exercise while on dobutamine. *Center,* Arteriovenous oxygen difference at rest and exhaustion. *Bottom,* Oxygen uptake at rest and exhaustion. $*p < 0.05$; $**p < 0.01$; $***p < 0.001$ (From Maskin et al,[66] with permission.)

amines,[73–75] thereby effectively limiting the ability of exogenous sympathomimetics to further augment inotropy. This effect may be accentuated by a lesser density of beta receptors in the failing myocardium and/or a decreased catecholamine sensitivity, as has been recently described by Bristow and associates[62] in failing human hearts. Although these findings demonstrated the inability of sympathomimetic agents to acutely augment maximum exercise capacity, they do not preclude a beneficial hemodynamic and metabolic effect during submaximal levels of activity when myocardial $beta_1$ receptors may not be fully saturated and/or when blood flow in the exercising circulations may not as yet be maximal.[76]

The role of oral catecholamines in the long-term management of congestive heart failure thus remains unclear, and they may indeed be of limited clinical benefit as primary therapeutic agents. Augmentation of cellular levels of 3′5′-cyclic AMP, and thus enhanced calcium availability for the contractile process, can, however, be accomplished in the absence of beta-adrenergic receptor stimulation. The potential limitations imposed by decreased receptor density and/or sensitivity, or by competition with endogenous catecholamines for receptor sites, might thereby be avoided.

XANTHINES

Methylxanthines such as theophylline and aminophylline represent interesting orally effective inotropic agents. Xanthines are phosphodiesterase inhibitors and increase myocellular levels of 3′5′-cyclic AMP[77,78] by decreasing its rate of degradation. Such effects potentiate the mechanical and biochemical actions of catecholamines[79,80] and may be most effective under conditions of enhanced sympathetic tone, as in severe heart failure and during exercise. Inhibition of phosphodiesterase also produces bronchodilation, similar to that produced by the $beta_2$ agonists discussed above. It appears that this old class of agents might be beneficial in the chronic treatment of heart failure and should be pursued.

GLUCAGON

Direct activation of adenyl cyclase will also increase levels of 3′5′-cyclic AMP, independent of the beta-adrenergic receptor, and can be induced by *glucagon,*[81] a pancreatic hormone. Intravenous administration of glucagon has, in fact, been shown to exert considerable inotropic effect when administered experimentally to animals as well as to humans.[82,83] However, the hemodynamic effects of glucagon are variable, and thus far its clinical usefulness has been limited to acute reversal of the anti-inotropic effects of beta-blocking agents in the failing heart. Furthermore, in vitro studies of both human[84] and animal papillary muscles[85] have suggested that in the presence of heart failure, glucagon fails to enhance levels of adenyl cyclase and augment contractility. Future development of agents with similar mechanisms of action may, however, prove clinically useful.

DIGITALIS GLYCOSIDES

Digitalis glycosides have, for nearly two centuries, been the principal orally effective inotropic agents available for use in humans and have been a mainstay in the treatment of heart failure. Their mechanism of action is believed to involve a partial inhibition of the Na^+-K^+–stimulated ATPase located on the sarcoplasmic reticulum.[86] It is postulated that extrusion of ionized calcium from the myocyte during diastole is thereby inhibited. Increased intracellular stores of calcium are thus available for the contractile process and tension development.

Although digitalis glycosides have been shown to be effective inotropic agents,[87–89] their ability to augment cardiac performance substantially and thus their clinical effectiveness are limited by the low toxic/therapeutic ratio. Increased toxicity, including malignant ventricular arrhythmia, bradyarrhythmia, and death, may occur when optimal inotropic drug effect is sought. Significant symptomatic benefit during long-term drug therapy has been questioned and may indeed vary with the stage of the disease. Furthermore, improvements in cardiac performance and functional capacity appear to be modest at best, and variable.[90–92] Acute improvement of exercise capacity and maximum oxygen uptake have not been described with digitalis glycosides, and only recently has improvement in hemodynamics during exercise been demonstrated.[93] Nevertheless, acute improvement in exercise capacity was not observed.

In most instances, the major beneficial effects of digitalis glycosides are the results of control of rapid heart rate in atrial fibrillation rather than increments in myocardial function.[92–94]

NEW AGENTS

Recent interest has focused on a new class of inotropic agents, the prototype of which is *amrinone*.[95] This newly synthesized dipyridine ring, which is neither a catecholamine nor a digitalis glycoside, has been demonstrated to have a potent inotropic effect as well as peripheral arteriolar dilating activity in animals (dog and cat). The mode of action of amrinone remains unknown, although it does enhance Ca^{++} movements in red cells.[96] Augmentation of Ca^{++} influx via the slow Ca^{++} current in guinea pig papillary muscles has been recently described[98,99] and may be involved in the inotropic action of amrinone. In the heart, it does not affect the Na^+-K^+–stimulated ATPase or enzymes associated with $beta_1$-receptor stimulation. In a recent study from our institution, phosphodiesterase inhibition has been demonstrated in a toad bladder preparation.[97] Indeed, a resultant increase in cellular levels of cyclic AMP could explain both enhanced myocardial contractility and reduced peripheral vascular resistance.

In humans with severe congestive heart failure, amrinone has been shown to substantially augment performance of the failing heart as evidenced by increased left ventricular dp/dt,[33] and by significant increases in cardiac output and reduction in left ventricular filling pressure without associated tachycardia or a change in arterial pressure.[33,100–103] Furthermore, these acute hemodynamic benefits appear to effect improvements in regional distribution of blood flow as evidenced by increased effective renal plasma flow and glomerular filtration rate.[103] To what extent these hemodynamic benefits are due to the inotropic or the vasodilating properties of amrinone is difficult to ascertain, and most probably both mechanisms are involved. Of special interest is the demonstration by Siskind and associates of an acute beneficial effect of amrinone therapy on both exercise hemodynamics and metabolism in patients with severe congestive heart failure (Fig. 3).[104] Consistent with these findings are the observations of increased maximum oxygen uptake during graded exercise as early as 1 week after initiation of amrinone therapy.[105] Thus, in contrast to other cardioactive agents, it appears that amrinone not only improves cardiac performance during exercise but also allows exercising muscle to benefit from the increased blood flow. However, the long-term clinical response to amrinone therapy has been variable, and similar to the experience with other cardioactive agents, the acute hemodynamic response is a poor predictor of the clinical response during chronic therapy.[27]

To further understand the long-term response during chronic amrinone therapy, we repeated the hemodynamic evaluation on maintenance therapy, as well as after withdrawal and resinstitution of the drug, in patients treated for an average of 41 weeks.[27] Indeed, sustained amrinone-dependent hemodynamic benefits without tachyphylaxis to the drug were demonstrated in every patient, as evidenced by the hemodynamic and clinical deterioration precipitated by withdrawal of therapy and reversed by readministration of amrinone (Fig. 4). Moreover, an interval progression of the underlying myocardial disease was suggested in all patients by the reduced stroke volume index and increased left ventricular filling pressure observed after withdrawal of amrinone, compared with values at initial presentation prior to therapy. Such a progression of the disease, which is indeed consistent with the progressive course of severe congestive heart failure,[106,107] may help to explain the worsening of symptoms and apparent loss of clinical benefit from amrinone observed in some patients.

Whether or not chronic inotropic stimulation with amrinone contributed to the progression of the disease, as has been suggested on theoretical grounds,[108] is unknown. Relevant to this issue, however, is the reduction in myocardial oxygen consumption observed in the failing canine left ventricle following amrinone administration, which was apparently related to a reduction in ventricular wall tension that more than offset the effect of increased contractil-

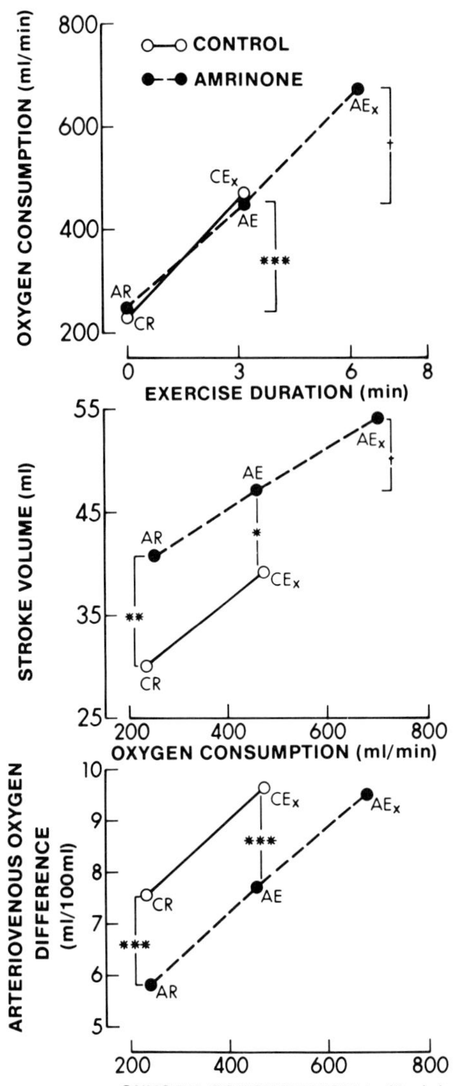

Figure 3. Hemodynamic and metabolic effects of amrinone administration during exercise. *Top,* Effects on oxygen consumption and exercise duration. *Center,* Effects on cardiac output as related to oxygen consumption. *Bottom,* Changes in arteriovenous oxygen difference as a function of oxygen consumption. CR = control period of exercise, resting state; AR = rest while on amrinone; CEx = control period exercise to exhaustion; AE = exercise on amrinone at a point equal to exhaustion during the control period; AEx = exercise to exhaustion while on amrinone. *p < 0.05; **p < 0.01; ***p < 0.001 (From Siskind et al,[104] with permission.)

ity,[109] as well as the beneficial effects on myocardial metabolism described in patients with severe chronic congestive heart failure.[33] Nonetheless, if the underlying disease was indeed progressive in our patients, it is somewhat discouraging that administration of amrinone was unable to arrest this process despite its sustained effect on cardiac performance. The role of amrinone on the course of the disease is difficult to approach inasmuch as the underlying cause of the myocardial depression per se is generally unclear. Most probably, only controlled and blinded studies will be able to adequately address and provide insight into these issues.

Unfortunately, the hemodynamic and clinical benefits of amrinone have been complicated by a variety of side effects, including gastrointestinal intolerance, dose-related thrombocytopenia, hepatotoxicity, and fever.[110] Of interest, therefore, is a recently synthesized analogue of amrinone, *WIN 47203,*[111,112] a nonglycosidic, nonadrenergic cardiotonic agent that also produces peripheral vascular dilatation. WIN 47203 appears to have potential advantages relative to amrinone in being 20 to 30 times more potent an inotropic agent in both *in vitro* and *in vivo* animal studies, while being apparently free of side effects. As with amrinone, the mechanisms of action of WIN 47203 remain unknown. While the drug also seems to inhibit phosphodiesterase, there appears to be temporal dissociation between inotropic effect and increased levels of cyclic AMP, suggesting that this activity is not causally related to its inotropic effect.

Recently, we have demonstrated that acute intravenous and oral administration of WIN 47203 to patients with severe congestive heart failure induces substantial improvements in cardiac performance.[113] Furthermore, no evidence of tachyphylaxis to the hemodynamic benefits of the drug could be demonstrated during monitoring of six consecutive doses, administered at 6-hour intervals. Similar to the experience with amrinone, these hemodynamic benefits were accompanied by improvements in exercise capacity and maximum oxygen uptake

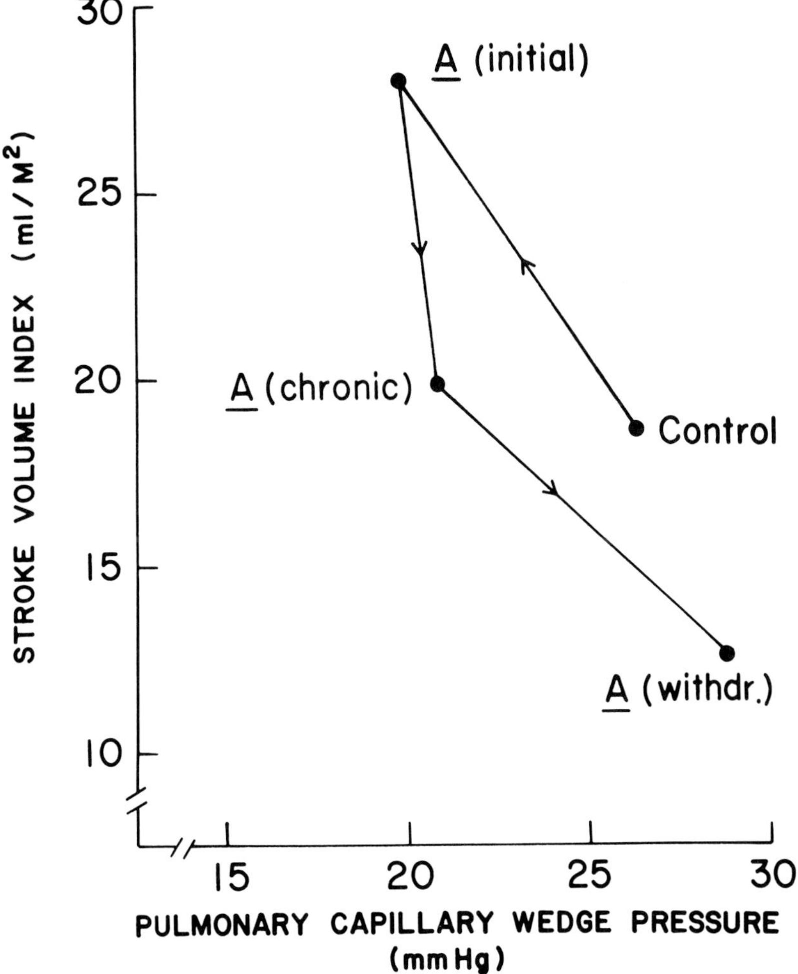

Figure 4. Acute and long-term effects of amrinone on stroke volume index and pulmonary capillary wedge pressure in patients with congestive heart failure. Although cardiac performance is worse at A (chronic) compared with A (initial), an interval progression of the underlying disease is suggested by the substantial worsening of hemodynamic status at A (withdr.) compared with Control. Withdrawal of long-term amrinone therapy resulted in hemodynamic deterioration in all patients; this was reversed following reinstitution of drug. C = control value prior to amrinone therapy; A (initial) = initial hemodynamic response to amrinone; A (chronic) = long-term response; A (withdr.) = value after late withdrawal of amrinone therapy. (From Maskin et al,[27] with permission.)

as early as 1 week after initiation of therapy, with further improvements observed in some during the ensuing 4 weeks.

During long-term therapy with WIN 47203, variable clinical responses have been observed, which, as in our experience with amrinone, could not be predicted by the magnitude of acute hemodynamic response. Indeed, whereas some patients maintained their initial functional improvements, others experienced a partial recrudescence of symptoms. Sustained and significant WIN 47203–dependent hemodynamic benefits without tachyphylaxis were, however, demonstrated by repeat hemodynamic evaluations during maintenance, withdrawal, and reinstitution of therapy.[114] Moreover, in those patients who had experienced some return of congestive symptoms, more dramatic hemodynamic and clinical decompensation was observed following withdrawal of WIN 47203, and parameters of cardiac performance after withdrawal of therapy were substantially worse than values at presentation, suggesting an interval progression of the underlying disease.

Presently, continued treatment with WIN 47203 for periods as long as 12 months has been free of side effects. If long-term administration remains well tolerated, this drug appears to be very promising for treatment of chronic and severe congestive heart failure, and long-term controlled double-blind studies should be pursued.

A new synthetic inotrope, *ARL 115BS,*[115] which is a benzimidazole derivative, is also under clinical investigation. Similar to amrinone and WIN 47203, its mechanism of action remains unclear. It is known to be neither a digitalis glycoside nor a beta-adrenergic agonist. In guinea pig and rat papillary muscles, ARL 115BS has been shown to be inotropic and to alter sarcolemmal Ca^{++} flux, thereby increasing intracellular Ca^{++} available to the contractile process.[116,117] Activity as a phosphodiesterase inhibitor has also been demonstrated *in vitro.* The clinical import of this agent is yet to be established.

MDL 17043, an imidazolone derivative, is another newly synthesized noncatecholamine, nonglycoside agent, which has recently been reported to possess inotropic activity *in vitro* (cat, guinea pig) and *in vivo* (dog) when administered intravenously and orally, as well as to be able to produce direct relaxation of vascular smooth muscle.[118] Although its mechanisms of action remain unclear, it is known to have phosphodiesterase inhibitory properties. Thus far, acute clinical studies suggest that in patients with severe heart failure the vasodilating effects of MDL 17043 predominate.[119] Indeed, owing to its effects on ventricular loading conditions, it has been difficult to determine the dose-response to its inotropic effects in man. The response to chronic administration of MDL 17043 is yet to be established.

In summary, although agents with inotropic activity are effective in stimulating the failing heart, their influence on the long-term outcome of severe heart failure is yet to be determined. What remains quite disturbing is the progressive downhill course observed in patients despite both initial and sustained benefits from drug therapy. Whether there is an early stage during which the progression of myocardial dysfunction can be reversed, that is, by improving cardiac performance and reducing left ventricular dilation, is yet to be defined. Whether inotropic stimulation of the failing heart might alter the pathophysiology is also unknown. The key challenge in the treatment of heart failure remains reversal of the underlying disease process. Nevertheless, palliation of symptoms is now possible and reasonable.

REFERENCES

1. Ross, J Jr, Gault, JH, Mason, DT, et al: *Left ventricular performance during muscular exercise in patients with and without cardiac dysfunction.* Circulation 34:597, 1966.

2. Epstein, SE, Beiser, GD, Stampfer, M, et al: *Characterization of the circulatory response to maximal upright exercise in normal subjects and patients with heart disease.* Circulation 35:1049, 1967.

3. Franciosa, JA, Zeische, S, and Wilen, M: *Functional capacity of patients with chronic left ventricular failure.* Am J Med 67:460, 1979.

4. Harvey, RM, Smith, WM, Parker, JO, et al: *The response of the abnormal heart to exercise.* Circulation 26:341, 1962.

5. Gelberg, HJ, Robin, SA, Ports, TA, et al: *Detection of left ventricular functional reserve by supine exercise hemodynamics in patients with severe chronic heart failure.* Am J Cardiol 44:1062, 1979.

6. Chidsey, CA, Sonnenblick, EH, Morrow, AG, et al: *Catecholamine excretion and cardiac stores of norepinephrine in congestive heart failure.* Am J Med 39:442, 1965.

7. Thomas, JA and Marks, BH: *Plasma norepinephrine and adrenaline in congestive heart failure.* Am J Cardiol 41:233, 1978.

8. Watkins, L, Burkin, JA, Haber, E, et al: *The renin-angiotensin aldosterone system in congestive heart failure in conscious dogs.* J Clin Invest 57:1606, 1976.

9. Curtiss, C, Cohen, JN, Viobel, T, et al: *Role of the renin-angiotensin system in the systemic vasoconstriction of chronic congestive heart failure.* Circulation 58:763, 1976.

10. Dzau, JV, Colucci, W, Hollingberg, NK, et al: *The renin-angiotensin aldosterone system in congestive heart failure: Relation to clinical states.* Circulation 63:645, 1981.

11. Braunwald, E, Ross, J Jr, and Sonnenblick, EH: *Mechanism of contraction of the normal and failing heart.* N Engl J Med 277:794, 853, 910, 962, 1012, 1967.

12. Sonnenblick, EH, Parmley, WW, and Urschel, CW: *The contractile state of the heart as expressed by force-velocity relations.* Am J Cardiol 23:488, 1969.

13. Factor, SM, Minase, T, and Sonnenblick, EH: *Clinical and morphological features of human hypertensive-diabetic cardiomyopathy.* Am Heart J 99:440, 1980.

14. Mason, DT, Spann, JF, Zelis, R, et al: *Alterations of hemodynamics and myocardial mechanics in patients with congestive heart failure: Pathophysiologic mechanisms and assessment of cardiac function and ventricular contractility.* Prog Cardiovasc Dis 12:507, 1970.

15. Dodge, HT and Baxley, WA: *Left ventricular volume and mass and their significance in heart disease.* Am J Cardiol 23:528, 1969.

16. Grossman, W: *Cardiac hypertrophy: Useful adaptation or pathologic process?* Am J Med 69:576, 1980.

17. Factor, SM, Minase, T, Cho, S, et al: *Microvascular spasm in the cardiomyopathic syrian hamster: A preventable cause of focal myocardial necrosis.* Circulation 66:342, 1982.

18. Sonnenblick, EH: *Force-velocity relations in mammalian heart muscle.* Am J Physiol 202:931, 1962.

19. Schwartz, F, Flameny, W, Schafer, J, et al: *Myocardial structure and function in patients with aortic valve disease and their relations to past operative results.* Am J Cardiol 44:661, 1978.

20. Spann, JF Jr, Covell, JW, Eckberg, DL, et al: *Contractile performance of the hypertrophied and chronically failing cat ventricle.* Am J Physiol 223:1150, 1972.

21. Dyke, SE, Urschel, CW, Sonnenblick, EH, et al: *Detection of latent function in acutely ischemic myocardium in dogs: Comparison of pharmacologic inotropic stimulation and post extrasystolic potentiation (PESP).* Circ Res 36:490, 1975.

22. Braunwald, E, Ross, J Jr, Frommer, PL, et al: *Clinical observations on paired electrical stimulation of the heart: Effects on ventricular performance and heart rate.* Am J Med 37:700, 1964.

23. Zelis, R, Delea, CS, Coleman, HN, et al: *Arterial sodium content in experimental congestive heart failure.* Circulation 41:213, 1970.

24. Zelis, R and Mason, DT: *Diminished forearm arteriolar dilator capacity produced by mineralocorticoid induced salt retention in man: Implications concerning congestive heart failure and vascular stiffness.* Circulation 41:589, 1970.

25. Zelis, R, Lee, F, and Mason, DT: *Influence of experimental edema on metabolically determined blood flow.* Circ Res 34:482, 1974.

26. Massie, B, Ports, T, Chatterjee, K, et al: *Long-term vasodilator therapy for heart failure: Clinical response and relationship to hemodynamic measurements.* Circulation 63:269, 1981.

27. Maskin, CS, Forman, R, Klein, NA, et al: *Long-term amrinone therapy in patients with severe heart failure.* Am J Med 72:113, 1982.

28. Weber, KT, Andrews, V, Janicki, JS, et al: *Pirbuterol, an oral beta-adrenergic receptor agonist in the treatment of chronic heart failure.* Circulation 66:1262, 1982.

29. Arnold, SB, Byrd, RC, Meister, W, et al: *Long-term digitalis improves left ventricular function in heart failure.* N Engl J Med 303:1443, 1980.

30. Covell, JW, Braunwald, E, Ross, J Jr, et al: *Studies on digitalis: XVI. Effects on myocardial oxygen consumption.* J Clin Invest 45:1535, 1966.

31. Graham, TP Jr, Covell, JW, Sonnenblick, EH, et al: *Control of myocardial oxygen consumption: Relative influence of contractile state and tension development.* J Clin Invest 47:375, 1968.

32. Kirk, ES, LeJemtel, TH, Nelson, GR, et al: *Mechanisms of beneficial effects of vasodilators and inotropic stimulation in the experimental failing ischemic heart.* Am J Med 65:189, 1978.

33. Benotti, JR, Grossman, W, Braunwald, E, et al: *Effects of amrinone on myocardial energy metabolism and hemodynamics in patients with severe congestive heart failure.* Circulation 62:28, 1980.

34. Rule, RT, Turi, Z, Brown, EJ, et al: *Acute effects of oral pirbuterol on myocardial oxygen metabolism and systemic hemodynamics in chronic congestive heart failure.* Circulation 64:139, 1981.

35. Timmis, AD, Bergman, G, Atkinson, L, et al: *Potential value of oral B_2 adrenoreceptor agonists in left ventricular failure.* Am J Cardiol 47:427, 1981.

36. Fowler, MB, Bergman, G, Timmis, AD, et al: *Is pirbuterol therapy in left ventricular failure associated with a positive inotropic action and what is its metabolic cost?* Circulation 66(Suppl II):II–137, 1982.

37. Wahr, D, Swedberg, K, Ports, T, et al: *Prenalteral, a new oral $beta_1$ selective adrenoreceptor agonist.* Circulation 66(Suppl II):II–137, 1982.

38. Katz, AM, Tada, M, and Kirchberger, MA: *Control of calcium transport in the myocardium by the cyclic AMP protein kinase system.* Adv Cyclic Nucleotide Res 5:453, 1975.

39. Goldberg, LI: *Cardiovascular and renal actions of dopamine: Potential clinical implications.* Pharmacol Rev 24:1, 1972.

40. Akhtar, N, Mikulic, E, Cohn, JN, et al: *Hemodynamic effect of dobutamine in patients with severe heart failure.* Am J Cardiol 36:202, 1975.

41. Sonnenblick, EH, Frishman, WH, and LeJemtel, TH: *Dobutamine: A new synthetic cardioactive sympathetic amine.* N Engl J Med 300:17, 1979.

42. Unverferth, DV, Blanford, M, Kates, RE, et al: *Tolerance to dobutamine after a 72 hour continuous infusion.* Am J Med 69:262, 1980.

43. Klein, NA, Siskind, SJ, LeJemtel, TH, et al: *Hemodynamic comparison of intravenous amrinone and dobutamine in patients with chronic congestive heart failure.* Am J Cardiol 48:170, 1981.

44. Unverferth, DV, Leier, CV, Magorien, RD, et al: *Improvement of human myocardial mitochondria after dobutamine: A quantitative ultrastructural study.* J Pharmacol Exp Ther 215:527, 1980.

45. Leier, CV, Huss, P, Lewis, RP, et al: *Drug induced conditioning in congestive heart failure.* Circulation 65:1382, 1982.

46. Moore, PF, Constantine, JW, and Barth, WE: *Pirbuterol, a selective $beta_2$ adrenergic bronchodilator.* J Pharmacol Exp Ther 297:410, 1978.

47. Sharma, B, Hoback, J, Francis, GS, et al: *Pirbuterol: A new oral sympathomimetic amine for the treatment of congestive heart failure.* Am Heart J 102:533, 1981.

48. Awan, NA, Everson, MK, Needkam, KE, et al: *Hemodynamic effects of oral pirbuterol in chronic severe congestive heart failure.* Circulation 63:96, 1981.

49. Sharma, B and Goodman, JF: *Beneficial effect of salbutamol on cardiac function in severe congestive cardiomyopathy: Effect on systolic and diastolic function of the left ventricle.* Circulation 58:449, 1978.

50. Awan, NA, Needham, K, Evenson, MK, et al: *Therapeutic efficacy of oral pirbuterol in severe heart failure: Acute hemodynamic and long-term ambulatory evaluation.* Am Heart J 102:555, 1981.

51. Colucci, WS, Alexander, RW, Mudge, GH, et al: *Acute and chronic effects of pirbuterol on left ventricular ejection fraction and clinical status in severe heart failure.* Am Heart J 102:564, 1981.

52. Colucci, WS, Alexander, W, Williams, GH, et al: *Decreased lymphocyte beta-adrenergic receptor density in patients with heart failure and tolerance to the beta-adrenergic agonist pirbuterol.* N Engl J Med 305:185, 1981.

53. Dawson, JR, Reuben, S, Poule-Wilson, PA, et al: *Acute and follow-up studies with pirbuterol in heart failure.* Am J Cardiol 47:492, 1981.

54. Pamelia, FX, Gheorghiade, M, Bishop, HL, et al: *Effects of oral pirbuterol in patients with severe congestive heart failure.* Circulation 64(Suppl IV):IV–295, 1981.

55. Stefoni, S, Coli, L, Mosconi, G, et al: *Ibopamine (SB 7505) in normal subjects and in chronic renal failure: A preliminary report.* Br J Clin Pharmacol 1:69, 1981.

56. Knaus, M, Pfister, B, Dubach, UC, et al: *Human pharmacology studies with a new, orally active stimulant of cardiac adrenergic beta receptors.* Am Heart J 95:602, 1978.

57. Waagstein, F, Reiz, S, Ariniego, R, et al: *Clinical results with prenalteral in patients with heart failure.* Am Heart J 102:548, 1981.

58. Kirklin, PC and Pitt, B: *Hemodynamic effects of intravenous prenalterol in severe heart failure.* Am J Cardiol 47:670, 1981.

59. Sharfe, N and Coxon, R: *Oral prenalterol in chronic heart failure.* Circulation 66(Suppl II):II–20, 1982.

60. Chidsey, CA and Braunwald, E: *Sympathetic activity and neurotransmitter depletion in congestive heart failure.* Pharmacol Rev 18:685, 1966.

61. Brauman, G, Riess, G, Erhardt, WD, et al: *Improved beta-adrenergic stimulation in the uninvolved ventricle post-acute myocardial infarction: Reversible defect due to excessive circulating catecholamine-induced decline in number and affinity of beta receptors.* Am Heart J 101:569, 1981.

62. Bristow, MR, Ginsburg, R, Minobe, W, et al: *Decreased catecholamine sensitivity and beta-adrenergic-receptor density in failing human hearts.* N Engl J Med 307:205, 1982.

63. Swedberg, K, Waagstein, F, Hjalmarson, A, et al: *Prolongation of survival in congestive cardiomyopathy by beta-receptor blockade.* Lancet 1:1374, 1979.

64. Vogel, JHK and Chidsey, CA: *Cardiac adrenergic activity in experimental heart failure assessed with beta receptor blockade.* Am J Cardiol 24:198, 1969.

65. Barlow, JJ, Main, BG, Moors, JA, et al: *The cardiovascular activity of ICI 118 587, a novel beta-adrenoreceptor partial agonist.* Br J Pharmacol 67:412P, 1979.

66. Maskin, CS, Forman, R, Sonnenblick, EH, et al: *Failure of dobutamine to increase exercise capacity despite hemodynamic improvement in severe chronic heart failure.* Am J Cardiol 51:177, 1983.

67. Maskin, CS, Sonnenblick, EH, Kugler, J, et al: *Contrasting effects of acute sympathetic stimulation and vasodilator therapy on cardiac performance during maximal exercise in severe heart failure.* Circulation 66(Suppl II):II–382, 1982.

68. Rubin, SA, Chatterjee, K, Ports, TA, et al: *Influence of short-term oral hydralazine therapy on exercise hemodynamics in patients with severe chronic heart failure.* Am J Cardiol 44:1183, 1979.

69. Rubin, SA, Chatterjee, K, Gelberg, HJ, et al: *Paradox of improved exercise but not resting hemodynamics with short-term prazosin in chronic heart failure.* Am J Cardiol 43:810, 1979.

70. Kugler, J, Maskin, CS, Frishman, WH, et al: *Regional and systemic metabolic effects of angiotensin-converting enzyme inhibition during exercise in patients with severe heart failure.* Circulation 66:1256, 1982.

71. Flaim, SF, Weitzel, RL, and Zelis, R: *Mechanism of action of nitroglycerine during exercise in a rat model of heart failure.* Circ Res 49:458, 1981.

72. LeJemtel, TH, Maskin, CS, Sinoway, L, et al: *Fixed vasodilating capacity in exercising leg muscles: A limitation of aerobic capacity in heart failure.* Clin Res 31:200A, 1983.

73. Chidsey, CA, Harrison, DC, and Braunwald, E: *Augmentation of the plasma norepinephrine response to exercise in patients with congestive heart failure.* N Engl J Med 267:650, 1962.

74. Francis, GS, Goldsmith, SR, Ziesche, SM, et al: *Response of plasma norepinephrine and epinephrine to dynamic exercise in patients with congestive heart failure.* Am J Cardiol 49:1152, 1982.

75. Silverberg, AB, Shah, SD, Hamond, MW, et al: *Norepinephrine: Hormone and neurotransmitter in man.* Am J Physiol 234:E252, 1978.

76. Zelis, R, Flaim, SF, Nellis, S, et al: *Autonomic adjustment to congestive heart failure and their consequences.* In Fishman, AP (ed): *Heart Failure.* Hemisphere Publishing, Washington, DC, 1978, p 237.

77. Marcus, ML, Skelton, CL, Graver, LE, et al: *Effects of theophylline on myocardial mechanics.* Am J Physiol 222:1361, 1972.

78. Blinks, JR, Olson, CB, Jewell, BR, et al: *Influence of caffeine and other methylxanthines on mechanical properties of isolated mammalian heart muscle: Evidence of a dual mechanism of action.* Circ Res 30:367, 1972.

79. Rall, TW and West, TC: *The potentiation of cardiac inotropic responses to norepinephrine by theophylline.* J Pharmacol Exp Ther 134:269, 1963.

80. Marcus, ML, Skelton, CL, Prindle, KE, et al: *Potentiation of the inotropic effects of glucagon by theophylline.* J Pharmacol Exp Ther 179:331, 1971.

81. Parmley, WW and Sonnenblick, EH: *Glucagon: A new agent in cardiac therapy.* Am J Cardiol 27:298, 1971.

82. Parmley, WW, Gluck, G, and Sonnenblick, EH: *Cardiovascular effects of glucagon in man.* N Engl J Med 279:12, 1968.

83. Levey, GS, Prindle, KH Jr, and Epstein, SE: *Effects of glucagon on adenylcyclase activity in the left and right ventricles and liver in experimentally produced isolated right ventricular failure.* J Mol Cell Cardiol 1:403, 1970.

84. Goldstein, RE, Skelton, L, Levey, GS, et al: *Effects of chronic heart failure on the capacity of glucagon to enhance contractility and adenocyclase activity of human papillary muscles.* Circulation 44:638, 1971.

85. Gold, HK, Prindle, KH, and Levey, GS: *Effects of experimental heart failure on the capacity of glucagon to augment myocardial contractility and activate adenyl cyclase.* J Clin Invest 49:999, 1970.

86. Schwartz, A: *Is the cell membrane Na^+, K^+-ATPase enzyme system the pharmacologic receptor for digitalis?* Circ Res 39:2, 1976.

87. Braunwald, E, Bloodwell, RD, Goldberg, LI, et al: *Observations in man on the effects of digitalis preparations on the contractility of the nonfailing heart and on total vascular resistance.* J Clin Invest 40:52, 1961.

88. Hoeschen, RJ and Cuddy, TE: *Dose response relation between therapeutic levels of serum digoxin and systolic time intervals.* Am J Cardiol 35:469, 1975.

89. Ferrer, IM, Conroy, RJ, and Harvey, RM: *Some effects of digoxin upon the heart and circulation in man.* Circulation 21:373, 1960.

90. Cohn, K, Selzer, A, Kersh, ES, et al: *Variability of the hemodynamic responses to acute digitalization in chronic cardiac failure due to cardiomyopathy and coronary artery disease.* Am J Cardiol 35:461, 1975.

91. Murphy, GW, Schreiner, BF, Bleakley, PL, et al: *Left ventricular performance following digitalization in patients with and without heart failure.* Circulation 30:358, 1964.

92. Arnold, SB, Byrd, RC, Meister, W, et al: *Long-term digitalis therapy improves left ventricular function in heart failure.* N Engl J Med 303:1443, 1980.

93. Firth, BJ, Dehmer, GJ, Corbett, JR, et al: *Effect of chronic oral digoxin therapy on ventricular function at rest and peak exercise in patients with ischemic heart disease.* Am J Cardiol 46:481, 1980.

94. Johnston, GD and McDevitt, DG: *Is maintenance of digoxin necessary in patients with sinus rhythm?* Lancet 1:567, 1979.

95. Alousi, AA, Farah, AE, Lesher, GY, et al: *Cardiotonic activity of amrinone-WIN 40680 5-amino-3,4'-bipyridine-6(1H)-one.* Circ Res 45:666, 1979.

96. Parker, JC and Harper, JR Jr: *Effects of amrinone, a cardiotonic drug on calcium movements in dog erythrocytes.* J Clin Invest 66:254, 1980.

97. Levine, SD, Jacoby, M, Sariano, JA, et al: *The effects of amrinone in transport and cyclic AMP metabolism in toad urinary bladder.* J Pharmacol Exp Ther 216:220, 1981.

98. Adams, HR, Rhody, J, and Sutko, JL: *Amrinone activates K^+-depolarized atrial and ventricular myocardium of guinea pigs.* Circ Res 51:662, 1982.

99. Arlock, P and Katzung, B: *Effects of amrinone on transmembrane currents in ferret papillary muscle.* Fed Proc 41:1310, 1982.

100. Benotti, JR, Grossman, W, Braunwald, E, et al: *Hemodynamic assessment of amrinone.* N Engl J Med 299:1373, 1978.

101. LeJemtel, TH, Keung, E, Sonnenblick, EH, et al: *Amrinone: A new non-glycosidic nonadrenergic cardiotonic agent effective in the treatment of intractable myocardial failure in man.* Circulation 59:1098, 1979.

102. LeJemtel, TH, Keung, EC, Schwartz, WJ, et al: *Hemodynamic effects of intravenous and oral amrinone in patients with severe heart failure: Relationship between intravenous and oral administration.* Trans Assoc Am Physicians 92:325, 1979.

103. LeJemtel, TH, Keung, EC, Ribner, HS, et al: *Sustained beneficial effects of oral amrinone on cardiac and renal function in patients with severe congestive heart failure.* Am J Cardiol 45:123, 1980.

104. Siskind, SJ, Sonnenblick, EH, Forman, R, et al: *Acute substantial benefit of inotropic therapy with amrinone on exercise hemodynamics and metabolism in severe congestive heart failure.* Circulation 64:966, 1981.

105. Weber, KT, Andrews, V, Janicki, JS, et al: *Amrinone and exercise performance in patients with chronic heart failure.* Am J Cardiol 48:164, 1981.

106. Hatle, L, Orjavik, O, and Storstein, O: *Chronic myocardial disease.* Acta Med Scand 299:399, 1976.

107. Hamby, RI: *Primary myocardial disease: A prospective clinical and hemodynamic evaluation in 100 patients.* Medicine 3:227, 1970.

108. Katz, AM: *A new inotropic drug: Its promise and a caution.* N Engl J Med 299:1409, 1978.

109. Jentzer, JH, LeJemtel, TH, Sonnenblick, EH, et al: *Beneficial effect of amrinone on myocardial oxygen consumption during acute left ventricular failure in dogs.* Am J Cardiol 48:75, 1981.

110. *Clinical experience with amrinone—"overall summary for NDA amendment."* Sterling Winthrop Research Institute, Rensselaer, NY.

111. Alousi, AA, Helstosky, A, Monenaro, MS, et al: *Intravenous and oral cardiotonic activity of WIN 47203, a potent amrinone analogue in dogs.* Fed Proc 40:663, 1981.

112. *A summary of laboratory data on WIN 47203.* Sterling Winthrop Research Institute, Rensselaer, NY, 1981.

113. Maskin, CS, Sinoway, L, Chadwick, B, et al: *Sustained hemodynamic and clinical effects of a new cardiotonic agent WIN 47203 in patients with severe congestive heart failure.* Circulation 67:1066, 1983.

114. Maskin, CS, Sinoway, L, Chadwick, B, et al: *Chronic therapy with a new inotropic agent WIN 47203 in severe heart failure: Sustained drug dependent benefits and concomitant progression of the disease.* Clin Res 31:524A, 1983.

115. DIEDIEN, W AND WEISENBERG, H: *Studies on the mechanism of positive inotropic action of ARL-115 BS, a new cardiotonic drug.* Arzn Forschung Drug Res 3:129, 1981.

116. FROM, AHL AND PIERPOINT, GL: *Pharmacology of a new inotrope: AR-L 115BS.* Circulation 64(Suppl IV):IV–23, 1981.

117. FROM, AHL AND PIERPOINT, GL: *AR-L 115BS increases action potential dependent Ca^{++} influx.* Circulation 66(Suppl II):II–56, 1982.

118. ROEBEL, LE, DAGE, RC, CHENG, HC, ET AL: *Characterization of the cardiovascular activities of a new cardiotonic agent MDL 17043 (1,3-dihydro-4-methyl-5-[4-(methylthio)-benzoyl]-2H-imidazol-2-one).* J Cardiovasc Pharm 4:721, 1982.

119. URETSKY, BF, GENERALOVICH, T, REDDY, PS, ET AL: *The acute hemodynamic effects of a new agent, MDL 17043, in the treatment of congestive heart failure.* Circulation 67:823, 1983.

Concepts of Peripheral Circulatory Control: Implications for Vasodilator Therapy in Heart Failure

Stanley A. Rubin, M.D. and H. J. C. Swan, M.D., Ph.D.

Cardiac and peripheral vascular functions are mutually interdependent. "Any doubts concerning the surprising fact that the heart alone cannot greatly increase cardiac output (are) put to rest by . . . (replacing) the heart of an anesthetized dog with a roller pump and (observing) that turning up the pump collapses the great veins but causes little increase in blood flow."[1] What we accept as important determinants of cardiac function—preload and afterload—are mainly determined by the peripheral circulation; two further determinants of cardiac function—rate and contractility—are strongly influenced by neurohumoral effectors located in the peripheral circulation. Two developments have prompted us to review the peripheral circulation despite the availability of many excellent summaries.[2,3] First, despite the dramatic clinical growth of the use of vasodilators during the past 10 years,[4] we believe that their fundamental mechanisms of action in heart failure are poorly understood. Second, over this same period, there has been a growth of concepts concerning control of the peripheral circulation.[5]

PROPERTIES OF THE BLOOD VESSELS

Systems that carry fluid flow (hydraulic systems) can be characterized by two physical properties—fluid storage (or capacitance) and fluid flow resistance (impedance or energy dissipation).

Storage

The venous bed—especially the venules, as well as the sinusoids of the liver and spleen—is the principal site of fluid storage, whereas the arterial tree contains lesser storage sites located principally in the Windkessel vessels (proximal larger arteries). Concepts of storage capacity and changes in storage capacity have been investigated over a number of years. The small veins and sinusoids contain approximately 45 percent of the intravascular volume, whereas the central venous reservoirs of vena cavae and large veins hold about 18 percent of the blood volume.[5] The storage properties of these vessels are determined by absolute shape and size, and the latter can be modified by long-term processes—such as growth, external compression, or intraluminal obstruction and obliteration. Of greater importance to circulatory homeostasis is the amount of volume that can rapidly be mobilized. This mobilization is influenced by position within the gravitational field and by neurohumoral effects on vascular smooth muscle. In the anesthetized dog, Drees and Rothe reported that the maximal reflexogenic change in volume storage was about 7 ml/kg, or approximately 10 percent of the intravascular volume.[6]

Recognizing the elastic nature of the peripheral vascular bed, Shoukas and Sagawa investigated *steady-state* elastic properties of the vascular bed based on two concepts: the relationship of volume to pressure in a hollow elastic structure, and a model of the behavior of the storage sites of the peripheral circulation.[7] Most of the vascular volume is stored as *unstressed vascular volume,* that is, the volume that fills the blood vessels under the minimal hydrostatic pressure consistent with the hollow shape of the blood vessels. A smaller part of the vascular volume is stored as *stressed vascular volume,* that is, the volume that pressurizes the vascular system apart from pressure associated with flow (Fig. 1). The *compliance* is the slope of the *stressed vascular volume* part of the volume-pressure relationship. In a later paper, Shoukas and Sagawa summarized their concepts on changes in vascular capacity (amount of blood held by the systemic vascular bed at a specific pressure): "When a given change in blood volume or cardiac output passively expands or shrinks the vascular system, the determinant of the resultant pressure change is the compliance. However, when a reflex mechanism modifies vascular elastic properties, the resultant change in vascular pressure depends on whether the reflex affects the unstressed vascular volume, the compliance, or both."[8] Shoukas and Sagawa reported changes in capacity for the carotid sinus baroreceptor reflex and found that as isolated baroreceptor pressure decreased from 200 to 75 mm Hg, vascular capacity decreased about 7.5 ml/kg,[8] similar to the maximal reflexogenic change reported by Drees and Rothe.[6] Because compliance did not change, Shoukas and Sagawa inferred that the

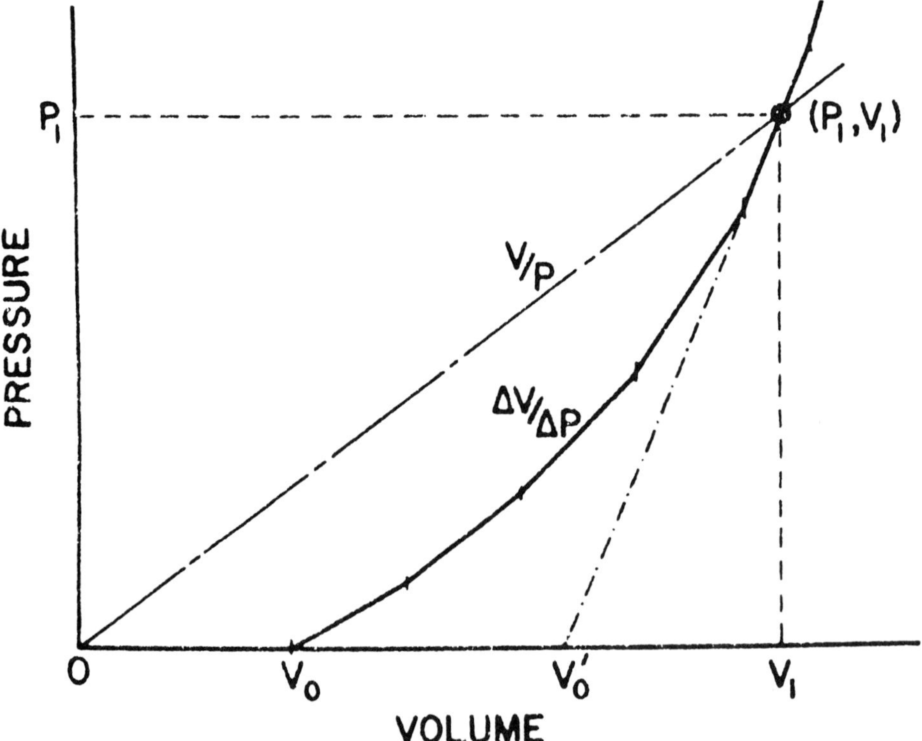

Figure 1. Volume-pressure relationship in the systemic vascular bed. Volume is stored, in part, as unstressed (Vo) and, in part, as stressed. The compliance expresses the slope of the volume-pressure relationship of the stressed vascular volume. Estimation of compliance as the V/P ratio requires assumptions that are probably not correct: that the relationship is linear and that the slope passes through the origin. A true estimate of the slope ($\Delta V/\Delta P$) requires determination over a segment of the relationship. (From Shoukas and Sagawa,[7] with permission.)

carotid sinus reflex changed vascular capacity by a change in *unstressed vascular volume.* We used the concepts, model, and preparation described by Shoukas and Sagawa and found in the dog that enormous doses of nitroprusside (up to 360 μg/min) produced graded increases in vascular capacity up to about 15 ml/kg—or twice that of maximal reflex changes.[9] Because nitroprusside did not change compliance, we also inferred that vascular capacity increased because of a change in *unstressed vascular volume.*

Where does this volume come from or go to when there are changes in the *unstressed vascular volume?* In the aforementioned experiments, this volume transfers to and from an external reservoir. However, in the intact animal, it would add to or subtract from the *stressed vascular volume* and would therefore change the pressure in the vascular system. Thus, these data are compatible with the classic viewpoint that the sympathetic nervous system and certain drugs influence the venous smooth muscle and change the storage capacity of the veins. Further, they are compatible with Guyton's concept of the pivotal role of the mean circulatory pressure as a determinant of venous return.[10] The mean circulatory pressure is the driving pressure to venous return: it is the pressure that occurs as a result of the volume-pressure relationship (compliance) of the *stressed vascular volume.* At any level of total vascular volume, the mean circulatory pressure changes as volume is transferred between stressed and unstressed storage.

When *unstressed vascular volume* decreases, as it does with increasing activity of the baroreceptors, *stressed vascular volume* increases and causes mean circulatory pressure to rise with subsequent effect on venous return and cardiac output. When *unstressed vascular volume* increases, as it does with nitroprusside, *stressed vascular volume* decreases and causes mean circulatory pressure to fall with subsequent effect on venous return and cardiac output.

Resistance

The property of a hydraulic system to dissipate energy of fluid flow is called hydraulic resistance or, if pulsatile, hydraulic impedance.

In the simplest model (analogy) of resistance, there is steady flow of fluid down a long tube in a nonturbulent manner. The parameters in the mathematical model of resistance were described by Pouiselle. If the properties of the blood and length of the tube are constant, then resistance is inversely proportional to the fourth power of the radius. When tubes are joined to form a circuit, the resistances of tubes arranged in series are added, and resistance increases as the sum of the individual resistances; the resistances of tubes arranged in parallel are added as their inverses, and resistance decreases in inverse proportion to the sum of the inverses of the individual resistances. The vascular tree is a series-parallel network in which some segments are large-bore single tubes (aortic arch and vena cavae) connected in series to parallel systems with increasing numbers of branches as flow goes toward the capillaries, and decreasing numbers of branches as one goes away from the capillaries. From an anatomic standpoint, the small arteries and arterioles are the sites of greatest resistance. This can be inferred from measurements of pressure drop in the vascular system. Because the major segments are arranged in series (that is, the total flow goes through each segment), pressure drop is proportional to resistance; the small arteries and arterioles account for about 60 percent of the circuit resistance because, compared with other vascular segments, they have relatively small radii in comparison with relatively few parallel branches (Fig. 2).

Analogous to our statements on storage, for purposes of circulatory homeostasis the emphasis is not only on that portion of the circulation that contains the site of the numerically greatest resistance, but rather on the site that can rapidly change its resistance. Because of their content of vascular smooth muscle and the richness of their connections to and receptors for neurohumoral influences, the small arteries and arterioles have a dominant role in changes of vascular resistance.

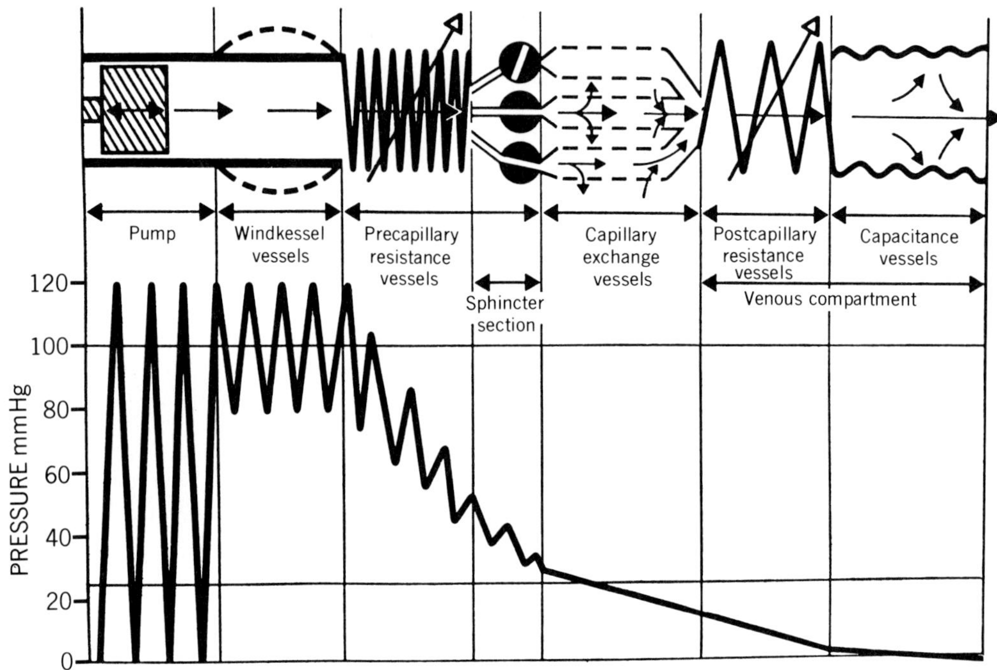

Figure 2. Pressures in the systemic vascular bed. Pressure and pressure pulsation are high in the proximal arterial tree. There is a large decrease in pressure and pressure pulsation in the resistance vessels—the small arteries and arterioles. (From Mellander and Johansson,[2] with permission.)

Because the vascular system is pulsatile, it is important to consider other system properties of energy dissipation apart from resistance. These properties are roughly twofold: the energy dissipation in the pulsation of the proximal arterial walls as the stroke volume is cyclically ejected into this elastic system, and the energy dissipation as a result of backward-traveling waves from the peripheral into the central circulation.

Characteristic impedance (Zo) is impedance in the absence of wave reflection and probably occurs in vivo because the elastic walls of the great vessels store part of the energy of the ejected stroke volume during systole and return a lesser portion during diastole. In mathematical models (analogies) of *characteristic impedance,* elasticity is an important determinant such that Zo is inversely proportional to vascular compliance (slope of the volume-pressure relationship). Arterial compliance is changed when vascular smooth muscle contracts or relaxes, and when the composition of the wall changes, perhaps because of alteration of the amount of an existing element (like collagen or fluid) or the addition of a new element (like atheroma or amyloid). Thus, when the vessel wall stiffens or constricts, Zo increases; and when the vessel dilates, Zo decreases. In addition, because of the curvilinear shape of the volume-pressure relationship of the proximal arterial tree such that the curve is bent toward the pressure axis, compliance decreases as pressure increases, and vice versa, with the expected increases in Zo.

The *reflection coefficient* (R) is the measure of wave reflection and probably occurs in vivo as reflected waves return from distal sites into the central vasculature. Wave reflections occur at discontinuities, especially at sites of tapering and branching. In vivo, the arterioles are probably the major sites of wave reflection because of the sudden drop in pressure (discontinuity) between the large arteries and the arterioles. This concept of discontinuity as the major source for wave reflection receives further support from drug experiments that change vascular resistance; vasodilation of the peripheral bed decreases wave reflection, whereas vasoconstriction enhances it. Effects of vasodilators are more marked than those of vasoconstrictors because of normally high levels of resting basal vasoconstrictor tone.

The parameters that govern Zo and R cannot be directly measured without a geometric and physical description of the vascular system. Nevertheless, it is possible to predict changes in behavior of the intact vascular system caused by changes in arterial pressure, arterial disease, and vasodilator drugs (vide supra). Also, estimates of Zo, R, and vascular resistance can be made from the impedance spectrum.[12] The impedance spectrum is derived from a

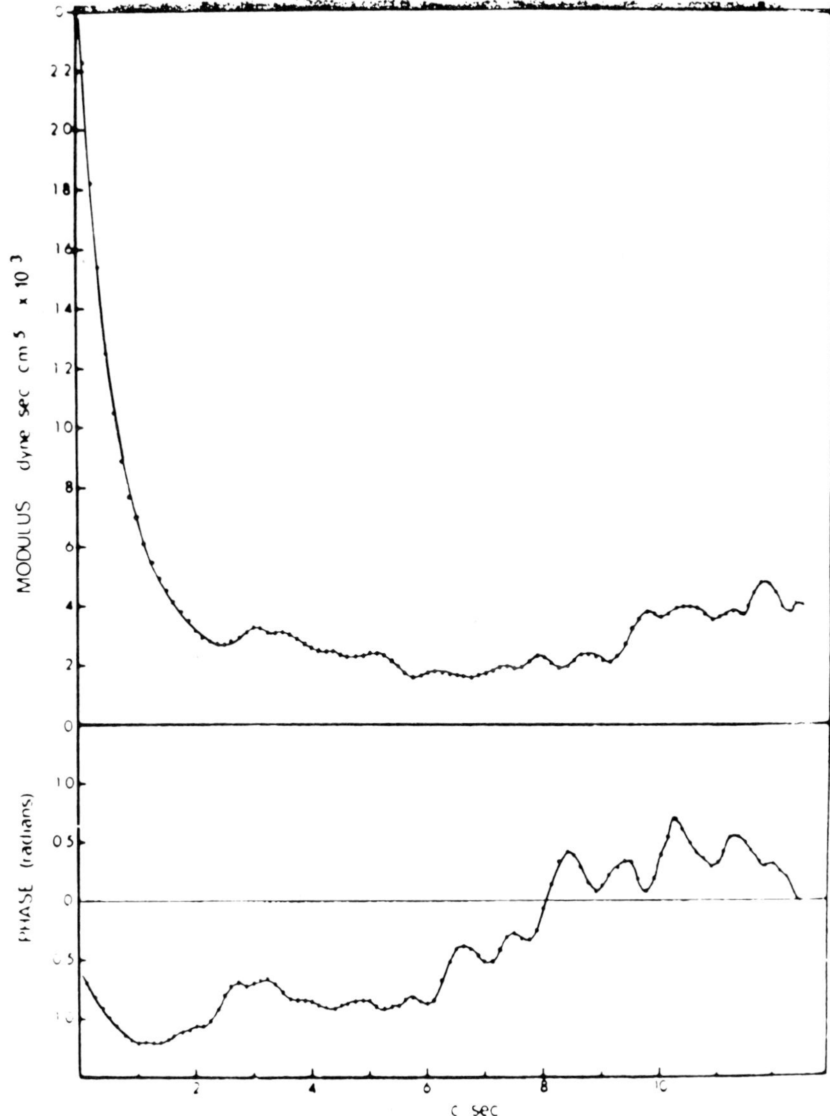

Figure 3. Impedance spectrum. Plots of modulus at the top (ratio of amplitudes of pressure to flow harmonics) and phase at the bottom (angular difference between pressure and flow harmonics). Both are plotted against frequency. From the impedance spectrum, estimates can be made of arterial properties such as resistance, characteristic impedance, and the index of wave reflection. For details, see text. (From Taylor, MG: *Use of random excitation and spectral analysis in the study of frequency-dependent parameters of the cardiovascular system.* Circ Res 18:585, 1966, with permission.)

numerical analysis of matched frequency components of the pulsatile pressure and flow waves. The spectrum contains two plots (Fig. 3): modulus (amplitude of pressure at a frequency divided by amplitude of flow or velocity at the same frequency) against frequency, and phase (angular difference of pressure minus flow at the same frequency) against frequency. The term at zero frequency in the modulus plot is the resistance (mean pressure divided by flow). This term is nonpulsatile and has a zero phase angle. Inasmuch as the impedance spectrum relates information about vascular properties, it is not surprising that the term changes depending on where measurements in the vascular system are taken. In the ascending aorta, the modulus of the mean term (vascular resistance or term at zero frequency) is 10 to 20 times larger than any other modulus. The moduli at increasing frequencies rapidly decrease to a minimum and tend to successively rise and fall with increasing frequency. The phase above this mean term is initially negative (flow leads pressure), rises and crosses zero at about the same frequency of the modulus minimum, and then oscillates about zero at higher frequencies.

Using the impedance spectrum, calculation of the *resistance* term is straightforward except that it differs from the usual formula in that downstream pressure is not subtracted. In the systemic bed, the downstream pressure (right atrial pressure) is usually small compared with the arterial pressure, and therefore errors are not great. In the pulmonary circuit, neglecting the downstream pressure may introduce serious error. *Characteristic impedance* (Zo) is calculated from the average of the impedance moduli above those frequencies thought to be "contaminated" by wave reflection—that is, above those frequencies on the steeply falling portion of the curve. An index of the *coefficient of wave reflection* (R) is calculated as the difference between relative minima and maxima at these higher frequencies. Changes in the impedance spectrum with changes in pressure, disease states, exercise, and drugs have pretty much followed those predicted for the behavior of vascular resistance, Zo, and R.[12]

What is the relationship between vascular impedance and cardiac function? It has been argued that vascular impedance measured in the aortic root is ventricular afterload.[13] Vascular properties strongly determine ventricular systolic function; and because the parameters of vascular impedance are representative of vascular properties, impedance is afterload. Heart failure is associated with increased vascular resistance, Zo, and R, and therefore cardiac function is decreased not only by cardiac disease but also by increased impedance. Vasodilation by drugs has the predicted effects outlined above, and ventricular function improves.

INTERACTION BETWEEN STORAGE AND RESISTANCE PROPERTIES

It had been customary to believe that changes in storage of the peripheral circulation required active changes in the storage vessels—the veins—until Caldini and colleagues presented evidence that changes in resistance could lead to changes in storage.[14] In 1912, the Scandinavian physiologist Krogh presented a two-compartment model of the circulation, with each compartment containing an upstream resistance and a downstream storage site. This model (Fig. 4) is not surprising inasmuch as it appears anatomically correct—arterioles (resistance) in front of venules (storage), and the entire circuit arranged with parallel branches. What is novel is the way Caldini and colleagues collected and interpreted their data in a canine preparation similar to that described for Shoukas' experiment. They inferred that changes in flow distribution among the compartments resulting from changes in upstream resistance could change storage *without* an active change in storage properties. Consider the following: Suppose total blood flow and venous pressure were constant in a circulation with two different compartments (see Fig. 4). Suppose an intervention (e.g., a drug) increased the upstream resistance in one compartment that initially had a large volume contained in its downstream storage element. As with all elastic storage elements, it is pressurized and contains a *stressed vascular volume* (vide supra) dependent on what pressure the upstream resistance permits in this storage site. If this drug intervention *increases* upstream resistance, then

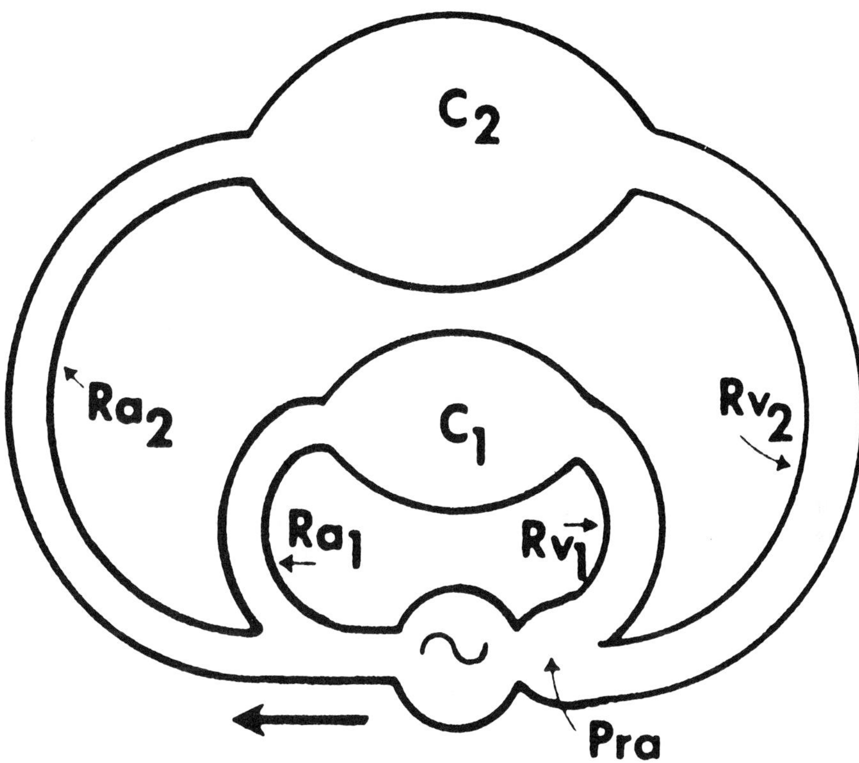

Figure 4. Two-compartment models of the systemic vascular bed. Each compartment has an upstream resistance element (Ra), a storage element (C), and a downstream resistance element (Rv). Even without an active change in properties of the storage elements, volume changes can occur by changes in upstream (arteriolar) resistance accompanied by changes in arteriolar inflow. (From Caldini et al,[14] with permission.)

downstream pressure in the area of the storage element *decreases,* and the storage element discharges some of its volume as predicted from its compliance (and perhaps further modified by changes in downstream resistance). This effect is the dominant part of a more complex effect that was found when epinephrine was given; additional changes in storage occurred because of changes in compliance and changes in unstressed vascular volume.[14] The authors found that a minimum of two vascular compartments were necessary to explain this effect: one compartment with a higher compliance, and one compartment with a lower compliance. Reinterpretation of preceding work suggested to them that the splanchnic vascular bed was the region most likely to charge and discharge a large volume following changes in arteriolar inflow; subsequent work has supported that contention.[15]

From this model, we learn that changes in blood flow distribution, which are a function of resistance and therefore arteriolar tone, can affect blood volume storage, which is usually believed to require changes in venous tone; it is also likely to some small extent that the inverse is true (storage affects resistance), although no experimental data exist to the point. The importance of this concept is that disease states, neurohumoral changes, or drugs could alter flow distribution patterns caused by changes in *arteriolar tone* that are virtually unmeasurable in humans, whereas our easily observed parameters, such as cardiac filling pressures, are erroneously interpreted to suggest changes in *venous tone.*

Two examples that may be illustrative of this point are offered, even though no data exist. Increased central blood volume and filling pressures in heart failure are attributed, in part, to increased venous tone. From the above discussion, it might be suggested that increased splanchnic arteriolar tone (by neurohumoral mechanisms) has decreased splanchnic storage and redistributed blood volume without a change in venous tone.

Another example may be the unsettled issue of why filling pressures decrease after drug blockade of the renin-angiotensin system, inasmuch as there are no known angiotensin receptors in the veins. It is likely that changes in arteriolar tone alter blood flow distribution and increase splanchnic inflow and result in a passive increase in venous storage. Similar effects may exist with other drugs that affect arteriolar tone and do so in such a manner as to alter the distribution of blood flow.

MODIFYING INFLUENCES ON THE PERIPHERAL CIRCULATION IN HEART FAILURE

This section will review the effects on the peripheral circulation that accompany heart failure.

Cardiac Effects

The potential changes that the peripheral circulation experiences in heart failure as a result of decreased cardiac function are decreases in blood pressure and cardiac output and increases in venous pressure.

The decrease in flow and arterial pressure results in absolute and relative changes in flow distribution. Such could be anticipated based on the above discussion of the physical properties of the circulation but, of course, the flow distribution is strongly modified by neurohumoral and local metabolic influences in the tissues.

The work of Wade and Bishop demonstrated the preservation of resting coronary, cerebral, and skeletal muscle blood flow in an absolute sense and, because cardiac output is decreased in heart failure, a relative increase in these circulations.[16] The inverse comments are true for splanchnic, renal, and skin blood flow. An additional redistribution occurs—and a potentially adverse conflict of blood flow needs arises—when there is an increased metabolic need such as in exercise (Fig. 5).[3] Under this circumstance, for example, the splanchnic bed may be entirely stripped of flow. The short- and long-term consequences of this redistribution and collision of blood flow requirements have been speculated about: many symptoms and signs of heart failure are at the peripheral tissue level probably as a result of this shift.

This effect of an increase in venous pressure is to imbalance the hydrostatic forces responsible for fluid filtration in the capillary,[2] with consequent increases in extravascular fluid volume and edema formation. The organ effects that occur range from cosmetic to serious functional derangement. Serious problems may occur in the lung and in the gut. The consequences of an increase in lung water include changes in ventilation/perfusion ratios of lung units, which may increase wasted ventilation and decrease arterial oxygenation. Another consequence of increased pulmonary venous pressure is increased pulmonary artery pressure, and it is probably this pressure per se rather than edema formation that causes a decrease in pulmonary compliance and triggers receptors ("J" receptors) as part of breathlessness symptoms.

The consequences of splanchnic edema have not been well defined; and clinically, the overlap that occurs between low splanchnic blood flow states and passive congestion may not allow a differentiation. Hepatocellular dysfunction and altered foodstuff absorption and metabolism may accompany the familiar symptoms of nausea, nondescript abdominal pain and fullness, and right upper quadrant tenderness.

Impaired renal handling of electrolytes and water may be due to both decreased blood flow and increased venous pressures and is further affected by neurohumoral events.

Still another tissue in which functional performance may be modified by edema is the wall of the blood vessels.[3] The changes may be caused by two different mechanisms. The increase

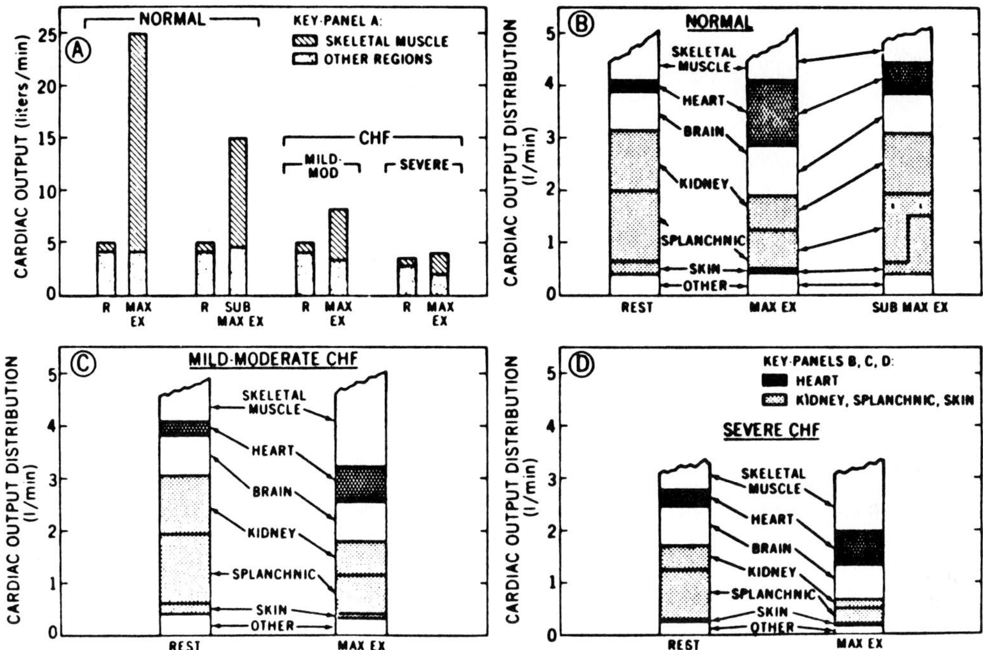

Figure 5. Distribution of cardiac output. *A*, Skeletal muscle blood flow is small at rest (R) but accounts for a progressively increased fraction of total cardiac output reserve, whereas skeletal muscle fraction is lower than normal during exercise in heart failure. More detailed data on distribution of cardiac output to non–skeletal muscle circulations is shown in normal persons (*B*), those with moderate heart failure (*C*), and those with severe heart failure (*D*). (From Zelis and Flaim,[3] with permission.)

of fluid in the vessel wall may change the physical properties of the blood vessels by stiffening the vessels and by encroaching on their lumen; or the electrolyte composition of the vessel wall may change with consequent effect on vascular smooth muscle via excitation–contraction coupling and tension development. Increases in resistance and decreases in storage of the vascular tree occur in heart failure; although it is difficult to separate these vascular effects from those caused by neurohumoral effects, it has been reported that diuresis partly reverses this abnormality, increasing the suspicion of the direct adverse effects of edema.

Neurohumoral Effects

The availability of accurate assays for the blood-borne humors of neurohumoral systems has promoted the concept of excess activity of vasoconstrictors in heart failure. Despite high circulating levels, however, a key unresolved issue is the activity of these hormones at the tissue level. Therefore, in addition to hormone concentration, the metabolism, the number, and the responsiveness of vascular receptors or active sites and their effect on vascular smooth muscle require further elucidation. This work has been hampered by the virtual inability to study these questions in vivo and the lack of suitable isolated systems or models of heart failure.

Sympathetic peripheral nerve terminal activity is believed to be excessive in patients with heart failure because of clinical and physiologic findings compatible with increased activity (e.g., sweating, tachycardia, increased peripheral resistance). Interpretation of clinical evidence is confounded by failure to identify other neurohumors that might have similar effect. Also, some information appears to be in conflict. Although resting values of physiologic activity are increased, clinical evaluation of stress-response relationships appear blunted. For example, stress maneuvers such as exercise, hypotension induced by amyl nitrite, and Valsalva's maneuver show normal or blunted responsiveness of blood pressure and heart rate.

Nerve terminal activity is also believed to be increased in heart failure because of increased circulating norepinephrine,[17,18] but there are considerable problems in interpreting these data. Catecholamine metabolism data are lacking in heart failure: data on production steps and sites, distribution, receptor number and activity, and catabolism and excretion are not described. Even though circulating levels of norepinephrine are increased, maximum levels achieved during exercise are decreased. A key enzyme in the production pathway (dopamine beta-hydroxylase) has been reported to be decreased. Tissue measurements of catecholamines have been reported as showing increased, normal, or decreased concentrations. And receptor number and activity may be decreased. The actual circulating level of catecholamines, even when extremely elevated in heart failure, is just barely at the threshold of physiologic response.

With newer assays for dopa, dopamine, and epinephrine, additional information suggests the adrenal gland as a site of excessive production of dopamine and epinephrine and the kidney as a site for excessive conversion of dopa to dopamine.

Our comments concerning the sympathetic nervous system can be transferred in parallel to the renin-angiotensin system. Early studies of circulating hormone and precursor levels emphasized normal values before diuretic treatment for patients in heart failure; increased levels were found after chronic treatment. It is no wonder that given the types of treatment, the duration of heart failure, and the condition of the patient with heart failure, more recent investigations have described low, normal, or elevated levels of renin and angiotensin. It has also become readily accepted that when beneficial effects occur after blockade of a neurohumoral system, that in turn demonstrates the important excess activity of that system. Pharmacologic testing and responsiveness offer only a very limited insight into physiologic behavior.

Other hormonal systems have been mentioned as possibly showing excessive activity in heart failure. The only other direct vasoconstrictor is vasopressin-ADH; circulating levels are not impressively elevated, but tissue-level effects may be important—especially renal effects on salt and water metabolism. Proof of the existence of a natriuretic factor has been elusive; recent evidence suggests that it exhibits digoxin-like (Na^+-K^+ ATPase) activity, which is an interesting twist on the renal and vascular effects of digoxin. The activity of this hormone may have very important effects on salt and water metabolism and vascular smooth-muscle tone in heart failure.

The bradykinin and prostaglandin systems are widely heralded as tissue-level systems with important effects on vascular tone. The production cascade of these systems is linked to the renin-angiotensin system through converting enzyme. The probable importance of local concentration rather than circulating concentration has made study difficult.

In summary, as opposed to other disease states with well-defined excess activity of neurohumors and clinical consequences—hyperthyroidism, hypercortisolism, pheochromocytoma—the syndrome of heart failure has not been defined to include excessive neurohumoral activity. Beneficial effect of vasodilator treatment, especially those treatments that block neurohumoral activity, does not necessarily indicate the excessive role of that hormone in heart failure.

REFERENCES

1. Riley, RL: *A postscript to circulation of the blood: Men and ideas.* Circulation 66:683, 1982.
2. Mellander, S and Johansson, B: *Control of resistance, exchange, and capacitance functions in the peripheral circulation.* Pharmacol Rev 20:117, 1968.
3. Zelis, R and Flaim, SF: *Alterations of vasomotor tone in congestive heart failure.* Prog Cardiovasc Dis 24:437, 1982.

4. SWAN, HJC AND RUBIN, SA (EDS): *Chronic Heart Failure and Vasodilator Therapy.* American College of Cardiology, Bethesda, 1980.
5. GOW, BS: *Circulatory correlates: Vascular impedance, resistance and capacity.* In BOHR, DF, SOMLYO, AP, AND SPARKS, HV (EDS): *Handbook of Physiology, Sec. 2, Vol. 2, The Cardiovascular System.* American Physiological Society, Bethesda, 1980, p 353.
6. DREES, JA AND ROTHE, CF: *Reflex venoconstriction and capacity vessel pressure-volume relationships in dogs.* Circ Res 34:360, 1974.
7. SHOUKAS, AA AND SAGAWA, K: *Total systemic vascular compliance measured as incremental volume-pressure ratio.* Circ Res 28:277, 1971.
8. SHOUKAS, AA AND SAGAWA, K: *Control of total systemic vascular capacity by the carotid sinus baroreceptor reflex.* Circ Res 33:22, 1973.
9. RUBIN, SA, MISBACH, G, LEKVEN, J, ET AL: *Resistance and volume changes caused by nitroprusside in the dog.* Am J Physiol 237:H99, 1979.
10. GUYTON, AC: *Venous return.* In HAMILTON, WF AND DOW, P (EDS): *Handbook of Physiology, Sec. 2, Vol. 2, Circulation.* American Physiological Society, Washington, 1963, p 1099.
11. HAMILTON, WF: *The patterns of the arterial pressure pulse.* Am J Physiol 141:235, 1944.
12. O'ROURKE, MF: *Vascular impedance in studies of arterial and cardiac function.* Physiol Rev 62:570, 1982.
13. MILNOR, WR: *Arterial impedance as ventricular afterload.* Circ Res 36:565, 1975.
14. CALDINI, P, PERMUTT, S, WADDELL, JA, ET AL: *Effect of epinephrine on pressure, flow and volume relationships in the systemic circulation of dogs.* Circ Res 34:606, 1974.
15. MITZNER, W AND GOLDBERG, H: *Effects of epinephrine on resistive and compliant properties of the canine vasculature.* J Appl Physiol 39:272, 1975.
16. WADE, OL AND BISHOP, JM: *Cardiac output and regional blood flow.* Blackwell Scientific, Oxford, 1962.
17. THOMAS, JA AND MARKS, BH: *Plasma norepinephrine in congestive heart failure.* Am J Cardiol 41:233, 1978.
18. RUTENBERG, HL AND SPANN, JF JR: *Alterations of cardiac sympathetic neurotransmitter activity in congestive heart failure.* Am J Cardiol 32:472, 1973.

Clinical Pharmacology of Diuretic Drugs

Albert N. Brest, M.D.

Although the potential exists for newer agents,[1] the currently available diuretic drug armamentarium has undergone few changes during the past decade. Recent additions include only the potassium-sparing agent amiloride and the loop diuretic bumetanide. In part, this lack of new diuretic drugs represents reasonable satisfaction with the present diuretic armamentarium. Indeed, it is possible currently to control most cases of cardiac edema and to achieve significant blood pressure reduction in most instances of sodium-dependent hypertension. However, as with all drug groups, successful application of diuretic therapy requires a thorough knowledge of clinical pharmacology, including potential untoward effects and their management.

PHARMACODYNAMIC EFFECTS

Diuretic drugs promote urine flow by inhibiting the renal tubular reabsorption of sodium or its accompanying anions, chloride and bicarbonate.[2,3] Thus, diuresis and natriuresis are inextricably linked. However, the ultimate diuretic effect depends on the potency of the drug's inhibitory effect on electrolyte reabsorption, on its site of action within the nephron, and on extrarenal influences (such as aldosterone, ADH, and effective circulating blood volume) that can counter diuretic drug actions by enhancing reabsorption of salt and water.

With regard to diuretic potency, it is well established that carbonic anhydrase inhibitors and potassium-sparing agents are substantially less potent than thiazide diuretics, whereas loop diuretics exhibit greater natriuretic and diuretic effects. Regarding diuretic site of action, it is noteworthy that 60 to 70 percent of the glomerular filtrate is reabsorbed in the proximal tubule, 15 to 30 percent in the thick ascending limb of the loop of Henle, and 10 to 15 percent in the distal convoluted tubule and the early collecting duct. Thus, drugs that act in the distal portions of the nephron, for example, thiazides and potassium-sparing agents, induce less diuresis than those that act more proximally, for example, loop diuretics. Reduction of effective blood volume may be related to the underlying condition, for example, congestive heart failure, or to the diuresis per se.[4] Decreased effective blood volume enhances proximal tubular reabsorption of sodium and water, thereby reducing urine flow and natriuresis. Hypovolemia also stimulates the renin-angiotensin-aldosterone mechanism, and the ensuing hyperaldosteronism increases distal tubular reabsorption of sodium in exchange for potassium and hydrogen. Finally, decreased effective blood volume stimulates ADH secretion, which facilitates water reabsorption. Thus, the ultimate diuretic and natriuretic effects exhibited by a given diuretic, or a combination of diuretic agents, depend on the interplay of a variety of pharmacodynamic and pathophysiologic actions.

Carbonic Anhydrase Inhibitors

Carbonic anhydrase inhibitors, such as acetazolamide, exert their principal diuretic effects at the proximal tubule. Specifically, these drugs block the reabsorption of sodium in exchange for hydrogen generated in the tubular cells by the hydration of carbon dioxide. Decreased reabsorption of sodium and bicarbonate is accompanied by significant kaliuresis and the development of metabolic acidosis. Unfortunately, drug tolerance ordinarily develops after 2 to 3 days of continuous administration. Thus, these drugs can be used only intermittently. In addition, side effects due to their sulfonamide structure may be encountered. As a result of these factors and the availability of more potent diuretics, carbonic anhydrase inhibitors are now rarely employed as single agents in the treatment of heart failure. Nonetheless, these drugs are occasionally useful temporarily in special situations because significant potentiated effects may be achieved sometimes by combining a carbonic anhydrase inhibitor with other more distally active agents, for example, thiazide diuretics.

Loop Diuretics

These drugs interfere with sodium chloride reabsorption in the ascending limb of the loop of Henle. The three loop diuretics that are commercially available, furosemide, ethacrynic acid, and bumetanide, are chemically different, but their pharmacodynamic effects are remarkably similar.[5,6] The onset of action after oral administration of these drugs occurs in about 1 hour, and their duration of action extends for 4 to 8 hours (Table 1). In contrast, onset of action starts within 5 to 15 minutes, and peak natriuretic and diuretic effects occur within the first hour of intravenous administration. Total duration of action extends about 3 hours after parenteral administration.

The major adverse effects encountered with loop diuretics are due to their marked diuretic potency. In the presence of adequate filtered loads of sodium chloride, massive diuresis may be induced. In addition, the large amounts of sodium presented to the distal sites of potassium-sodium exchange may result in severe kaliuresis. These drugs may induce diuresis despite volume and electrolyte depletion, thereby further aggravating these conditions. Furthermore, the loop diuretics seriously impair free water clearance. Thus, potential untoward effects include marked hyponatremia, hypokalemia, and hypochloremic alkalosis. Excessive diuresis may result in dehydration and reduction in blood volume, causing orthostatic hypotension, hemoconcentration, and the possibility of vascular thrombosis and embolism. Other untoward effects include hyperuricemia, hyperglycemia, and acute transient hearing loss. Deafness is particularly apt to occur when large doses are used in patients with decreased renal function. Furosemide is a sulfonamide and therefore may exhibit cross-hypersensitivity reactions in common with the thiazides and their congeners. Bumetanide is a metanilimide derivative, and patients allergic to sulfonamides may also show hypersensitivity to bumetanide. Conversely, ethacrynic acid is chemically unrelated to other available diuretics and can be prescribed for patients who exhibit hypersensitivity reactions to sulfonamides.

In contrast to the thiazide diuretics, the loop diuretics exhibit a much steeper dose-response curve. Moreover, these drugs may be remarkably effective even when renal function is substantially impaired. Their ability to reduce renal vascular resistance and to readjust blood flow within the renal parenchyma (from the inner cortex and outer medulla to the outer cortical region) apparently accounts, at least in part, for the beneficial activity of the loop diuretics under conditions of reduced renal function. Whereas the thiazides are cortically active with respect to the nephron, the loop diuretics are primarily medullary with respect to the concentration gradient.[1] It is noteworthy that the renal origin of the prostaglandins is medullary, and the prostaglandins exert their principal actions on the countercurrent mechanism of the loop of Henle and on the vasa recta. Perhaps the aforementioned renal blood flow

Table 1. Commonly employed oral diuretics

Diuretic	Dosage (mg)			Duration of Action (hr)
	Minimal	*Usual*	*Maximal*	
Thiazides and thiazide-type diuretics				
Bendroflumethiazide	2.5 o.d.	5 o.d.	10 o.d.	18–24
Benzthiazide	50 o.d.	50 o.d.	100 o.d.	12–18
Chlorothiazide	500 o.d.	500 o.d.	1,000 b.i.d.	6–12
Chlorthalidone	25 o.d.	50 o.d.	100 o.d.	48–72
Cyclothiazide	1 o.d.	2 o.d.	4 o.d.	18–24
Hydrochlorothiazide	50 o.d.	50 b.i.d.	100 b.i.d.	12–18
Hydroflumethiazide	50 o.d.	50 b.i.d.	100 b.i.d.	18–24
Methyclothiazide	2.5 o.d.	5 o.d.	10 o.d.	24
Metolazone	2.5 o.d.	5 o.d.	10 o.d.	12–24
Polythiazide	1 o.d.	2 o.d.	4 o.d.	24–48
Quinethazone	50 o.d.	100 o.d.	200 o.d.	18–24
Trichlormethiazide	2 o.d.	4 o.d.	8 o.d.	24
Loop diuretics				
Ethacrynic acid	50 o.d.	50 b.i.d.	200 b.i.d.	6–8
Furosemide	40 o.d.	40 b.i.d.	300 b.i.d.	6–8
Bumefanide	0.5 o.d.	1 b.i.d.	5 b.i.d.	4
Potassium-sparing diuretics				
Amiloride	5 o.d.	10 o.d.	20 o.d.	24
Spironolactone	25 b.i.d.	50 b.i.d.	100 b.i.d.	48–72
Triamterene	50 b.i.d.	100 b.i.d.	150 b.i.d.	12–16

changes induced by the loop diuretics may be intertwined with drug-induced alterations in the prostaglandins.

In titrating the dosage of oral loop diuretics, incremental increases should be made at 6- to 8-hour intervals. If a given dose does not induce the desired effect, the dosage rather than the frequency of administration should be increased.

Because of their marked potency, use of the loop diuretics is preferred in patients with cardiac edema that is refractory to treatment with less potent diuretic agents. Also, they may be uniquely useful in the presence of coexistent renal failure, whether the heart failure is mild or severe. In addition, because of their rapid onset of activity and great diuretic potency, these diuretics administered parenterally have become the diuretics of choice in the treatment of acute pulmonary edema.

Thiazides and Related Drugs

These drugs act at the distal cortical diluting segment of the nephron. They inhibit sodium reabsorption and, like the loop diuretics, interfere with the generation of free water. However, because of the lesser absorption of sodium that ordinarily occurs in the distal nephron, the thiazides and thiazide-type drugs exhibit less natriuretic potency than the loop diuretics, which act more proximally. Conversely, the thiazides and their congeners are more potent than the potassium-sparing drugs that act even more distally in the nephron.

The numerous thiazide and thiazide-type (phthalimidine and quinazoline) diuretics differ with regard to milligram potency and duration of action, but their pharmacodynamic actions, effects on electrolyte excretion, and clinical applications are similar.[7] All these drugs are absorbed rapidly from the gastrointestinal tract, with onset of natriuretic and diuretic actions ordinarily exhibited within the first 1 to 2 hours after oral administration. Duration of action ranges from 6 hours to more than 24 hours for the various preparations (see Table 1). Potassium depletion and metabolic alkalosis are common consequences of both loop diuretic and thiazide diuretic therapy. The kaliuresis is not a primary action of either drug group but results instead from the increased sodium load presented to the more distal tubular sites for potassium-sodium exchange. Other thiazide-induced electrolyte alterations include increased urinary loss of magnesium and decreased calcium excretion. Additional potential biochemical alterations include hyperuricemia, hyperglycemia, and hyperlipidemia.

A variety of untoward systemic and hematologic effects have been encountered with thiazides and related drugs.[8] These untoward effects include thrombocytopenic and nonthrombocytopenic purpura, glomerulonephritis, pancreatitis, vasculitis, hepatic injury, photosensitivity, and skin rashes of various types. These reactions may be due to hypersensitivity or idiosyncrasy. Although not all of these adverse reactions have been reported with each drug in this group, their occurrence should be considered to be possible with any of these agents.

The thiazides and related duiretics are considered by many physicians to be the cornerstone of therapy for hypertension. In addition, these compounds are the agents of choice in the management of cardiac edema of mild to moderate severity, except in the presence of significant renal functional impairment. Thiazides and thiazide-like drugs are relatively ineffective when used alone in patients with renal insufficiency. In this regard, metolazone is the one exception in that it may induce diuresis even in patients with glomerular filtration rates below 20 ml/min.[9] The effectiveness of metolazone in this situation is probably due to its more powerful inhibitory effects in the proximal tubules, in comparison with related compounds. Apart from the latter exception, maximal effective doses of these various compounds are approximately equipotent, at equivalent milligram dosages.[7] Moreover, there are no additive effects to be achieved by combining any of the thiazides and related compounds. If additional diuretic effect is needed, once maximal dosages are reached, either more potent diuretics or combination diuretic therapy should be employed.

Potassium-Sparing Drugs

The potassium-sparing diuretics (triamterene, spironolactone, and amiloride) block potassium-sodium exchange in the distal portions of the nephron (distal convoluted tubule and early collecting duct), thereby conserving potassium while promoting sodium excretion.[10] Triamterene and amiloride interfere directly with potassium-sodium exchange (in the presence or absence of aldosterone), whereas spironolactone is a competitive antagonist of aldosterone. Despite these differences in mechanism of action, the clinical efficacy of these three drugs is similar.

Diuresis may be observed with triamterene and amiloride within 2 hours after an oral dose. The duration of diuretic effect extends for 12 to 16 hours with triamterene, and about 24 hours with amiloride (see Table 1). In contrast, spironolactone has a relatively slow onset of action and must be continued for at least 2 days for substantial effect. Optimal response to triamterene and spironolactone requires twice-daily dosing, whereas amiloride can usually be given once daily.

The most important potential untoward effect encountered with these agents is hyperkalemia. In the presence of significantly impaired renal function, potassium supplementation should not be given concomitantly with these agents. Likewise, patients should be counseled against the concomitant use of foods that are high in potassium content and of salt substitutes that contain large amounts of potassium.[11] In all cases, serum potassium concentration should be monitored periodically.

Side effects of triamterene can include nausea and vomiting, diarrhea, headache, and weakness. Amiloride may cause nausea, anorexia, abdominal pain, flatulence, and skin rash. Drowsiness, mental confusion, and gastrointestinal irritation have been reported with administration of spironolactone. In addition, spironolactone may cause gynecomastia in males and menstrual disturbances or lactation in women.

Because they act distally after most of the sodium has been reabsorbed, the potassium-sparing agents exhibit only mild diuretic action when used alone. In order to achieve substantial diuresis, these drugs must be used in combination with other, more potent diuretic agents. When potassium-sparing drugs are administered with thiazides or loop diuretics, the diuretic response to the latter agents is substantially enhanced, probably because the effects of secondary hyperaldosteronism are largely blocked. Consequently, combined therapy not only reduces potassium excretion and minimizes alkalosis, but it is also quite effective in mobilizing refractory edema fluid.

Combination Diuretic Drug Therapy

There are no convincing data to indicate that the combination of two thiazides or thiazide-like drugs will yield any greater diuretic effect than that induced by administering maximal dosage of any single agent from this drug category. However, the diuretic efficacy of thiazides and related compounds can be enhanced by the concomitant use of a potassium-sparing agent, loop diuretic, or carbonic anhydrase inhibitor. Moreover, the triple drug regimen of thiazide, potassium-sparing drug, and loop diuretic may induce diuretic and natriuretic effects that exceed the additive effects obtained when these drugs are administered separately. The potentiated effects of these regimens are achieved because of their concomitant actions at different sites in the nephron and by their differing mechanisms of action.

In the presence of substantial renal impairment, potassium-sparing agents generally should be avoided. However, in the latter situation, metolazone in combination with a loop diuretic may be effectively employed. Although other thiazide-type drugs are generally ineffective when administered alone in the presence of low glomerular filtration rates, these agents too may at times be useful in this situation in combination with a loop diuretic.[12]

COMPLICATIONS OF DIURETIC DRUG THERAPY

As already indicated, diuretic drug therapy may induce a wide variety of untoward reactions.[13] Some of these side effects are uniquely linked to individual drugs, whereas others reflect the diuresis per se and its accompanying biochemical alterations.

Diuresis leads directly to intravascular volume depletion. A modest, slow reduction in ventricular filling pressure may either improve cardiac function or occur without causing any significant change in cardiac stroke volume. However, an abrupt, excessive reduction in intravascular volume may result in clinically significant decreases in filling pressure, stroke volume, and cardiac output.[14] Thus, diuretic-induced hypovolemia may at times exaggerate the clinical manifestations of low cardiac output syndromes. For example, in the presence of a myocardial infarction with low cardiac output, the accompanying hypotension may worsen and, in the extreme case, cardiogenic shock may follow. In the patient with chronic congestive heart failure, excessive diuresis may shift ventricular function to the steep descent of the Starling curve, resulting in exaggerated signs of systemic hypoperfusion with further reduction of renal function (oliguria) and cerebral blood flow (mental confusion). In the latter instance, the duiretic should be discontinued, and small aliquots of saline or plasma infused (preferably with concomitant monitoring of pulmonary artery pressure to guide the volume repletion). In general, one should aim to achieve a slow, smooth diuresis in the patient with congestive heart failure who is not in pulmonary edema.

Dilutional hyponatremia may sometimes accompany congestive cardiac failure. Conversely, rapid excessive natriuresis accompanying diuretic drug therapy may result in temporary depletional hyponatremia. The latter is especially apt to occur with overly brisk diuresis plus markedly restricted dietary salt intake and/or undue extrarenal losses of sodium due, for instance, to vomiting or diarrhea. More commonly, however, the use of loop diuretics and/or thiazides may cause or exaggerate dilutional hyponatremia because each of these drug groups can seriously impair free water clearance. Dilutional hyponatremia calls for severe fluid restriction (600 ml per day or less).

Hypokalemia induced by loop diuretics or thiazides is caused by the increased delivery of sodium to the distal sites of potassium-sodium exchange and to the presence of increased circulating aldosterone. Mild hypokalemia is not necessarily associated with any symptoms, but it poses the threat of digitalis intoxication in patients receiving digitalis and can induce serious arrhythmias in the patient with myocardial disease.[15] Additionally, neuropsychiatric symptoms, constipation, and anorexia may be encountered, and prominent skeletal muscle weakness, abdominal distention, and paralytic ileus may occur in the presence of marked potassium depletion.

Because serious and at times even fatal events may follow diuretic-induced hypokalemia, thoughtful steps should be taken to prevent, minimize, or correct this disorder. This end may be achieved by dietary measures, administration of potassium chloride supplements, and/or concomitant use of a potassium-sparing drug together with the potassium-wasting diuretic. Adequate dietary intake of potassium is not always feasible, especially if the potassium loss is high. Supplementation of the daily diet with an additional 80 mEq of potassium requires the patient to eat six medium-sized bananas or to drink six cups of orange juice or their equivalent. It should be remembered also that high sodium intake may exaggerate potassium loss (because more sodium is presented to the distal tubule for potassium-sodium exchange); therefore, sodium abuse must be avoided. Indeed, dietary salt intake should ordinarily be restricted when these drugs are employed.[16] Orally administered potassium supplements, including salt substitutes, also may be employed to offset the urinary loss of potassium during diuretic therapy. Although several salts are available, potassium chloride is preferred because the chloride is useful in correcting the associated alkalosis. The concomitant use of a potassium-sparing drug is often the most effective means for maintaining serum potassium concentrations during diuretic therapy. However, in the presence of renal functional impairment, potassium supplements and potassium-sparing diuretics both must be used with great caution, including frequent monitoring of serum potassium.

Potassium depletion also may induce glucose intolerance. The associated hyperglycemia may develop because of delayed insulin release. Potassium supplementation or concomitant use of a potassium-sparing drug will often reverse or attenuate the hyperglycemia.

Diuretic-induced hyperuricemia may result from enhanced proximal tubular reabsorption of uric acid due to blood volume contraction. The hyperuricemia often occurs without associated symptoms, but acute gouty attacks occasionally will be precipitated. These attacks abate with colchicine or other antigout measures, and the hyperuricemia generally can be reversed by the concomitant use of allopurinol or a uricosuric drug such as probenecid. Hypercalcemia, like hyperuricemia, also may be caused by extracellular fluid volume depletion. The hypercalcemia results from increased proximal tubular reabsorption of calcium. Treatment of the hypercalcemia involves restoration of blood volume. Although thiazides are contraindicated in hypercalcemic patients, it is noteworthy that loop diuretics can increase calcium excretion if extracellular fluid volume depletion is avoided.[17]

Loop diuretics and thiazides also may induce significant urinary loss of magnesium. Hypomagnesemia tends to promote a loss of myocardial cellular potassium and, as a result, cardiac arrhythmias may follow. Likewise, hypomagnesemia increases the risk of digitalis intoxication in patients taking digitalis preparations. Treatment of this disorder involves temporary discontinuation of diuretic therapy and repletion of magnesium stores.

CLINICAL USE OF DIURETICS IN CARDIAC FAILURE

Diuretic therapy is obviously a powerful tool in the management of cardiac edema. It is evident from the preceding comments, however, that equally powerful side effects may be induced. Moreover, exaggerated diuresis ("overdiuresis") may aggravate low cardiac output syndromes. Thus, the use of these drugs calls for broad knowledge and appropriate clinical respect for their potent effects.

Fundamental clinical goals in the management of heart failure include (1) recognition and specific treatment (whenever possible) of the underlying cardiac disorder, and (2) correction of any contributory extracardiac conditions (such as anemia, hypertension, electrolyte imbalance, thyroid dysfunction, and pulmonary disease).

Diuretic therapy mainly affects preload, which is just one of several factors affecting cardiac performance. Clearly, optimal therapy for cardiac failure can be achieved best by concomitant attention to all factors involved, not simply preload. The other major factors involved in cardiac functional capacity are myocardial contractility, heart rate and rhythm, and afterload.

In addition to diuretic drug therapy, reduction in preload is amplified by dietary salt restriction and administration of nitrates. The decrease in preload results in a decline in pulmonary artery pressure and pulmonary congestion. Concomitant improvement in cardiac output is best achieved by combining diuretics (and other preload reduction measures) with inotropic drugs and/or arterial dilators. Myocardial contractility can be improved directly by inotropic agents such as digitalis and catecholamines. Arterial dilators (e.g., hydralazine) may exhibit beneficial effects by decreasing impedance to left ventricular ejection, thereby facilitating ventricular emptying. The effects of the augmented renin-angiotensin-aldosterone mechanism in cardiac failure can be blunted by the use of a converting enzyme inhibitor (i.e., captopril). Finally, it should be remembered that cardiac arrhythmias, including conduction defects, may seriously compromise cardiac failure and, thus, it follows that any accompanying cardiac dysrhythmias must be treated concomitantly to achieve optimal control of heart failure. In summary, optimum management of cardiac decompensation requires knowledgeable application of a wide variety of therapeutic interventions.

REFERENCES

1. Beyer, KH Jr: *Diuretics in the 1980s.* Clin Ther 5:3, 1982.
2. Seely, JF and Dirks, JH: *Site of action of diuretic drugs.* Kidney Int 11:1, 1977.
3. Jacobson, HR and Kokko, JP: *Diuretics: Sites and mechanisms of action.* Annu Rev Pharmacol Toxicol 16:201, 1976.
4. Porter, GA: *The role of diuretics in the treatment of heart failure.* JAMA 244:1614, 1980.
5. Brest, AN, Onesti, G, Seller, R, et al: *Pharmacodynamic effects of a new diuretic drug, ethacrynic acid.* Am J Cardiol 16:99, 1965.
6. Brest, AN, Seller, R, Ramirez, O, et al: *Comparative diuretic efficacy of furosemide.* J New Drugs 5:329, 1965.
7. Swartz, C, Seller, R, Fuchs, M, et al: *Five years' experience with the evaluation of diuretic agents.* Circulation 28:1024, 1963.
8. Brest, AN and Moyer, JH: *Untoward effects of diuretic drugs.* J Med Assoc Penna 66:27, 1963.
9. Lowenthal, DT and Shear, L: *Use of a new diuretic agent (metolazone) in patients with edema and ascites.* Arch Intern Med 132:39, 1973.
10. *Potassium-sparing diuretics: Spironolactone, triamterene and amiloride.* Curr Ther Bull 4:30, 1972.
11. Sopko, JA and Freeman, RM: *Salt substitutes as a source of potassium.* JAMA 238:608, 1977.
12. Wollam, GL, Tarazi, RC, Bravo, EL, et al: *Diuretic potency of combined hydrochlorothiazide and furosemide therapy in patients with azotemia.* Am J Med 72:929, 1982.
13. Plumb, VJ and James, TN: *Clinical hazards of powerful diuretics.* Mod Concepts Cardiovasc Dis 47:91, 1977.
14. Giles, TD: *Problems in the management of edema in the patient with chronic congestive cardiac failure.* Practical Cardiology 7:79, 1981.
15. Holland, OB, Nixon, JV, and Kuhnert, L: *Diuretic-induced ventricular ectopy. Am J Med 70:762, 1981.*
16. Wilcox, CS, Mitch, WE, Kelly, RA, et al: *Effect of salt intake on sodium homeostasis during furosemide administration.* Kidney Int 21:160, 1982.
17. Kelly, RA, Wilcox, CS, and Mitch, WE: *Diuretics: An update.* J Cardiovasc Med 7:1153, 1982.

Adrenergic Receptors: New Concepts and Implications for Cardiovascular Therapeutics

Wilson S. Colucci, M.D., and Eugene Braunwald, M.D.

All direct cardiovascular effects of the adrenergic nervous system are mediated through the interaction of catecholamines with alpha- or beta-adrenergic receptors. Because they possess highly specific structural requirements for the recognition of hormones and drugs, adrenergic receptors provide an important site for the pharmacologic manipulation of the cardiovascular system. Thus, as opposed to sympatholytic drugs such as guanethidine or reserpine that globally depress adrenergic function, drugs that act on adrenergic receptors can be used selectively to inhibit or stimulate specific portions of the cardiovascular system. For instance, beta-adrenergic receptor antagonists directly reduce the inotropic and chronotropic states of the heart without reducing systemic vascular tone, whereas alpha-adrenergic receptor antagonists cause vasodilation and consequent reduction of arterial pressure but have little direct effect on myocardial function. Our basic understanding of adrenergic receptors has grown rapidly as a result of the development of compounds that exhibit unique affinities for these receptors both as agonists (stimulants) and antagonists, and this new information is having a growing impact on clinical practice. The purpose of this review is to summarize our understanding of adrenergic receptors and to consider the current role of adrenergic receptor pharmacology in cardiovascular medicine.

ADRENERGIC RECEPTOR CLASSIFICATION

The initial classification of adrenergic receptors stemmed from the observation by Raymond P. Ahlquist in 1948 that the order of potency of the catecholamines norepinephrine, epinephrine, and isoproterenol varies from tissue to tissue.[1] For instance, in the myocardium, isoproterenol is the most potent inotropic and chronotropic stimulant, whereas in blood vessels, epinephrine and norepinephrine (NE) are both more potent than isoproterenol in causing constriction. Indeed, isoproterenol is a vasodilator. Consequently, Ahlquist proposed that contraction of vascular smooth muscle and myocardium is mediated by two different receptors, which he termed alpha and beta, respectively. The order of potency of catecholamines at alpha receptors is epinephrine $>$ NE $\gg$ isoproterenol, whereas the order at beta receptors is isoproterenol $\gg$ epinephrine $\geq$ NE. These observations have facilitated greatly the classification of both adrenergic agonists and antagonists.

The basic concept of differentiation of receptors into alpha and beta types has stood the test of time and is supported by several lines of physiologic, pharmacologic, and biochemical evidence. However, as our understanding of adrenergic receptors has increased, so too has the complexity of the initial classification system. First, two subtypes of each basic receptor are now recognized, termed $alpha_1$, $alpha_2$, $beta_1$, and $beta_2$. Second, it is apparent that alpha- and beta-adrenergic receptors exist not only on end-organs within the cardiovascular system but also on adrenergic nerve endings and within cardiovascular regulatory centers of the brain stem. Finally, considerable data indicate that adrenergic receptors are important loci for the regulation of end-organ responsiveness.

Thus, adrenergic receptors are involved at three different levels in the regulation of cardiovascular function. First, *postsynaptic* alpha- and beta-adrenergic receptors, located on the surface of cardiac and vascular smooth muscle cells, serve as the interface between the sympathetic nervous system and cardiovascular end-organs. Strategically located on the effector cell membrane, postsynaptic receptors determine the neurohumoral response pattern of the cell and, in addition, provide a locus at which cellular responsiveness to specific stimuli may be regulated. Second, alpha- and beta-adrenergic receptors located on peripheral neurons (i.e., *presynaptic* receptors) are part of a feedback mechanism that provides local modulation of neurotransmitter release. Finally, adrenergic receptors located within the *central nervous system* are involved in the overall regulation of sympathetic outflow to the cardiovascular system. In addition to their role in cardiovascular regulation, alterations in the behavior of adrenergic receptors at each of these sites can be responsible for the development of organ dysfunction, and pharmacologic manipulation of these receptors can be used therapeutically.

Alpha-Adrenergic Receptor Subtypes

Traditionally, the physiologic description of alpha-adrenergic receptors has been based on catecholamine-induced contraction of vascular smooth muscle which can be blocked by the antagonist phentolamine. However, over the last few years, a number of compounds (Table 1) have been identified that exhibit an even higher degree of specificity for alpha receptors than do the catecholamines and phentolamine. Through the use of these agents in both physiologic systems and radioligand-binding assays, it is now apparent that there are two basic types of alpha-adrenergic receptors, termed $alpha_1$ and $alpha_2$.[2]

Presynaptic Versus Postsynaptic Alpha Receptors

The recognition of two physiologic types of alpha receptors was based largely on the observation that the release of NE, the endogenous adrenergic neurotransmitter, from peripheral adrenergic nerve terminals can be modulated by the action of alpha-adrenergic agents at "presynaptic" alpha-adrenergic receptors. As shown in Figure 1, adrenergic agonists and NE itself inhibit the release of the neurotransmitter. Thus, the release of NE from the preganglionic fiber has two effects: (1) it acts on the postsynaptic receptor on the effector cell, for example, a vascular smooth muscle cell; and (2) simultaneously, the released NE also acts on presynaptic receptors on the sympathetic nerve fiber, inhibiting the release of more NE and thereby reducing the quantity of neurotransmitter released for any given level of nerve

Table 1. Alpha-adrenergic receptor subtype selectivity of various agonists and antagonists

	$Alpha_1$	*Nonselective*	*$Alpha_2$*
Agonists	Phenylephrine Methoxamine	Norepinephrine Epinephrine	Clonidine Alpha-methylnorepinephrine Guanabenz
Antagonists	Prazosin Trimazosin Indoramin	Phentolamine Phenoxybenzamine	Yohimbine

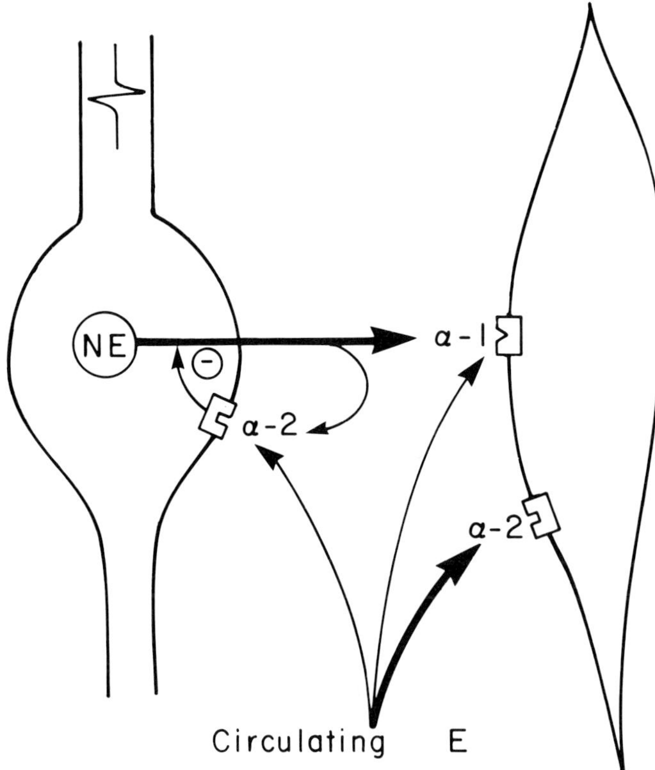

Figure 1. Schematic representation of presynaptic and postsynaptic alpha-adrenergic receptors located on an adrenergic nerve varicosity and vascular smooth muscle cell, respectively. Norepinephrine (NE) released from the nerve varicosity stimulates postsynaptic $alpha_1$ receptors resulting in vascular smooth muscle contraction, and presynaptic $alpha_2$ receptors which have an inhibitory influence on further NE release. An $alpha_1$ selective antagonist (e.g., prazosin) blocks primarily the postsynaptic receptor, whereas a nonselective antagonist (e.g., phentolamine) also blocks the presynaptic $alpha_2$ receptor, thereby resulting in increased NE release. Postsynaptic $alpha_2$ receptors that mediate contraction are present in some vessels and may be acted on primarily by circulating or exogenous catecholamines. Stimulation of presynaptic beta-adrenergic receptors on the nerve varicosity (not shown) causes an increase in NE release, and stimulation of postsynaptic $beta_2$ receptors on the vascular smooth muscle cells (not shown) results in vascular relaxation. (Adapted from Langer.[3])

impulse traffic in the sympathetic fibers. Following the recognition that stimulation of presynaptic alpha-adrenergic receptors results in a reduction in neurotransmitter release, it became apparent that the order of potency for certain alpha-adrenergic agonists and antagonists at the presynaptic receptor differed markedly from the order of potency at postsynaptic alpha-adrenergic receptors on blood vessels.[2–4] For example, the alpha-adrenergic agonists phenylephrine and methoxamine are more potent than clonidine with regard to contraction of vascular smooth muscle, that is, activation of postsynaptic receptors; whereas clonidine is a more potent inhibitor of neurotransmitter release, that is, activation of presynaptic receptors. Likewise, prazosin is more potent than yohimbine with regard to inhibition of catecholamine-induced contraction of vascular smooth muscle, whereas yohimbine is more potent than prazosin with regard to stimulation of neurotransmitter release. The endogenous agonists NE and epinephrine are equipotent at presynaptic and postsynaptic sites, as is the antagonist phentolamine.

Table 2. Classification of alpha-adrenergic receptors

Location	*Function*	*Subtype*
Postsynaptic		
Vascular smooth muscle	Contraction	$Alpha_1$, $Alpha_2$
Myocardium	Increase inotropy	$Alpha_1$
	Decrease chronotropy	$Alpha_1$
Presynaptic		
Peripheral nerve terminals	Decrease norepinephrine release	$Alpha_2$
Central nervous system	Decrease sympathetic outflow	$Alpha_2$
	Increase parasympathetic outflow	$Alpha_2$

$Alpha_1$ Versus $Alpha_2$ Receptors

The relative potencies of the aforementioned agonists and antagonists with regard to neurotransmitter release and contraction of vascular smooth muscle have provided the basis for the pharmacologic classification of alpha-adrenergic receptors as $alpha_1$ or $alpha_2$.[2] If the potency of an agonist or antagonist is greater in vascular smooth muscle, that is, if it resembles NE in the case of an agonist or prazosin in the case of an antagonist, the drug in question is classified as acting on $alpha_1$ receptors. If the drug resembles clonidine in the case of an agonist or yohimbine in the case of an antagonist, it is classified as acting on $alpha_2$ receptors. Conversely, one can classify alpha-adrenergic receptors by their response to these agonists and antagonists. If they are more potently antagonized by prazosin than yohimbine, they are termed $alpha_1$ receptors; the opposite obtains for $alpha_2$ receptors. The development of alpha-adrenergic receptor subtype-selective compounds based on this physiologic classification system has provided a powerful tool for the study of alpha receptors both in physiologic systems and by means of radioligand-binding methods.

Although it initially was thought that all postsynaptic receptors were of the $alpha_1$ subtype and all presynaptic receptors were of the $alpha_2$ subtype, this generalization is now known to be only partially correct. Whereas *presynaptic* receptors appear to be exclusively of the $alpha_2$ subtype, *postsynaptic* receptors may be either $alpha_1$ or $alpha_2$, and in any given tissue, the postsynaptic receptors may be entirely $alpha_1$, entirely $alpha_2$, or a mixture of both subtypes[2] (Table 2). For instance, there is evidence that in some blood vessels, a variable degree of catecholamine-induced contraction is mediated by $alpha_2$ receptors. Thus, it has been demonstrated in vivo in pithed rats and dogs that a component of the alpha-adrenergic-mediated pressor response is resistant to the $alpha_1$ selective antagonist prazosin, but blocked by the $alpha_2$ selective antagonist yohimbine.[5–8]

Beta-Adrenergic Receptor Subtypes

In 1967, Lands and coworkers demonstrated that beta-adrenergic receptors could be classified into two types; $beta_1$ receptors, which mediate cardiac stimulation and lipolysis, and $beta_2$ receptors, which mediate relaxation of vascular and bronchial smooth muscle[9] (Tables 3, 4). The order of catecholamine potency at $beta_1$ receptors is isoproterenol $\gg$ NE = epinephrine, whereas at $beta_2$ receptors the order is isoproterenol $\gg$ epinephrine $>$ NE. A number of beta-adrenergic antagonists such as metoprolol, atenolol, and practolol subsequently have been developed that preferentially block $beta_1$ receptors. These drugs are *relatively* free of effects on bronchial smooth muscle at concentrations that reduce myocardial inotropy and chronotropy and, clinically, are the preferred beta blockers for patients with pulmonary dis-

Table 3. Beta-adrenergic receptor subtypes

	$Beta_1$	*$Beta_2$*
Potency Order	Isoproterenol≫ epinephrine = norepinephrine	Isoproterenol≫ epinephrine> norepinephrine
Function	Increase myocardial inotropy, automaticity	Relax vascular and bronchial smooth muscle, ? increase cardiac chronotropy

ease. Thus, in addition to supporting the validity of the concept of beta-receptor subtypes, the "cardioselective" agents have proven to be of clinical value.

Recently, it has been suggested that $beta_1$-adrenergic receptors are located on effector cells in proximity to adrenergic synapses (i.e., intrasynaptic), whereas $beta_2$ receptors are located at some distance from the synapses (i.e., extrasynaptic).[10] According to this theory, $beta_1$ receptors respond primarily to neuronally released NE, whereas $beta_2$ receptors respond preferentially to circulating epinephrine from the adrenal medulla, or to exogenously injected agonists. Also, as in the case of alpha-adrenergic receptors, beta-adrenergic receptors located presynaptically on the nerve fiber regulate NE release. However, as opposed to presynaptic alpha-receptors, which have an inhibitory role, stimulation of presynaptic beta receptors augments NE release.[3]

Biochemical Coupling of Adrenergic Receptors (Fig. 2)

Beta-Adrenergic Receptors

As initially shown by Sutherland and coworkers, stimulation of beta-adrenergic receptors stimulates the activity of the membrane enzyme adenylate cyclase and, consequently, an increase in intracellular cyclic AMP.[11] Acting as a "second messenger," cyclic AMP results in the typical beta-adrenergic effects by activating protein kinases, which in turn phosphorylate various substrates. The activation of adenylate cyclase by beta-receptor stimulation appears to require at least two other components; a "catalytic moiety" and a guanine nucleotide regulatory protein, or "G-protein." Occupancy of the receptor by a beta-adrenergic agonist induces "coupling" of the receptor–catalytic moiety–guanine nucleotide regulatory protein–adenylate cyclase complex, and hence, activation of adenylate cyclase.[12] The degree to which an agent induces coupling of these components is related to its "intrinsic activity," or the maximal physiologic effect obtainable with a high concentration of the agent. Full agonists induce a high degree of coupling, full antagonists attach to the receptor and prevent agonists from doing so but induce no coupling, and partial agonists have a mixed function.

Several beta-adrenergic receptor–blocking drugs such as pindolol and practolol are partial rather than full antagonists. Although these partial agonists bind to the beta receptor with

Table 4. Subtype selectivity of beta-adrenergic agents

	$Beta_1$ Selective	*Nonselective*	*$Beta_2$ Selective*
Agonists	Dobutamine Prenalterol	Isoproterenol Norepinephrine Epinephrine	Terbutaline Salbutamol
Antagonists	Practolol Metoprolol Atenolol	Propranolol Nadolol Pindolol	Butoxamine

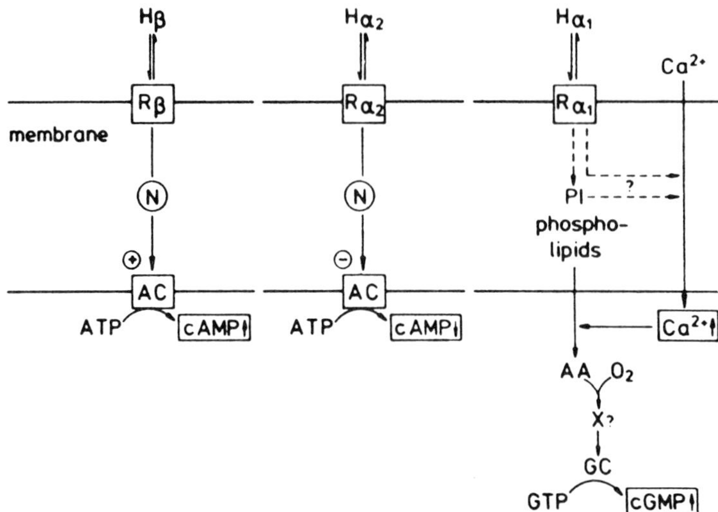

Figure 2. Proposed mechanisms by which adrenergic receptors are coupled to intracellular events. Stimulation of $beta_1$ and $beta_2$ receptors causes an increase in adenylate cyclase activity and an increase in cAMP, whereas stimulation of $alpha_2$ receptors causes inhibition of adenylate cyclase and a reduction in cAMP. Although the mechanism of $alpha_1$ coupling is not known, one possibility involves changes in phosphotidylinositol metabolism, which subsequently alter calcium transmembrane influx and/or intracellular mobilization. H = hormone; R = receptor; N = guanine nucleotide regulatory protein; AC = adenylate cyclase; PI = phosphotidylinositol; AA = arachidonic acid; GC = guanylate cyclase. (Adapted from Jakobs and Schultz.[15])

high affinity, thereby blocking the receptor to the action of agonists, they also result in partial coupling of the receptor–adenylate cyclase complex, and therefore are said to possess "intrinsic sympathomimetic activity." The net effect of a partial agonist depends on a balance between its degree of intrinsic sympathomimetic activity and the existing level of sympathetic tone, that is, the level of NE in the vicinity of the receptor. Thus, when sympathetic tone is high as during exercise or emotional stress, the overall effect is beta blockade. Alternately, when sympathetic tone is low, beta blockers with intrinsic sympathomimetic activity may result in weak sympathetic stimulation and less potent beta blockade than drugs without intrinsic sympathomimetic activity. It has been suggested that beta-adrenergic blockers with intrinsic sympathomimetic activity may result in less depression of resting heart rate and a lower incidence of atrioventricular conduction disturbances and bronchospasm, although a clear clinical advantage of these agents has not been established.[13]

Although the large majority of beta receptor–activated processes are mediated by cyclic AMP, there is some evidence that beta-adrenergic receptor stimulation may result in other direct, cyclic AMP–*independent* changes in plasma membrane properties which potentially may affect cell function.[14]

$Alpha_2$ Receptors

Simulation of $alpha_2$ receptors in several tissues results in a *fall* in intracellular cyclic AMP concentration owing to inhibition of the enzyme adenylate cyclase. As with beta-adrenergic receptors, the coupling of $alpha_2$ receptors to adenylate cyclase requires the presence of guanine nucleotides, thereby suggesting the involvement of a guanine-nucleotide regulatory protein.[14,15] Because relaxation of vascular smooth muscle by beta-adrenergic stimulation appears to be mediated, at least in part, by an increase in cyclic AMP, it is possible that a reduction in cyclic AMP due to $alpha_2$-adrenergic receptor stimulation could cause contraction of vascular smooth muscle that possesses $alpha_2$ receptors.

Alpha$_1$ Receptors

Much less is known about the way in which alpha$_1$-adrenergic receptors are coupled to subsequent contractile events. Most evidence supports the view that the main consequence of alpha$_1$-receptor stimulation is an increase in the cytosolic calcium concentration due to influx of calcium and/or mobilization of calcium from intracellular storage sites.[15] The increase in cytosolic calcium concentration, in turn, results in contraction of vascular smooth muscle and, hence, in vasoconstriction. One hypothesis is that the alpha$_1$-stimulated increase in cytosolic calcium is mediated by an increase in the turnover of phosphotidylinositol (PI), a phospholipid component of the inner plasma membrane.[16]

RADIOLIGAND STUDIES OF ADRENERGIC RECEPTORS

The recent development of methods for measuring directly the density and binding characteristics of adrenergic receptors with radiolabeled ligands has resulted in considerable progress in the biochemistry and physiology of adrenergic receptors.[17] These techniques, reviewed elsewhere,[18,19] have made it possible to determine the density of receptors and their affinity for hormones and drugs. In general, these experiments use compounds labeled with tritium (^{3}H) or iodine (^{125}I) that bind with high affinity and specificity to the receptor of interest. Compounds used for labeling beta-adrenergic receptors include ^{3}H-dihydroalprenolol, ^{125}I-pindolol, and ^{125}I-cyanopindolol. Alpha-adrenergic receptors have been labeled with the non-subtype-selective ligand ^{3}H-dihydroergocryptine; the alpha$_1$-selective ligands ^{3}H-prazosin, ^{3}H-WB-4101, and ^{125}I-BE-2254; and the alpha$_2$-selective ligands ^{3}H-clonidine and ^{3}H-yohimbine. In all cases, it is necessary to demonstrate that the labeled compound fulfills specific criteria for the identification of a receptor.[17] These criteria include (1) appropriate kinetics of binding, (2) reversibility of binding, (3) high-affinity binding, (4) saturability of binding sites, (5) displacement of the radioligand by unlabeled agonists and antagonists in the appropriate order of potency, and (6) stereospecificity of binding.

Receptor Regulation

A large body of evidence indicates that one way in which the responsiveness or sensitivity of a tissue to catecholamines may be altered is by a change in receptor number (density) or binding affinity.[17] An increase in receptor density and/or affinity is commonly referred to as "up-regulation," and a decrease as "down-regulation." Regulation of both number and affinity has been observed in cardiovascular tissues, and in many cases the type of receptor regulation (i.e., number or affinity) induced by a given factor appears to be tissue, species, or receptor-subtype dependent. For instance, in human platelets, estrogens result in an increase in alpha$_2$-adrenergic receptor *density*,[20] whereas in rat mesenteric artery, the effect of estrogens is to increase the *affinity* of alpha$_1$ receptors for agonists without an effect on density.[21] For this reason, generalizations should be avoided when considering the regulation of adrenergic receptors.

Vascular Adrenergic Receptors

The direct characterization of vascular adrenergic receptors is made difficult by the small amounts of smooth muscle available from most vessels and by contamination by elastic and connective tissue. Nevertheless, a number of investigators have successfully applied radioligand methods to canine, bovine, and rat vessels for the identification of alpha-[22–24] and beta-[25] adrenergic receptors. Alpha$_1$ and, in some cases, alpha$_2$ receptors have been identified in these vessels. Vascular beta receptors have received much less attention. A single study reported their presence in rat aorta and demonstrated a lower density in vessels from spontaneously hypertensive rats compared with normotensive controls.[25]

Cardiac Adrenergic Receptors

Myocardial beta-adrenergic receptors and, to a lesser extent, alpha-adrenergic receptors have been studied extensively by radioligand techniques. Whereas ventricular receptors are exclusively $beta_1$,[26] radioligand studies indicate that approximately 25 percent of atrial receptors are of the $beta_2$ subtype. As discussed below, atrial $beta_2$ receptors, presumably located within the sinoatrial node, may mediate the chronotropic effects of catecholamines on the heart. The subtype of myocardial alpha-adrenergic receptors is somewhat controversial, although most evidence favors the presence of only $alpha_1$ receptors.[27] In addition to adrenergic receptors on the myocardium, the coronary vessels also possess alpha and $beta_2$ receptors (see below), and therefore, the net effect on the heart of any adrenergic agonist or antagonist is the sum of its effects on working myocardial cells, specialized automatic tissue, and coronary vessels.

VASCULAR ADRENERGIC RECEPTORS

Most blood vessels contain both alpha-adrenergic receptors ($alpha_1$ and in some cases $alpha_2$) that mediate contraction (i.e., vasoconstriction) and $beta_2$-adrenergic receptors that mediate relaxation (i.e., vasodilation). Therefore, the *net* response (contraction versus relaxation) depends on the alpha versus beta selectivity of the agonist, the relative numbers of alpha and beta receptors in the particular vessel, and the efficiency of receptor coupling to subsequent mechanisms. Although the response of the vast majority of vessels to the endogenous neurotransmitter NE is contraction, one component of its action is beta receptor–mediated relaxation. This is evident from the fact that beta-adrenergic blocking agents result in increased vascular tone, a situation commonly referred to as "unopposed alpha-tone." Likewise, even though the usual response to NE is contraction, following alpha-adrenergic blockade the response to NE may become vasodilation due to the "unmasking" of the beta-adrenergic vasodilator effect. In contrast to the large majority of peripheral vessels in which NE is a potent constrictor, the net response to NE of certain vessels (such as coronary arterioles) is vasodilation, suggesting that in these vessels beta-adrenergic receptors predominate over alpha-adrenergic receptors.[28]

Coronary Vascular Adrenergic Receptors

Although local metabolic factors are the major determinants of coronary vascular tone, there is evidence that adrenergic receptor–mediated stimuli may contribute significantly to coronary vascular tone, both at rest and during various forms of stress. As mentioned above, the coronary vasculature differs from other peripheral vessels in response to adrenergic stimulation. Depending on the species and size of the coronary vessel studied, the response to NE may be constriction (in large vessels) or dilation (in small arteries and arterioles).[28,29] A vasodilator response to NE occurs in smooth muscle from small coronary arteries studied in vitro, indicating that the vascular relaxation is not due simply to metabolic factors related to increased myocardial oxygen needs.[29,30] The ability of neuronally released NE to cause constriction of large (conductive) coronary vessels may be particularly important when adrenergic activity is increased, or when coronary vasodilator reserve is reduced by fixed (organic) coronary artery obstruction and/or treatment with beta blockers. Thus, in patients with obstructive coronary artery disease, the cold pressor test (immersion of the hand in ice water) results in an alpha receptor reflexly mediated increase in coronary vascular resistance, whereas this response is not observed in patients with normal coronary arteries.[31] In the latter case, the capacity for vasodilation on a metabolic basis exists, thus counteracting the alpha-adrenergically induced coronary constriction. The increase in coronary vascular resistance during the cold pressor stimulus can be blocked by the $alpha_1$-selective antagonist trimazosin, suggesting that alpha receptors in human coronary arteries are of the $alpha_1$ subtype.[32] Likewise, there are considerable physiologic data pointing to the importance of $beta_2$-adrenergic receptors in the coronary circulation; and a clinically significant role in humans is suggested by the observation in patients with coronary artery disease that the intravenous administration of propranolol, a noncardioselective agent that blocks vascular ($beta_2$) as well as myocardial ($beta_1$) receptors, potentiates the cold pressor–induced increase in coronary vascular resistance, presumably due to the development of "unopposed" alpha-adrenergic tone.[33] Coronary artery spasm can be provoked in some patients with ischemic heart disease by the administration of ergonovine, which may act as an alpha-adrenergic agonist. Thus, alpha- and beta-adrenergic receptors within the coronary arterial tree appear to play a significant role in the modulation of coronary blood flow, particularly in the setting of coronary artery disease, beta blockade, and/or increased adrenergic activity. Further study is needed to evaluate the clinical relevance of this modulation, which potentially may be involved in the pathogenesis of coronary spasm and the determination of collateral blood flow and infarct size.

Vascular Alpha-Adrenergic Receptors

As already mentioned, recent data suggest that in some cases constriction of blood vessels may be mediated, in part, by postsynaptic $alpha_2$ receptors. These observations, as well as the differential effects of subtype-selective agents on the pressor responses to circulating versus neuronally released catecholamines has led to the hypothesis that alpha-adrenergic receptors located on vascular smooth muscle within the area of the nerve synapse (intrasynaptic) are of the $alpha_1$ subtype, whereas receptors located on vascular smooth muscle at some distance from the synapse (extrasynaptic) are of the $alpha_2$ subtype.[5,6,10] It has been suggested that the relative proportions of $alpha_1$ and $alpha_2$ receptors in a given vessel may relate to the density of innervations: $alpha_1$ receptors predominating in heavily innervated vessels, and $alpha_2$ receptors predominating in sparsely innervated vessels. Consistent with this suggestion is the observation that contraction of the rabbit aorta, which is innervated, is mediated by $alpha_1$ receptors; whereas contraction of the rat aorta, which is not innervated, appears to be mediated by $alpha_2$ receptors.[5] Further evidence that the alpha receptor subtypes differ in various vessels comes from direct radioligand-binding studies that have demonstrated $alpha_2$ receptors in canine aorta,[24] but not in the heavily innervated rat mesenteric artery.[23]

Vascular Beta-Adrenergic Receptors

Although frequently overlooked, there is considerable evidence that beta-adrenergic receptors contribute significantly to the *net* response of blood vessels to catecholamines. Whereas the net response of most vessels to a nonselective agonist such as NE is vasoconstriction, beta-adrenergic selective agonists often result in blood vessel dilation.[28] As already discussed, vascular beta receptors are predominantly, if not solely, of the $beta_2$ subtype. In contrast to alpha-mediated vascular constriction, which is relatively stable over time, the vasodilator response to beta-adrenergic stimulation may be more transient, thereby suggesting that vascular beta receptors are prone to "desensitization." For instance, the vasodilator action of isoproterenol (a catecholamine that is predominantly a beta-adrenergic agonist, but that also possesses alpha-agonist properties) can be converted to an alpha-mediated vasopressor response by pretreatment of the animal with high doses of catecholamines, a phenomenon referred to as "isoproterenol reversal."[34] Also in contrast to alpha-mediated vasoconstriction, beta-mediated vasodilation appears to decrease with advancing age,[35,36] which may be due to an age-related decrease in vascular beta receptor density, and it has been suggested that an age-related reduction in vascular beta receptors may play a role in the essential hypertension commonly observed with advancing age.

Regulation of Vascular Adrenergic Receptors

The modulation of vascular sensitivity to adrenergic agonists may occur by prejunctional (i.e., presynaptic) or postjunctional (i.e., postsynaptic) mechanisms.[37] *Prejunctional* modulation of sensitivity is due to changes in the delivery and/or disposition of neurotransmitter. Thus, substances that block the re-uptake of NE by adrenergic nerves (such as cocaine) result in an increase in the sensitivity of NE-induced vascular smooth muscle contraction, as shown by a leftward shift of the NE dose-response relationship. The exact locus at which *"postjunctional"* or postsynaptic sensitivity is modulated is not known, but may be at the level of the membrane adrenergic receptor in the coupling of receptor to the contractile proteins, or in the contractile proteins themselves. It is likely that in some cases more than one of these mechanisms may be involved.

Denervation Supersensitivity

A reduction in the level of adrenergic tone induced by any of several methods (surgical sympathectomy, 6-hydroxydopamine, or depletion of neurotransmitter by reserpine) results in an *increase* in the sensitivity of vascular smooth muscle to contraction by alpha-adrenergic agonists.[37,38] For instance, after catecholamine depletion by reserpine, the sensitivity of rabbit aorta to contraction by NE is increased approximately twelvefold.[38] Likewise, reserpine treatment induces a marked increase in alpha-adrenergic receptor binding affinity as demonstrated by radioligand binding methods.[39] This increase in the binding affinity of the receptor for agonists closely parallels the increase in physiologic sensitivity both in time course and magnitude of shift, and suggests that it is responsible, at least in part, for the phenomenon of vascular denervation supersensitivity to alpha-adrenergic agonists.

There is evidence that vascular denervation supersensitivity occurs in patients with the Shy-Drager syndrome, a neurologic disorder in which sympathetic tone is markedly reduced. In these patients, the pressor responsiveness to an infused alpha-adrenergic agonist is greatly increased. Although direct assay of vascular alpha-adrenergic receptors in humans is not feasible, the density of platelet alpha$_2$-adrenergic receptors is strikingly elevated in patients with the Shy-Drager syndrome,[40] a finding that supports the hypothesis that vascular supersensitivity is related to an alteration in vascular alpha receptors.

Subsensitivity

After exposure to elevated levels of catecholamines, the responsiveness of isolated vascular smooth muscle to NE is reduced.[37,41] Likewise, in patients with pheochromocytoma in whom circulating catecholamines are markedly elevated, the vasopressor response to exogenously administered norepinephrine is markedly attenuated in comparison to the responsiveness in normal subjects.[40] Radioligand-binding experiments have shown that the density of alpha-adrenergic receptors in the rat mesenteric artery is significantly decreased following 48 hours of constant exposure to high levels of epinephrine,[39] and suggest that "down-regulation" of vascular alpha-adrenergic receptors may be involved in the loss of responsiveness with prolonged exposure of blood vessels to catecholamines.

Sex Hormones

In experimental animals, vascular sensitivity to alpha-adrenergic stimulation is increased in females compared with males,[42] and in males after administration of estrogen.[43] Estrogen adminstration to male rats results in a dose-related threefold to sixfold *increase* in the affinity of the mesenteric artery alpha-adrenergic receptor for epinephrine, as determined by radioligand binding.[21] Likewise, vascular alpha-adrenergic receptor affinity is increased in female rats compared with males, and after oophorectomy, the vascular alpha-adrenergic receptor affinity in females decreases. Potentially, these experimental observations may be related to the development of hypertension in women receiving estrogen-containing birth control pills, and the much higher occurrence of Raynaud's phenomenon in females than in males.

Hypertension

A role for vascular alpha and/or beta receptors in the pathogenesis of hypertension is suggested by studies that show a reduction in the vasodilator response to beta agonists[36] as well as a hypersensitivity of the vasculature to NE[44] in patients and experimental animals with hypertension compared with normotensive controls. In support of this possibility is the finding of a decrease in the density of beta-adrenergic receptors as measured by radioligand binding in the aortas of spontaneously hypertensive rats.[25] The available evidence does not make it possible to localize the site of the NE hypersensitivity, which may be at the level of the vascular postsynaptic alpha receptor, or at a more distal step in the contractile process.

MYOCARDIAL ADRENERGIC RECEPTORS

The adrenergic nervous system exerts a major direct influence on cardiac function. The overall effect of catecholamines is to increase the inotropic (contractile), chronotropic (heart rate), and dromotropic (conduction velocity) states of the heart. Although these effects are substantial, it appears that adrenergic tone is not essential for the maintenance of cardiac function in normal, resting subjects.[45] For instance, in the normal heart, beta-adrenergic blockade with propranolol has little effect on stroke volume at rest; and likewise, adequate resting myocardial function is demonstrated by the denervated hearts of cardiac transplant recipients. In contrast, the adrenergic nervous system plays an important role in response to the stress of exercise, or to abnormally increased workloads as may occur with valvular heart disease and in the presence of myocardial failure. Thus, beta blockade can impair the response of the normal heart to exercise[46] and can have deleterious effects in patients with otherwise compensated heart failure.[47]

Myocardial Beta-Adrenergic Receptors

The effects of catecholamines on the contractile and electrical properties of the heart are mediated predominantly by beta-adrenergic receptors. As determined by physiologic and radioligand-binding studies, the large majority of myocardial beta receptors are of the $beta_1$ subtype; and likewise, the inotropic effects of beta-adrenergic agonists are mediated predominantly, if not exclusively, by $beta_1$ receptors. However, there is evidence that the chronotropic response of the heart may not be mediated entirely by $beta_1$ receptors. Thus, a number of $beta_1$- and $beta_2$-selective agonists and antagonists have been shown to exert differential effects on inotropy and chronotropy, respectively.[48,49] Based on these observations, it has been suggested that chronotropy may be mediated by $beta_2$ receptors, presumably located in the sinoatrial node.[48] In support of this hypothesis, quantitative subtype analysis of radioligand binding in guinea pig and rat hearts indicates that although ventricular myocardium contains only $beta_1$ receptors, about 25 percent of atrial beta receptors are of the $beta_2$ subtype.[26]

Dobutamine is a synthetic sympathomimetic amine whose principal action is to stimulate myocardial contractility with only a modest effect on heart rate. This relative lack of chronotropic effect has been attributed to its selectivity for $beta_1$ receptors.[50] An alternate hypothesis is that the overall effect of dobutamine is influenced by its actions on myocardial $alpha_1$ receptors, a possibility that is supported by the demonstration with radioligand methods that dobutamine binds with high affinity to myocardial $alpha_1$ receptors.[50] The negative chronotropic effect of myocardial alpha-receptor stimulation, discussed below, potentially may counteract the beta-mediated positive chronotropic effect, thereby resulting in an apparently greater effect of dobutamine on inotropy. Prenalterol, an orally active catecholamine analog, also has been observed to have a greater effect on inotropy than on chronotropy,[51] and similar mechanisms may be involved. A third explanation for the differential inotropic and chronotropic effects of some beta-adrenergic agonists is that two *sub*-subtypes of $beta_1$ receptors exist that mediate inotropy and chronotropy, respectively. Resolution of this issue may have important implications for cardiovascular therapeutics.

Myocardial Alpha-Adrenergic Receptors

A growing body of evidence suggests that catecholamines exert at least some of their effects through myocardial alpha-adrenergic receptors. As with myocardial beta-adrenergic receptors, stimulation of myocardial alpha receptors augments myocardial contractility.[52–55] However, as alluded to above, in contrast to beta-receptor stimulation, stimulation of myocardial alpha receptors results in a *decrease* in chronotropy.[56]

Because the original physiologic classification of adrenergic receptors assumed that the myocardial effect of catecholamines is mediated exclusively by beta-adrenergic receptors, it is not surprising that the potential role of myocardial alpha receptors has received relatively little attention. The demonstration of alpha-mediated effects on the myocardium of humans or intact animals is complicated by alpha-mediated systemic vasoconstriction that inhibits cardiac performance by increasing cardiac afterload, reducing adrenergic stimulation of the heart due to activation of baroreflexes, and inducing coronary vasoconstriction. However, when these problems are avoided by the use of in vitro systems such as isolated myocardial strips or a preparation in which hemodynamics are controlled, alpha-receptor stimulation can be shown to stimulate myocardial contractility.[52–54] A number of observations suggest that the molecular mechanism by which alpha-adrenergic receptors exert a positive inotropic effect is different from that of beta receptors.[55] Whereas stimulation of beta-adrenergic receptors increases intracellular cyclic AMP, which is thought to mediate subsequent events, stimulation of alpha-adrenergic receptors has no effect on cyclic AMP production in myocardium. Also, alpha receptor–mediated effects on inotropy are more sensitive to the extracellular calcium concentration or blockade of calcium influx by calcium-channel blockers than are beta-mediated effects. Based on these observations, it has been suggested that alpha-adrenergic receptors mediate an increase in inotropy primarily by means of an increase in calcium influx.[55]

The slowing of heart rate caused by alpha-receptor stimulation appears to be due to a decrease in the slope of phase-4 depolarization of sinoatrial nodal tissue.[56] Under normal conditions, the effect of catecholamines is to increase heart rate, indicating that the beta receptor–mediated effect predominates. However, it is possible that the alpha-mediated negative chronotropic effect may be more important in the presence of beta blockade or in conditions such as myocardial ischemia, which are associated with a relative increase in myocardial alpha receptors.[57]

Regulation of Myocardial Adrenergic Receptors

Thyroid Hormone

Thyroid hormone influences myocardial function in both man and experimental animals. Thus, hyperthyroidism is associated with a hypercontractile state, and hypothyroidism with depressed myocardial contractility. The hyperthyroid heart resembles one stimulated by catecholamines, whereas the hypothyroid heart resembles one subjected to adrenergic blockade. By radioligand binding it has been shown that myocardial beta-adrenergic receptor density is increased in hyperthyroidism and reduced in hypothyroidism, but the effects of the thyroid state on myocardial alpha receptors have varied from study to study.[58] Although the physiologic relevance of these changes in myocardial adrenergic receptor density remains to be determined, potentially they may relate to the abnormalities of cardiac function that occur in patients with thyroid disease.

Denervation and Chronic Receptor Blockade

After catecholamine depletion by reserpine, the myocardium exhibits postjunctional supersensitivity to the inotropic and chronotropic effects of several agents, including alpha- and beta-adrenergic agonists, histamine, and calcium.[59] Because this form of myocardial supersensitivity is not specific for adrenergic agonists, several mechanisms might be involved. Nevertheless, a potential role for adrenergic-receptor regulation is suggested by increases in the densities of rat myocardial alpha- and beta-adrenergic receptors after chronic "denervation" with 6-hydroxydopamine[60] or guanethidine.[61] After chronic therapy with the beta-adrenergic antagonist propranolol, there is a doubling in the density of beta-adrenergic receptors in rat myocardium.[62] Clinically, the abrupt discontinuation of beta-blocker therapy in patients has been associated, albeit infrequently, with the sudden intensification of myocardial ischemia, the precipitation of myocardial infarction, and a transient state of beta-receptor hypersensitivity.[63] Because there is a marked increase in the density of beta receptors in the myocardium of rats and on the white blood cells of patients during chronic beta blockade,[62–64] it seems reasonable to suggest that this "propranolol-withdrawal syndrome" may be related in part to an elevation in beta-receptor density following the disappearance of the beta blocker's pharmacologic action. An unmasking of the underlying ischemic disease that has progressed during beta blockade is another possible explanation.

Desensitization

Desensitization to the beta-adrenergic effects of catecholamines occurs in numerous biologic systems.[19] That desensitization can occur in human myocardium is suggested by the demonstration that the continuous infusion of the beta-adrenergic agonist dobutamine for 96 hours results in a 43 percent loss of the initial inotropic effect.[65] Likewise, in patients with congestive heart failure, treatment with the $beta_2$ selective agonist pirbuterol for 1 month resulted in an almost complete loss of the initial positive inotropic effect, and the latter was accompanied by a marked reduction in the density of beta receptors on circulating lymphocytes.[66]

The mechanism responsible for beta-adrenergic desensitization in myocardium has not been defined. Following the experimental production of left ventricular infarction in the rat, the contractile response of noninfarcted right ventricular myocardium to isoproterenol declines, a decline that is associated with reductions in beta-receptor density and isoproterenol-stimulated adenylate cyclase activity, whereas the effects of histamine on adenylate cyclase and contractility are preserved.[67] Because this rapid beta-adrenergic desensitization can be prevented by pretreatment with reserpine or metoprolol, it appears to be due to beta-adrenergic receptor stimulation by excessive levels of catecholamines during the peri-infarction period.[67] By 6 days postinfarction, the contractile response to isoproterenol, beta-receptor density, and adenylate cyclase activity have all returned to normal. In vitro studies in the chick embryo ventricle suggest that during the acute exposure to a desensitizing concentration of isoproterenol, there is an apparent functional "uncoupling" between the beta receptor and the adenylate cyclase complex[68] that may precede any decrease in receptor number.

Thus, desensitization of the myocardial beta-adrenergic pathway may have an important role in states characterized by elevated catecholamine levels such as acute myocardial infarction, treatment with sympathomimetic agents, and, as discussed below, congestive heart failure.

Congestive Heart Failure

It has been well established that chronic heart failure is associated with reduction in myocardial NE content.[69] A recent study performed on the failing hearts of cardiac transplant recipients demonstrated a 50 percent reduction in beta-receptor density.[70] This reduction corresponded to decreases in adenylate cyclase and contractile responses of the isolated papillary muscle to isoproterenol, but not histamine. The observed desensitization of the beta-adrenergic receptor pathway was attributed to high concentrations of circulating catecholamines. This study, carried out on the hearts of patients with chronic end-stage heart failure, contrasts with that of Karliner and associates, who examined the effect of chronic heart failure induced by aortic constriction on the density of $alpha_1$- and beta-adrenergic receptors in membranes prepared from guinea pig myocardium.[71] Eleven days to 2 months after aortic constriction, at a time when the animals had developed overt heart failure, there were *increases* in the densities of myocardial $alpha_1$- and beta-adrenergic receptors measured by radioligand binding.[71] Because cardiac catecholamine content was markedly reduced in this model of heart failure, it was suggested that the increases in adrenergic receptor densities might represent a compensatory response analogous to the response to denervation. Differences between the results of the two studies cited above may relate to a large number of factors, and emphasize the need for more information in this area.

Ischemia

In the cat, brief coronary artery occlusion results in ventricular irritability as manifested by a rapid idioventricular rate and the development of ventricular fibrillation.[72] Treatment with the alpha-adrenergic antagonist phentolamine or prazosin markedly reduces the degree of ventricular irritability and slows the idioventricular rate, whereas the beta-adrenergic antagonist propranolol has no effect. In a recent study, the densities of $alpha_1$- and beta-adrenergic receptors were measured in the myocardium at various times before, during, and after the production of myocardial ischemia.[57] There was a marked increase in the density of alpha receptors, which was maximal after 30 minutes of ischemia and gradually returned to baseline after 15 minutes of reperfusion. No changes occurred in beta-adrenergic receptor density or affinity. Although further studies are needed to clarify the relevance of alpha receptor–mediated arrhythmias during ischemia in man, these observations provide a potential therapeutic role for alpha-adrenergic blockade during periods of transient myocardial ischemia such as those caused by coronary artery spasm or transient coronary obstruction by platelet plugs.

CENTRAL ADRENERGIC RECEPTORS

The regulation of adrenergic outflow from the brain stem is a complex function influenced by input from both higher cortical centers and peripheral afferent sensory nerves. The integration of the various controlling factors appears to occur in discrete areas of the brain stem, particularly the nucleus of the tractus solitarius, the vasomotor center, and the nucleus of the vagus nerve.[73,74] Although both alpha- and beta-adrenergic receptors can be demonstrated within the central nervous system by radioligand-binding techniques, central adrenergic outflow appears to be controlled predominantly by alpha-adrenergic receptors. Thus, stimulation of central alpha-adrenergic receptors results in a *reduction* in adrenergic outflow and an increase in vagal tone and, consequently, reductions in systemic vascular resistance, heart rate, and myocardial contractility.

The antihypertensive agents clonidine, guanabenz, and alpha-methyldopa are thought to exert their actions by stimulation of central alpha-adrenergic receptors. Clonidine and guanabenz act directly on central alpha receptors, whereas alpha-methyldopa is first converted to its active metabolite, alpha-methylnorepinephrine, which is an $alpha_2$-adrenergic receptor agonist.[73] Although both $alpha_1$- and $alpha_2$-adrenergic receptors can be demonstrated within the central nervous system by radioligand-binding techniques, it appears that the central cardiovascular effects of clonidine, guanabenz, and alpha-methyldopa are mediated largely, if not exclusively, by $alpha_2$ receptors.[73,74] Furthermore, because destruction of presynaptic neurons by 6-hydroxydopamine does not abolish the effects of clonidine, it has been suggested that these central $alpha_2$ receptors are postsynaptic in location.[75]

A specific role for beta-adrenergic receptors in determining central adrenergic outflow, or for that matter in any central nervous system function, has not been identified. However, it is likely that neuropsychiatric side effects such as depression, insomnia, and nightmares caused in some patients by beta blockers are due to the ability of these drugs to cross the blood-brain barrier.[76] Not surprisingly, these central side effects are most prominent with lipophilic beta-adrenergic antagonists such as propranolol and less so with nonlipophilic antagonists such as atenolol.[76]

ALPHA-ADRENERGIC ANTAGONISTS

Advances in our appreciation of alpha-adrenergic receptor subtypes, and particularly of the role of presynaptic alpha-adrenergic receptors in the negative-feedback regulation of NE, have had a considerable impact on the clinical use of alpha-adrenergic antagonists. The major limitations in the use of non-subtype-selective alpha antagonists are tachycardia, persistent orthostatic hypotension, and in some cases, attenuation of the desired clinical effect.[77,78] In part, these problems are related to nonspecific blockade of presynaptic $alpha_2$ receptors.[77–79] The subsequent *increase* in NE release results in tachycardia and increased renin release due to stimulation of beta-adrenergic receptors, and in attenuation of the desired antihypertensive action due to stimulation of vascular postsynaptic $alpha_1$ receptors. Prazosin, an orally active $alpha_1$ antagonist in widespread clinical use, and other as-yet investigational $alpha_1$ selective antagonists are largely free of these undesirable effects.

Phentolamine, Tolazoline, and Phenoxybenzamine

In clinically relevant concentrations, phentolamine and phenoxybenzamine act predominantly as alpha-adrenergic antagonists, whereas the effects of tolazoline are probably only in small part due to blockade of alpha receptors. These drugs cause a fall in peripheral vascular resistance and cardiac stimulation, the latter caused by reflex baroreceptor activation and blockade of presynaptic $alpha_2$ receptors with subsequent neuronal release of NE, which then acts on cardiac beta receptors. Unlike phentolamine and tolazoline, which bind reversibly to alpha-adrenergic receptors, phenoxybenzamine binds irreversibly, probably by the formation of covalent bonds, and therefore its biologic half-life is much longer, in the range of 24 hours. Phentolamine is available for intravenous use, tolazoline for intravenous and oral use, and phenoxybenzamine only for oral administration.

Although these drugs have *not* been useful in the chronic therapy for patients with essential hypertension, both phenoxybenzamine and phentolamine have proven to be of value in the management of patients with pheochromocytoma. In the preoperative management of such patients, oral phenoxybenzamine can be begun in a dose of 10 mg every 12 hours with gradual increases until blood pressure is adequately controlled. Phenoxybenzamine may be continued on a chronic basis in inoperable patients. Phentolamine (2 to 5 mg, by intravenous bolus) may be administered both before and during operative removal of a pheochromocytoma. Alpha-adrenergic blockade should always be instituted *prior* to beta-adrenergic receptor blockade in patients with pheochromocytoma, because beta blockade alone may result in a further *increase* in blood pressure due to blockade of vascular $beta_2$ receptors leaving alpha-adrenergic receptors unopposed.

Phentolamine and tolazoline have been used with varying degrees of success in patients with primary pulmonary hypertension.[80] These agents have also been used effectively in patients with peripheral vasospasm due to Raynaud's disease. When used in patients with intermittent claudication due to peripheral vascular disease, these agents may cause an increase in resting blood flow, but generally have *little* effect during exercise. Both phentolamine and phenoxybenzamine have been used as vasodilator agents in patients with congestive heart failure,[81,82] although experience has been limited. Phentolamine may be infiltrated locally into skin and subcutaneous tissues to prevent the vasoconstriction and necrosis that frequently follow accidental extravasation of potent adrenergic vasoconstrictor agents.

Prazosin, Trimazosin, and Indoramin

In contrast to phenoxybenzamine and phentolamine, prazosin has proven to be of distinct value in the management of hypertension.[78,82] Due to its high degree of selectivity for $alpha_1$ receptors, prazosin results in little or no increase in heart rate, plasma renin activity, or peripheral NE release. Prazosin may be used alone in mild hypertension,[93] although in most cases it has been combined with a diuretic or other antihypertensive agents in the treatment of moderate or severe hypertension. Prazosin is an effective antihypertensive in patients with pheochromocytoma, as well as in patients with chronic renal failure, including those receiving hemodialysis. The major side effect of prazosin is postural hypotension after the first drug administration, the so-called "first-dose phenomenon." This effect can be prevented by initiation of therapy with a small dose (1 mg). Also, because this effect is more common in patients who are volume contracted, it is recommended that diuretics be withheld on the day prior to and the day of drug initiation. The maintenance dose of prazosin should be arrived at by gradual upward titration, and ranges from 2 to 20 mg per day in two to three divided doses. Attenuation of the antihypertensive effect has not been evident despite therapy for prolonged periods.[83] A growing body of data indicates that the therapy for hypertensive patients with prazosin results in reductions in serum cholesterol and triglyceride levels, and a small increase in the high-density lipoprotein fraction,[84] as opposed to therapy with beta antagonists and thiazide diuretics, which tend to affect serum lipid levels adversely.[84] The potential long-term value of prazosin's lipid-lowering effects remains to be evaluated.

In patients with congestive heart failure, oral prazosin produces balanced arterial and venous dilation similar to that produced by intravenous nitroprusside.[85] During short-term multiple administrations, various degrees of attenuation of some or all of the initial hemodynamic effects have been observed.[78,86] However, sustained symptomatic and hemodynamic improvement has been observed during long-term administration in many cases.[78,87–89] These beneficial effects are most evident during exercise when sympathetic activity is excessive in patients with heart failure.[78,89] Thus, it appears that initial hemodynamic attenuation, when it occurs, does not necessarily preclude long-term effectiveness. The mechanism responsible for this early hemodynamic attenuation is not known but may relate to alterations in the sympathetic nervous system, the renin-angiotensin system, or the vascular alpha-adrenergic receptor. In some patients, a tendency for increased fluid retention may blunt the therapeutic response during chronic therapy but is often reversible by increased diuresis, particularly with aldosterone antagonists.[78,90] The long-term effects of therapy with prazosin (or other vasodilators) on the survival of patients with heart failure are not known, and therefore the goal of therapy at present should be to improve clinical status.

Recent reports emphasize that prazosin may be effective in the therapy for peripheral vasospasm due to Raynaud's phenomenon or ergotamine overdose.[91,92] Animal experiments have also raised the possibility that prazosin may have antiarrhythmic effects in the setting of transient myocardial ischemia,[73] in line with the previously cited arrhythmogenic effects of alph-adrenergic stimulation.[57] However, this use has not yet been evaluated clinically.

Although prazosin is the only $alpha_1$ selective antagonist presently available for clinical use, considerable experience has accumulated with several investigational $alpha_1$ antagonists including trimazosin and indoramin, both of which have been shown to be effective antihypertensive agents.[94–96] Trimazosin has also been shown to have beneficial acute and chronic effects as a vasodilator in the therapy for congestive heart failure.[97,98] It is likely that in the future, clinicians will have available to them a variety of alpha-adrenergic antagonists with a range of pharmacologic characteristics from which to choose.

BETA-ADRENERGIC RECEPTOR ANTAGONISTS

Although the concept of two classes of adrenergic receptors was first proposed in 1948,[1] it was not until 10 years later that the first beta-adrenergic receptor–selective antagonist was developed, thereby confirming the original hypothesis and initiating a major development in cardiovascular therapeutics. Since that time, a large number of beta-adrenergic receptor antagonists with a wide range of pharmacologic traits have been developed and are now used extensively in therapy for angina pectoris, hypertension, cardiac arrhythmias, and hypertrophic cardiomyopathy. The clinical pharmacology of beta-adrenergic antagonists is considered elsewhere in this book.

CONCLUSIONS

Since the initial proposal of the theory of adrenergic receptors by Ahlquist, there have been major advances in the fields of adrenergic receptor physiology and pharmacology. These advances have resulted from two types of investigation: (1) the development of drugs, both agonists and antagonists, with selective pharmacologic actions, allowing a more precise dissection of receptor subtypes; and (2) the utilization of radioligand-binding techniques for the direct measurement of receptor density and binding properties. Although the field of adrenergic receptor pharmacology is becoming increasingly complex, much of this complexity can be turned to clinical advantage through improved understanding of basic physiologic and pathophysiologic mechanisms, and the development of therapeutic agents with more specific actions.

REFERENCES

1. Alhquist, RP: *Study of the adrenotropic receptors.* Am J Physiol 153:586, 1948.
2. Hoffman, BB and Lefkowitz, RJ: *Alpha-adrenergic receptor subtypes.* N Engl J Med 302:1390, 1981.
3. Langer, SZ: *Presynaptic regulation of catecholamines.* Pharmacol Rev 32:337, 1981.
4. Berthelsen, S and Pettinger, WA: *A functional basis for classification of alpha-adrenergic receptors.* Life Sci 21:595, 1977.
5. Ruffolo, RR Jr, Waddell, JE, and Yaden, EL: *Postsynaptic alpha adrenergic receptor subtypes differentiated by yohimbine in tissues from the rat. Existence of alpha-2 adrenergic receptors in the rat aorta.* J Pharmacol Exp Ther 217:235, 1981.
6. Yamaguchi, I and Kopin, IJ: *Differential inhibition of alpha-1 and alpha-2 adrenoceptor-mediated pressor responses in pithed rats.* Pharmacol Exp Ther 214:275, 1980.
7. Drew, GM and Whiting, SB: *Evidence for two distinct types of postsynaptic alpha-adrenoceptor in vascular smooth muscle in vivo.* Br J Pharmacol 67:207, 1979.
8. McGrath, JC: *Evidence for more than one type of post-junctional alpha-adrenoceptor.* Biochem Pharmacol 31:467, 1982.
9. Lands, AM, Arnold, A, McAuliff, JP, et al: *Differentiation of receptor systems activated by sympathomimetic amines.* Nature 214:597, 1967.

10. WILFFART, B, TUMMERMANS, PBMWM, AND VAN ZWIETEN, PA: *Extrasynaptic location of alpha-2 and non-innervated beta-2 adrenoceptors in the vascular system of the pithed normotensive rat.* J Pharmacol Exp Ther 221:762, 1982.

11. SUTHERLAND, EW AND RALL, TW: *The relation of adenosine-3′, 5′ phosphate and phosphorylase to the actions of catecholamines and hormones.* Pharmacol Rev 12:265, 1960.

12. ROSS, EM AND GILMAN, AG: *Biochemical properties of hormone-sensitive adenylate cyclase.* Annu Rev Biochem 49:533, 1980.

13. FRISHMAN, WH: *The significance of intrinsic sympathomimetic activity in beta adrenoceptor blocking drugs.* Cardiovasc Rev Reports 3:503, 1982.

14. RODBELL, M: *The role of hormone receptors and GTP-regulatory proteins in membrane transduction.* Nature 284:17, 1980.

15. JAKOBS, KH AND SCHULTZ, G: *Signal transformation involving alpha-adrenoceptors.* J Cardiovasc Pharmacol 4:563, 1982.

16. PUTNEY JW JR: *Recent hypotheses regarding the phosphotidylinositol effect.* Life Sci 29:1183, 1981.

17. LEFKOWITZ, RJ: *Direct binding studies of adrenergic receptors: Biochemical, physiologic, and clinical implications.* Ann Intern Med 91:450, 1979.

18. COLUCCI WS: *Alpha-Adrenergic receptors in cardiovascular medicine.* In HAFT, JI AND KARLINER, JS (EDS): *Receptor Science in Cardiology.* Futura Publishing, Mt Kisco, NY, 1983.

19. WILLIAMS, RS: *Beta-adrenergic receptors.* In HAFT, JI AND KARLINER, JS (EDS): *Receptor Science in Cardiology.* Futura Publishing, Mt Kisco, NY, 1983.

20. ROBERTS, JM, GOLDFIEN, RD, TSUCHIYA, AM, ET AL: *Estrogen treatment decreases alpha-adrenergic binding sites on rabbit platelets.* Endocrinol 104:722, 1979.

21. COLUCCI, WS, GIMBRONE, MA JR, MCLAUGHLIN, MK, ET AL: *Increased vascular catecholamine sensitivity and alpha-adrenergic receptor affinity in female and estrogen-treated male rats.* Circ Res 50:805, 1982.

22. TSAI, BS AND LEFKOWITZ, RJ: *^{3}H-Dihydroergocryptine binding to alpha adrenergic receptors in canine aortic membranes.* J Pharmacol Exp Ther 204:606, 1978.

23. COLUCCI, WS, GIMBRONE, MA JR, AND ALEXANDER, RW: *Characterization of postsynaptic alpha-adrenergic receptors by radioligand binding in muscular arteries from the rat mesentery.* Hypertension 2:149, 1980.

24. BOBIK, A: *Identification of alpha-adrenoceptor subtypes in dog arteries by ^{3}H-prazosin.* Life Sci 30:219, 1982.

25. LIMAS, CJ AND LIMAS, C: *Decreased number of beta-adrenergic receptors in hypertensive vessels.* Biochim Biophys Acta 582:533, 1979.

26. HEDBERG, A, MINNEMAN, KP, AND MOLINOF, PB: *Differential distribution of beta-1 and beta-2 adrenergic receptors in cat and guinea-pig heart.* J Pharmacol Exp Therap 213:503, 1980.

27. WILLIAMS, RS, DUKES, DF, AND LEFKOWITZ, RJ: *Subtype specificity of alpha-adrenergic receptors in rat heart.* J Cardiovasc Pharmacol 3:522, 1981.

28. BEVAN, JA, BEVAN, RD, AND DUCKLES, SP: *Adrenergic mechanisms of vascular smooth muscle.* In BOHR, DF, SOMOLYO, AP, AND SPARKS, HV JR (EDS): *The Cardiovascular System, Vol. 2, Vascular Smooth Muscle.* Williams & Wilkins, Baltimore, 1981.

29. ROSS, G: *Adrenergic responses of the coronary vessels.* Circ Res 39:461, 1976.

30. KLOCKE, FJ, KAISER, GA, ROSS, J JR, ET AL: *An intrinsic adrenergic vasodilator mechanism in the coronary vascular bed of the dog.* Circulation 16:376, 1965.

31. MUDGE, GH JR, GROSSMAN, W, MILLS, RM, ET AL: *Reflex coronary-artery vasoconstriction in patients with ischemic heart disease.* N Engl J Med 295:1333, 1976.

32. HOROWITZ, JD, KERN, MJ, GANZ, P, ET AL: *Selective alpha-1 adrenergic mediated coronary vasconstriction in coronary artery disease.* Circulation 66:II-249, 1982.

33. KERN, MJ, GANZ, P, HOROWITZ, JD, ET AL: *Potentiation of coronary vasoconstriction by beta-adrenergic blockade.* Circulation 67:1178, 1983.

34. WALZ, DT, KOPPANYI, T, AND MAENGWYN-DAVIES, GW: *Isoproterenol vasomotor reversal by sympathomimetic amines.* J Pharmacol Exp Ther 129:200, 1960.

35. FLEISCH, JH AND SPAETHE, SM: *Vasodilation and aging evaluated in the isolated perfused rat mesenteric vascular bed: Preliminary observations on the vascular pharmacology of dobutamine.* J Cardiovasc Pharmacol 3:187, 1981.

36. BERTEL, O, BUHLER, FR, KIOWSKI, W ET AL: *Decreased beta-adrenoceptor responsiveness as related to age, and catecholamines in patients with essential hypertension.* Hypertension 2:130, 1980.

37. FLEMING, WW: *Supersensitivity in smooth muscle.* Fed Proc 34:1969, 1975.

38. Hudgins, PM and Fleming, WW: *A relatively non-specific supersensitivity in aortic strips resulting from pretreatment with reserpine.* J Pharmacol Exp Ther 153:70, 1966.

39. Colucci, WS, Gimbrone, MA Jr, and Alexander, RW: *Regulation of the postsynaptic alpha-adrenergic receptor in rat mesenteric artery.* Circ Res 48:104, 1981.

40. Davies, G, Suders, D, Sagnella, G, et al: *Increased numbers of alpha receptors in sympathetic denervation supersensitivity in man.* J Clin Invest 69:779, 1982.

41. Carrier, O, Wedell, EK, and Barron, KW: *Specific alpha-adrenergic receptor desensitization in vascular smooth muscle.* Blood Vessels 15:247, 1978.

42. Altura, BM: *Sex and estrogens and responsiveness of terminal arterioles to neurohypophyseal hormones and catecholamines.* J Pharmacol Exp Ther 193:403, 1975.

43. Altura, BM: *Sex as a factor influencing the responsiveness of arterioles to catecholamines.* Eur J Pharmacol 20:261, 1972.

44. Windquist, RJ, Webb, C, and Bohr, DF: *Vascular smooth muscle in hypertension.* Fed Proc 41:2387,.

45. Epstein, SE and Braunwald, E: *The effect of beta adrenergic blockade on patterns of urinary sodium excretion. Studies in normal subjects and in patients with heart disease.* Ann Intern Med 75:20, 1966.

46. Epstein, SE, Robinson, BF, Kahler RL, et al: *Effects of beta-adrenergic blockade on the cardiac response to maximal and submaximal exercise in man.* J Clin Invest 44:1745, 1965.

47. Braunwald, E (ed): *Beta-Adrenergic Blockade—A New Era in Cardiovascular Medicine.* Excerpta Medica, New York, 1978.

48. Carlsson, E, Dahiot, CG, Hedberg, A, et al: *Differentiation of cardiac chronotropic and inotropic effects of beta adrenoceptor agonists.* Naunym Schmiedbergs Arch Pharmacol 300:101, 105, 1977.

49. Dreyer, AC and Offermeier, J: *Indications for the existence of two types of cardiac beta-adrenergic receptors.* Pharmacol Res Commun 7:151, 1975.

50. Williams, RS and Bishop, T: *Selectivity of dobutamine for adrenergic receptor subtypes.* J Clin Invest 67:1703, 1981.

51. Reiz, S, Waagstein, F, and Hjalmarson, A: *Clinical experience of a new inotropic agent—prenalterol—in hypotension and heart failure.* Clin Cardiol 3:96, 1980.

52. Grovier, WC: *Myocardial alpha-adrenergic receptors and their role in the production of a positive inotropic effect by sympathomimetic agents.* J Pharmacol Exp Ther 159:82, 1968.

53. Rabinowitz, B, Chuck, L, Kligerman, M, et al: *Positive inotropic effects of methoxamine: Evidence for alpha-adrenergic receptors in ventricular myocardium.* Am J Physiol 229:582, 1975.

54. Lee, JC, Fripp, RR, and Downing, SE: *Myocardial responses to alpha-adrenoceptor stimulation with methoxamine hydrochloride in lambs.* Am J Physiol 242:H405, 1982.

55. Wagner, J and Shumann, H-J: *Different mechanisms underlying the stimulation of myocardial alpha- and beta-adrenoceptors.* Life Sci 24:2045, 1979.

56. Luc-Rabine, L, Hardof, AJ, Bowman, FO, et al: *Alpha and beta adrenergic effects on human atrial specialized conducting fibers.* Circulation 57:84, 1978.

57. Corr, PB, Shayman, JA, Kramer, JB, et al: *Increased alpha-adrenergic receptors in ischemic cat myocardium: A potential mediator of electrophysiological derangements.* J Clin Invest 67:1232, 1981.

58. McConnaughey, M, Jones, LR, Watanabe, AM, et al: *Thyroxine and propylthiouracil effects on alpha- and beta-adrenergic receptor number, ATPase activities, and sialic acid content of rat cardiac membrane residues.* J Cardiovasc Pharmacol 1:609, 1979.

59. Meisheri, KD, Tenner, TE Jr, and McNeil, JH: *Reserpine-induced supersensitivity to the cardiac effects of agonists.* Life Sci 24:473, 480, 1979.

60. Yamada, S, Yamamura, HI, and Roeske, WR: *Characterization of alpha-1 adrenergic receptors in the heart using ^{3}H-WB-4101: Effect of 6-hydroxydopamine treatment.* J Pharmacol Exp Ther 215:176, 1980.

61. Glaubiger, G, Tsai, BS, Lefkowitz, RJ, et al: *Chronic guanethidine treatment increases cardiac beta-adrenergic receptors.* Nature 273:240, 1978.

62. Glaubiger, G and Lefkowitz, RJ: *Elevated beta-adrenergic receptor number after chronic propranolol treatment.* Biochem Biophys Res Comm 78:720, 1977.

63. Alderman, EL, Coltart, DJ, Wettach, GE, et al: *Coronary artery syndromes after sudden propranolol withdrawal.* Ann Intern Med 81:625, 1974.

64. Aarons, RD, Nies, AS, Gal, J, et al: *Elevation of beta-adrenergic receptor density in human lymphocytes after propranolol administration.* J Clin Invest 675:949, 1980.

65. Unverferth, DV, Blanford, M, Kates, RE, et al: *Tolerance to dobutamine after a 72-hour continuous infusion.* Am J Med 69:262, 1980.

66. Colucci, WS, Alexander, RW, Williams, GH, et al: *Decreased lymphocyte beta-adrenergic-receptor den-*

sity in patients with heart failure and tolerance to the beta-adrenergic agonist pirbuteral. N Engl J Med 305:185, 1981.

67. BAUMANN, G, RIESS, G, ERHARDT, WD, ET AL: *Impaired beta-adrenergic stimulation in the uninvolved ventricle post acute myocardial infarction.* Am Heart J 101:569, 1981.
68. MARSH, JD, BARRY, WB, NEER, EJ, ET AL: *Desensitization of chick embryo ventricle to the physiological and biochemical effects of isoproterenol.* Circ Res 47:492, 1980.
69. CHIDSEY, CA AND BRAUNWALD, E: *Sympathetic activity and neurotransmitter depletion in congestive heart failure.* Pharmacol Rev 18:685, 1966.
70. BRISTOW, MR, GINSBURG, R, MINOBE, W, ET AL: *Decreased catecholamine sensitivity and beta-adrenergic-receptor density in failing human hearts.* N Engl J Med 307:205, 1982.
71. KARLINGER, JS, BARNES, P, BROWN, M, ET AL: *Chronic heart failure in the guinea pig increases cardiac alpha-1 and beta adrenoceptors.* Eur J Pharmacol 67:115, 1980.
72. SHERIDAN, DJ, PENKOSKE, PA, SOBEL, BE, ET AL: *Alpha adrenergic contributions to dysrhythmias during myocardial ischemia and reperfusion in cats.* J Clin Invest 65:161, 1980.
73. VAN ZWIETEN, PA AND TIMMERMANS, PBMWM: *Basic pharmacology of centrally acting antihypertensive drugs.* Cardiovasc Rev Reports 3:1079, 1982.
74. HAUSLER, G: *Central alpha-adrenoceptors involved in cardiovascular regulation.* J Cardiovasc Pharmacol 4:S72, 1982.
75. KOBINGER, W: *Central alpha-adrenergic systems as targets for hypotensive drugs.* Rev Physiol Biochem Pharmacol 81:39, 1978.
76. CRUICKSHANK, JM: *The clinical importance of cardioselectivity and lipophilicity in beta blockers.* Am Heart J 100:160, 1980.
77. WEINER, N: *Drugs that inhibit adrenergic nerves and block adrenergic receptors.* In GILMAN, AG, GOODMAN, LS, AND GILMAN, A (EDS): *The Pharmacological Basis of Therapeutics,* ed 6. Macmillan, New York, 1980.
78. COLUCCI, WS: *Alpha-adrenergic receptor blockade with prazosin.* Ann Intern Med 97:67, 1982.
79. SAEED, M, SOMMER, O, HOLTZ, J, ET AL: *Alpha-adrenoceptor blockade by phentolamine causes alpha-adrenergic vasodilation by increased catecholamine release due to presynaptic alpha blockade.* J Cardiovasc Pharmacol 44:44, 1982.
80. RUSKIN, JN AND HUTTER, AM JR: *Primary pulmonary hypertension treated with oral phentolamine.* Ann Intern Med 90:772, 1979.
81. MAJID, PA, SHARMA, B AND TAYLOR, SH: *Phentolamine for vasodilator treatment of severe heart failure.* Lancet 2:719, 1971.
82. KOVICK, RB, TILLISCH, JH, BERENS, SC, ET AL: *Vasodilator therapy for chronic left ventricular failure.* Circulation 53:322, 1976.
83. WALKER, RG, WHITWORTH, JA, SAINES, D, ET AL: *Long-term treatment of moderate and severe hypertension and lack of "tolerance."* Med J Aust 2:146, 1981.
84. LEREN, P, HELGELAND, A, HOLME, I, ET AL: *Effect of propranolol and prazosin and blood lipids. The Oslo study.* Lancet 2:406, 1980.
85. MEHTA, J, IACONA, M, FELDMAN, RL, ET AL: *Comparative hemodynamic effects of intravenous nitroprusside and oral prazosin in refractory heart failure.* Am J Cardiol 41:925, 1978.
86. PACKER, M, MELLER, J, GORLIN, R, ET AL: *Hemodynamic and clinical tachyphylaxis to prazosin-mediated afterload reduction in chronic congestive heart failure.* Circulation 59:531, 1979.
87. COLUCCI, WS, WYNNE, J, HOLMAN, BL, ET AL: *Long-term therapy of heart failure with prazosin. A randomized double-blind trial.* Am J Cardiol 45:337, 1980.
88. BERTEL, O, BURKART, F, AND BUHLER, FR: *Sustained effectiveness of chronic prazosin in severe chronic congestive heart failure.* Am Heart J 101:529, 1981.
89. GOLDMAN, SA, JOHNSON, LE, ESCALA, E, ET AL: *Improved exercise ejection fraction with long-term prazosin therapy in patients with heart failure.* Am J Med 68:36, 1980.
90. AWAN, NA, NEEDHAM, KE, EVENSON, MK, ET AL: *Therapeutic application of prazosin in chronic refractory congestive heart failure.* Am J Med 71:153, 1981.
91. HARPER, FE AND LEROY, EL: *Raynaud's phenomenon: An update on treatment.* J Cardiovasc Med 7:282, 1982.
92. COBAUGH, DS: *Prazosin treatment of ergotamine-induced peripheral ischemia.* JAMA 244:1360, 1980.
93. OKUN, R: *Effectiveness of prazosin as initial antihypertensive therapy.* Am J Cardiol 51:645, 1983.
94. CHRYSANT, SG, ET AL: *Systemic and renal hemodynamic effects of trimazosin: A new vasodilator.* J Cardiovasc Pharmacol 2:205, 1980.

95. Chrysant, SG, et al: *Long-term hemodynamic and metabolic effects of trimazosin in essential hypertension.* Clin Pharmacol Ther 30:600, 1981.

96. Klahr, L, Salazar, A, Almeida, D, et al: *The effects of indoramin in essential arterial hypertension: A placebo-controlled trial.* Curr Med Res Opin 3:685, 1976.

97. Awan, NA: *Cardiocirculatory effects of afterload reduction with oral trimazosin in severe chronic heart failure.* Am J Cardiol 44:126, 1979.

98. Weber, KT, et al: *Long-term vasodilator therapy with trimazosin in chronic cardiac failure.* N Engl J Med 303:242, 1980.

The Clinical Pharmacology of Beta-Adrenergic Blockers

David T. Lowenthal, M.D.

Presently, there are more than 20 beta-adrenergic blocking drugs (BABD) on the market in Western Europe. There are seven on the market in Canada, and the United States now has six approved BABD. The clinical indications for their usage include hypertension, arrhythmias, ischemic heart disease, thyrotoxicosis, migraine headaches, glaucoma, and anxiety states. The purpose of this chapter is to review the clinical pharmacologic aspects of this group of drugs and, hopefully, to delineate some differences that subserve their raison d'etre. In general, the pharmacodynamic effects of these drugs are quite similar, yet the properties of biotransformation, including pharmacokinetics, tend to be salient distinguishing features.

RECEPTOR PHARMACOLOGY

Since Ahlquist's original paper wherein he postulated the "tentative" existence of receptor sites, much has been learned concerning alpha and beta receptors.[1] Alpha receptors have been subdivided into $alpha_1$ and $alpha_2$ receptors. The $alpha_1$ receptors, which are located postsynaptically on the vascular smooth muscle wall, cause vasoconstriction when stimulated. The prototype agonists for $alpha_1$ receptors are phenylephrine and methoxamine. $Alpha_2$ receptors are presynaptic and are located on the sympathetic neuron terminal; when stimulated, a feedback system is invoked in that release of norepinephrine from the nerve terminal is inhibited. Phentolamine and phenoxybenzamine, prototype alpha-adrenergic inhibitors, stimulate both $alpha_1$ and $alpha_2$ receptor sites. Consequently, both tachycardia and orthostatic hypotension occur. Prazosin,[2] which is an atypical alpha receptor–blocking drug, acts only at the $alpha_1$ locus, and therefore there is no reflex tachycardia. Although beyond the scope of this discussion, alpha receptors exist within the central nervous system, as best exemplified by the action of centrally acting antihypertensives, for example, clonidine and guanabenz, wherein central alpha-agonist stimulation results in a decrease in sympathetic outflow to the periphery.[3]

More germane to the discussion is that the beta receptors, $beta_1$ and $beta_2$, play a major role in the response to the stimulation and inhibition of the sympathetic nervous system.[4] Since $beta_1$-receptor pharmacology relates to the heart, kidney, and eye, stimulation of such receptors results in positive inotropic and chronotropic effects, renin release, and an increase in aqueous humor production, respectively. On the other hand, when $beta_2$ receptors are stimulated, there is relaxation of vascular smooth muscle in skeletal muscle circulation resulting in vasodilatation, and relaxation of bronchial, uterine, and gastrointestinal smooth muscle. Biochemically, stimulation of $beta_2$ receptors results in lipolysis, glycogenolysis, insulin release, and lactic acid production. The prototype pure beta agonist is isoproterenol. It affects both $beta_1$ and $beta_2$ receptors, resulting in tachycardia and relaxation of bronchial smooth muscle. $Beta_2$ agonists are best exemplified by terbutaline, isoetharine, metaproterenol, and salbutamol. Finally, it is noteworthy that tissues such as the heart that possess predominantly $beta_1$ receptors also contain some $beta_2$ receptors. Thus, tissue selectivity is not absolute.

PROPERTIES COMMON TO BETA ANTAGONISTS[5]

Central effects, for example, sedation, depression, and sleep disturbances, are often encountered with beta antagonists, especially the more lipophilic drugs (i.e., propranolol, metoprolol, pindolol). These annoyances are especially common in elderly persons and in those patients whose renal function is somewhat compromised.

Central and peripheral effects of beta antagonists on beta receptors in the kidney result in a marked *reduction in renin activity or concentration,* and consequently in aldosterone, to degrees greater than the suppression observed with central alpha agonists. Likewise, there is a more sustained *reduction in cardiac hemodynamics* (i.e., declines in cardiac output, stroke volume, and heart rate, with an early rise in peripheral resistance and an eventual but predictable autoregulatory decrease in vascular resistance), in direct contrast to the central alpha agonists, which more promptly reduce peripheral vascular resistance without substantial impairment of cardiac hemodynamics.

The *propensity for the withdrawal syndrome,* especially in patients with ischemic heart disease, can lead to further embarrassment of cardiac function. This problem of a rebound hyperdynamic circulatory state is related to changes in central and peripheral beta-receptor sensitivity to catecholamines,[4] wherein beta agonists decrease and beta antagonists increase the number of receptor sites.[6] When propranolol is abruptly discontinued, there are more receptor sites available to "accommodate" circulating catecholamines. The result is an increase in myocardial oxygen demand, and symptoms of myocardial ischemia can result.[7]

There is a general *blunting of the exercise response.* It is well established that beta blockade, regardless of genre (cardioselective or nonselective, presence of intrinsic sympathomimetic activity or not), suppresses the exercise response. Extended types of physical activity (distance running, cycling, swimming, walking) depend on free fatty acids, that is, the process of lipolysis, for energy. The latter is inhibited by beta blockade but not by central alpha agonists. Moreover, when compared with the usual increase in potassium during dynamic physical activity, there is a substantially greater rise in plasma potassium level in patients taking metoprolol, atenolol, or propranolol.[8] The latter effect is probably not related to renin and aldosterone suppression but more likely to a direct effect on the cellular membranes, resulting in an efflux of potassium from the cell. Based on short-term and long-term studies comparing the potassium response in the presence of centrally acting drugs such as methyldopa, clonidine, and propranolol, it is evident that there is a significantly greater increase in potassium at peak levels of dynamic (treadmill) exercise under the influence of propranolol (80 mg, single dose) in contrast to single doses of clonidine or methyldopa.[9] When propranolol is given for a week or more, there does not seem to be any significantly greater rise in potassium at low dosage (40 mg bid), whereas at higher dosage, the drug produces greater increases in potassium. After chronic dosing with clonidine (0.1 mg bid) and methyldopa (250 mg bid) for 1 week, plasma potassium does not increase adversely. These drug-exercise interactions can be important in patients with cardiac arrhythmias, or those with mild to moderate degrees of renal insufficiency, who like to perform some form of physical activity. Appropriate drug selection may prevent adverse hyperkalemic responses.

Because of the altered hemodynamic profile induced by beta antagonists and the blunted sympathetic responses encountered in the elderly, beta antagonists are of *limited usefulness in treatment of hypertension in the geriatric population.*[10] Hypertension in elderly persons classically is predominantly systolic hypertension, characterized by fixed, rigid type of peripheral vasculature that would not respond to beta blockade.

In the absence of cardiac and renal disease, there is *no marked sodium retention.* However, a decrease in renal hemodynamics with long-term propranolol treatment has been described.[11]

Table 1. Recommended BABD for patients with brochospastic disorders

Metoprolol (cardioselective)
Atenolol (cardioselective)
Pindolol (ISA)

ISA = intrinsic sympathomimetic activity

Finally, beta blockade is *useful in the management of hyperkinetic hypertension,* that is, neurogenic hypertension encountered in young persons. There are data, however, demonstrating similar beneficial effects with central alpha agonists in the same syndrome.[12]

CLASSIFICATION OF BETA-ADRENERGIC BLOCKING DRUGS[5,13,14]

The six general categories by which BABD are classified are (1) beta-blocker potency, (2) cardioselectivity, (3) intrinsic sympathomimetic activity, (4) membrane-stabilizing activity, (5) lipophilicity, and (6) pharmacokinetics.

Beta-Blocker Potency

The potency of BABD does not refer to antihypertensive or antianginal activity. Instead, this category considers the response to the prototype beta agonist, isoproterenol, which when given intravenously can produce an increase in heart rate. Under controlled conditions, a patient is given a dose sufficient to increase the heart rate by 25 beats per min, both before and after the administration of a beta blocker. The extent of beta blockade can then be expressed as a "dose-ratio," or ratio of the dose of isoproterenol required before beta blockade to that required after beta blockade. The literature relates potency of BABD to propranolol, which is given the rating 1. In this regard, timolol and pindolol, which are the most potent agents milligram for milligram, are rated at eight and six times the potency of propranolol, respectively. Metoprolol, nadolol, and atenolol are all equivalent to propranolol. Acebutolol, alprenolol, and labetalol have one third the potency of propranolol.

Cardioselectivity

Metoprolol[15] and atenolol[16] have beta_1 cardioselectivity. This implies that at low doses these drugs affect the heart primarily, with very little effect on extracardiac tissues such as bronchial smooth muscle. All of the other currently available BABD are nonselective. In low dosage, atenolol and metoprolol can be used not only in the presence of well-controlled bronchospastic disorders but also may be used in patients with insulin-dependent diabetes, with a greater degree of safety than with nonselective BABD (Tables 1 and 2). It has been demonstrated that the increase in heart rate response to hypoglycemia may still be intact in the presence of a beta_1 cardioselective inhibitor[17,18]; this is because there is less peripheral vasoconstriction and a greater degree of vasodilatation when the catecholamine response to hypo-

Table 2. Recommended BABD for patients with insulin-dependent diabetes mellitus

Metoprolol Atenolol Labetalol	Less peripheral vasoconstriction; better likelihood for reflex increase in heart rate during hypoglycemia

glycemia ensues. Thus, the increase in heart rate is a direct response to the catecholamine stimulation during insulin-induced hypoglycemia. Labetalol, which is nonselective and reduces peripheral resistance, may provide a similar benefit in patients with diabetes.[19] Overall, however, this issue of BABD contraindication in persons with insulin-dependent diabetes is greatly exaggerated. Conversely, once the higher doses of the $beta_1$ cardioselective drugs are reached, bronchospasm may exacerbate in patients with asthma.

Intrinsic Sympathomimetic Activity (Partial Agonist Activity)[20]

Intrinsic sympathomimetic activity (ISA) has been observed with pindolol, a noncardioselective BABD with six times the potency of propranolol. The term "partial agonist activity" implies a bit of a paradox in that the drug inhibits some actions and yet stimulates other functions involving beta receptors. In animal models whose autonomic response has been attenuated by adrenalectomy or by catecholamine depletion using reserpine, it is possible to demonstrate that some BABD have ISA in addition to beta-antagonist properties. Even though partial agonist activity such as cardiac stimulation can be demonstrated, it is still much less intense than that exhibited with isoproterenol.

The overall clinical significance of BABD that possess ISA is still an enigma. Although some investigators believe that ISA protects against myocardial depression, bronchospasm, and peripheral vasoconstriction, evidence to support these claims is as yet inconclusive. It is known that beta blockers with ISA (e.g., pindolol, oxprenolol) produce smaller increases in cardiopulmonary volume and either do not affect or may actually lower pulmonary capillary wedge pressure, as contrasted to beta blockers without ISA, which produce an increase in wedge pressure and cardiopulmonary blood volume. Nevertheless, even though there may be some cardiac stimulation with BABD possessing ISA when used in a catecholamine-depleted preparation, these BABD with ISA as well as those without both blunt the exercise response. Finally, pindolol may be somewhat more bronchoprotective in patients who are intolerant to propranolol because of bronchospasm. Yet there is inadequate evidence to substantiate clearly that beta blockers with ISA are indeed safer in patients with bronchospastic disorders.

Membrane-Stabilizing Activity ("Quinidine-Like" Activity)[21–23]

Propranolol has electrophysiologic properties unrelated to its antagonism of beta-adrenergic receptors. Propranolol slows the rate of rise of the cardiac action potential, whereas resting potential and duration of the spike potential are unchanged. This has also been shown to occur with oxprenolol and alprenolol. The effects are observed in vitro at very high concentrations of propranolol (10,000 ng/ml), whereas arrhythmia suppression and the inhibition of exercise-induced tachycardia occur at levels of only 100 ng/ml. In essence, this property may be of only theoretical importance since the "quinidine-like" activity occurs at doses greater than those used clinically.

Lipophilicity (Lipid Solubility)[24]

The most lipophilic of the BABD is propranolol. This property implies its avidity for the central nervous system. Lipophilic drugs are almost completely metabolized by the liver. As lipid solubility decreases, more drug tends to be excreted unchanged by the kidney. It is likely that the reason for the effectiveness of propranolol in migraine headache and in various anxiety states may be related to its ability to penetrate the blood-brain barrier. Conversely, patients who develop sleep disorders while on lipophilic agents may benefit by taking a beta blocker which is less lipid soluble and therefore excreted by the kidney. Labetalol is weakly lipid soluble and thus does not penetrate the blood-brain barrier to any appreciable degree. Atenolol and nadolol, which are eliminated by the kidney, have low partition coefficients (ratio in octanol to water), indicating that their solubility in water is greater than in alcohol, a prototype lipid solvent.

Pharmacokinetics of Beta-Adrenergic Blocking Drugs[25,26]

The processes of drug biotransformation include absorption, distribution (plasma protein binding), metabolism, and elimination.

ABSORPTION. The absorption of all BABD varies. Between 90 and 100 percent of propranolol, timolol, metoprolol, and pindolol are absorbed. In contrast, absorption of nadolol is only 15 to 25 percent and atenolol 46 to 62 percent. The percentage of the dose of an orally administered drug that reaches the systemic circulation is an index of bioavailability. However, the systemic bioavailability of BABD for pharmacologic activity is not necessarily related to the degree of absorption. For example, the systemic availability of alprenolol and propranolol, owing to first-pass metabolism, is only 10 percent and 30 percent, respectively; timolol, on the other hand, had a 75 percent bioavailability, pindolol greater than 90 percent, metoprolol 50 percent, and atenolol approximately 55 percent. Thus, larger doses of alprenolol and propranolol, initially, *may* be necessary to achieve pharmacologic effects similar to those that lower doses of pindolol could accomplish.

DISTRIBUTION. Drugs are bound mainly to plasma albumin. Propranolol is the most avidly protein-bound of all of the BABD, that is, greater than 90 percent. In contrast, atenolol, timolol, and metoprolol are minimally protein-bound, that is, 5 percent, 10 percent, and 12 percent, respectively. Nadolol is bound only about 25 to 30 percent.

METABOLISM. Propranolol, metoprolol, and timolol are metabolized extensively in the liver. Propranolol is the only one of these three BABD that gives rise to an active metabolite, 4-hydroxypropranolol. The dosages of these drugs have to be reduced in patients with impaired liver function, whereas the dosage may not need to be altered from that given to normal persons should renal impairment exist. On the other hand, atenolol and nadolol are minimally metabolized by the liver and depend on the intact kidneys for their elimination (Table 3). Thus, for patients with imparied renal function, the doses of atenolol and nadolol need to be reduced. Pindolol is about 60 percent metabolized in the liver, and 40 percent is excreted unchanged by the kidneys.

ELIMINATION. Since propranolol is the most extensively metabolized BABD, very little of the drug is eliminated unchanged. On the other hand, most of the dosage of atenolol and nadolol is eliminated unchanged by the kidney. Therefore, the half-lives of atenolol and nadolol of 6 to 7 hours and 12 to 24 hours, respectively, are prolonged in patients with impaired renal function. In contrast, only small amounts of the absorbed doses of timolol and metoprolol are excreted unchanged in the urine.

Factors other than renal and liver disease may affect the biotransformation of drugs. It is now widely established that elderly persons may suffer a higher incidence of adverse drug reactions than young persons. This difference may be due to an alteration of the elimination process by both hepatic and renal mechanisms. For example, it has been demonstrated that following 80 mg every 8 hours of propranolol, blood levels were substantially greater in

Table 3. Recommended BABD for patients with acute and chronic hepatic insufficiency (CHI)

Drug	*T½ (hr)*	*T½ (CRF)*	*Dosage Alterations in CHI*
Nadolol	17–24	Prolonged	None
Atenolol	10	Prolonged	None

CRF = chronic renal failure

patients over age 35 compared with those under age 35. Besides age, smoking has a substantial effect on the plasma concentrations of propranolol. It has been found that smokers have significantly reduced blood levels of propranolol in comparison with nonsmokers. In smokers receiving propranolol, it was found that there was an age-related effect of smoking. Smoking increased the ability of the liver to eliminate propranolol only in the young, whereas the elderly demonstrated resistance to this effect. Owing to the fact that hepatic blood flow falls with age in both smokers and nonsmokers, there appears to be little effect of smoking on the age-related reduction in hepatic blood flow per se.[27–29]

Renal function also decreases with age. For every decade beyond age 35 there is a 6 to 10 percent decrement in glomerular filtration rate and renal plasma flow. Thus, the dosage of those drugs that depend on renal elimination, for example, atenolol and nadolol, should be reduced in the elderly, whether or not underlying renal parenchymal disease exists.

SOME APPLICATIONS RELATED TO BIOTRANSFORMATION AND DISEASE

Propranolol, a nonselective beta-adrenergic antagonist, is used primarily in the treatment of hypertension, angina pectoris, and cardiac arrhythmias. When administered orally, propranolol undergoes first-pass hepatic extraction with a high extraction ratio of 0.6 to 0.8. Propranolol is metabolized (hydroxylation) by the hepatic oxidative pathway to 4-hydroxypropranolol,[30] an active metabolite. The hepatic clearance of propranolol is proportional to hepatic blood flow and, therefore, sensitive to factors that alter this flow.[31] Owing to the avid hepatic uptake, oral doses result in lower plasma concentrations than do equivalent intravenous doses. Long-term administration of propranolol to normal individuals results in saturation of hepatic uptake and metabolic processes, and hence plasma concentrations and a prolongation of the biologic half-life.[32] There is significant interindividual variability[33] in the plasma concentration–dose relationship as well as significant intraindividual[34] variability in plasma propranolol concentrations. Technical interference by Vacutainer-type tubes[35] as well as by heparin[36] may contribute to the variability in propranolol plasma levels that often results in reports of low plasma concentrations.

Previous studies[37] in our laboratory have not demonstrated an impairment of propranolol absorption in patients with chronic renal disease. However, significantly higher plasma concentrations of propranolol 1.5 hours after the administration of 80 mg occurs when patients with renal failure are compared with normal control subjects.[37] In patients with renal failure, the dose per kilogram was significantly greater, yet the metabolic clearance was lower when compared with the control group. Elimination half-life and the elimination rate constant of propranolol were not significantly altered by renal failure.[37] Yet, because of the significantly higher plasma concentrations of propranolol, the area under the curve (AUC) was threefold greater in renal failure. These observations suggest an impairment in the first-pass effect of propranolol in renal insufficiency.[37,38] We have also found a decrease in volume of distribution of propranolol in two patients with end-stage renal disease.[39] Because propranolol is largely extracted by the liver, severe hepatic disease with diminished hepatic blood flow and drug extraction efficiency would also be expected to result in higher blood levels.

In contrast to normal individuals, when long-term maintenance doses of propranolol (that is, 40 to 80 mg every eight hours) are given to patients with renal failure, the elimination half-life is shorter than when the drug is given in single doses.[40] There is evidence that some drugs, such as antipyrine,[41] phenytoin,[42] and pentobarbital,[43] which, like propranolol, are metabolized by oxidation processes, have accelerated rates of metabolism and shortened biologic half-lives in patients with end-stage renal disease. It is likely that the chronic administration of propranolol may also be associated with increased metabolism when the drug is given over a long period. This effect may reflect an increase in the activity of the microsomal oxidative system in chronic renal failure.

Table 4. BABD for patients with chronic renal failure (CRF)

Drug	$T^{1/2}$*(hr)*	*Protein binding changes in CRF*	*Dialyzability*	*Dosage alterations in CRF*
Propranolol	3–4	None	Poor	None
Metoprolol	4	None	Unknown	None
Timolol	5	None	Poor	None
Pindolol	3–4	Unknown	Unknown	None
Labetalol	4	Unknown	Unknown	None

In summary, propranolol dosage should be carefully monitored in patients with kidney disease. Careful attention must be paid to blood pressure and pulse rate change as a result of the early elevated plasma concentrations. However, the increased plasma propranolol level is transient, and, generally, no accumulation of propranolol occurs when long-term dosing is prescribed. Although 4-hydroxypropranolol, naphthoxylactic acid, and naphthoxyacetic acid accumulation may occur, these substances do not result in adverse or overt hemodynamic alterations.[44,45] Therefore, dosage alteration is unnecessary for chronic propranolol therapy in patients with advanced renal disease (Table 4).

Protein-binding studies in our laboratory with radioactive carbon (^{14}C)–labeled propranolol or unlabeled drug, by means of ultracentrifugation and equilibrium dialysis, demonstrate that the binding of propranolol is not impaired in patients with renal insufficiency. However, when patients are treated with long-term peritoneal dialysis, the binding of propranolol is significantly reduced; this effect is probably due to the loss of albumin during the peritoneal dialysis procedure. Because of its avid protein binding of 90 percent or greater, it can be predicted that the dialyzability of propranolol is small. Previous work has demonstrated that this indeed is the case with propranolol.[37]

Changes have been reported in the distribution and disposition of intravenous propranolol in patients with cirrhosis and chronic active hepatitis compared with normal subjects.[46] The clearance of propranolol decreases as the severity and derangement of hepatic function increases.[46] The average clearance and volume of distribution of propranolol are 0.44 L/min and 448 L, respectively, in patients with hepatic disease as compared with 0.92 L/min and 220 L in normal subjects. There is an increase in free propranolol concentration in patients with chronic liver disease. It is difficult to extrapolate these data generated by the intravenous administration of propranolol to chronic oral dosing because of the unknown effect of chronic liver disease on hepatic exzyme activity (intrinsic hepatic clearance), hepatic blood flow, and volume of distribution. However, because of the increase in the free fraction of propranolol in patients with impaired hepatic function, oral doses should be increased with caution. Interestingly, in patients with portacaval shunt, high plasma concentrations occur because the oral dose circumvents the avid hepatic extraction process. Branch and coworkers[46] have found an eightfold increase in propranolol half-life in patients with cirrhosis with hypoalbuminemia even though hepatic clearance is reduced to only one third of normal. This is probably related to the fact that there is a significant increase in the volume of distribution of propranolol, as noted previously.

Timolol[47] is six times as potent as propranolol with regard to beta-adrenergic blocking activity, and the drug has no cardiac selectivity or membrane-stabilizing activity. Timolol is only 10 percent protein bound. The elimination half-life of timolol in patients with renal disease is 4 hours, which is similar to the half-life in patients with normal renal function.[47] However, following 20 mg of timolol given in single dose, there does seem to be a prolongation of the blood pressure response as well as heart rate response, with the systolic and diastolic pressures and heart rate very gradually returning to predosing levels by 24 hours. When given prior to hemodialysis, the drug induces significant hemodynamic effects leading to hypotension, bradycardia, nausea, and sweating. These effects contraindicate the use of timolol prior to dialysis. Timolol does not give rise to active metabolites, in contrast to propranolol. No data exist concerning the pharmacodynamics or biotransformation of timolol in patients with acute or chronic liver disease.

Labetalol possesses alpha- and beta-adrenoreceptor blocking properties. It is extensively metabolized in the liver and less than 5 percent is excreted unchanged in the urine. Based on this fact, it would be safe to give to patients with chronic renal disease. However, in patients with chronic liver disease, bioavailability studies with labetalol demonstrate increased bioavailability owing to a reduction in first-pass metabolism.[48] This effect correlated negatively with serum albumin concentrations. In addition, the decrease in heart rate and blood pressure was greater after oral administration, suggesting an exaggerated response due to the increased bioavailability. Similar results have been reported with increased bioavailability for propranolol. Oxprenolol, alprenolol, and metoprolol, which also have high hepatic extraction, have not yet been studied in this setting of chronic hepatic disease, but similar results must be anticipated.

Pindolol is six times as potent as propranolol as a beta-adrenergic antagonist. Another major difference is that it has significant partial agonist activity. Its half-life in normal renal function is 3 to 4 hours, and 40 percent of a single dose of pindolol is recovered unchanged in the urine.[49,50] Nevertheless, there has not been any correlation found between the overall elimination rate constant of pindolol and endogenous creatinine clearance. Ohnhaus and associates[49] concluded that the extrarenal elimination rate constant was increased in chronic renal failure. However, Oie and Levy[50] found a statistically significant positive correlation between the renal clearance of pindolol and creatinine.

Sotalol is approximately one tenth as potent as propranolol and has no cardioselectivity, partial agonist activity, or membrane-stabilizing activity. Sotalol is excreted mainly by the kidneys as unchanged drug. In patients with end-stage renal disease, the plasma half-life is approximately 42 hours, as compared with 5 hours in normal subjects.[51] Thus, significant dosage reduction and lengthening of dosing interval are suggested in patients with renal failure.

Nadolol is a noncardioselective beta-adrenergic blocking drug and can be administered once daily. It is two to four times as potent as propranolol as a beta-adrenergic antagonist. Nadolol is only about 30 percent protein bound, and more than 90 percent is recovered unchanged in the urine and feces.[52,53] No active metabolites have been identified. Nadolol has a half-life in patients with normal renal function of 17 to 24 hours following a single oral dose. The renal clearance of nadolol has been found to correlate directly with creatinine clearance. As a consequence, the plasma half-life is prolonged in patients with impaired renal function. Therefore, dosing intervals should be lengthened in patients with decreased renal function receiving nadolol. Hemodialysis can effectively reduce serum concentrations of the drug and, thus, be useful as a means of treating nadolol intoxication. When creatinine clearance is below 50 ml/min, the dosage can be reduced by 50 percent and the dosing interval can be widened to every other day.

Metoprolol acts as a cardioselective beta-adrenergic blocking agent when administered at lower doses (less than 150 mg/day). It is 12 percent protein bound, and primarily undergoes hepatic biotransformation with some first-pass effect. The half-life of oral metoprolol in normal persons is 3 to 4 hours, and about 3 percent of a single dose is recovered unchanged in the urine. There are no known active metabolites. There is no need to alter the dosage in patients with impaired renal function.[15] Interestingly, about 95 percent of an oral or intravenous dose of metoprolol is recovered in the urine over a period of 72 hours. Whereas the elimination half-life of the total metabolites after oral administration is about 3 hours, it is about 5 hours after an intravenous dose. This finding indicates that the route of administration might influence the metabolic pathways of metoprolol, which results in 50 percent of administered dose reaching the systemic circulation. The first-pass process may be impaired in chronic hepatic disease, resulting in an enhanced bioavailability and pharmacodynamic effect of metoprolol.

When compared with propranolol, alprenolol has less bioavailability (10 percent) and is avidly protein bound with an elimination half-life similar to that of propranolol. Less than 1 percent of the drug is excreted unchanged, and like propranolol, it too has active metabolites. Alprenolol is nonselective and equipotent to propranolol, but it has partial agonist activity. Although the pharmacokinetics of alprenolol have not been delineated in patients with impaired renal function, the fact that hepatic biotransformation gives rise to an active metabolite suggests that a dosage reduction should be recommended in order to avoid significant accumulation of the active metabolite. This recommendation would apply in patients with advanced renal failure. In patients with chronic liver disease, a decreased first-pass effect may result in increased bioavailability and enhanced pharmacologic effect.

Atenolol has an elimination half-life in subjects with normal renal function of 6 to 9 hours.[54] This property is prolonged as renal function decreases.[55] It is equipotent to propranolol and is cardioselective, and it may be the only adrenoreceptor blocker that does not cross the blood-brain barrier. There are no active metabolites, and approximately 40 percent of atenolol is recovered unchanged in the urine after a single dose. Therefore, some dosage reduction must be considered if atenolol is given to patients with impaired renal function. However, it is noteworthy that the drug is dialyzable.[56]

CONCLUSIONS

There are significant pharmacokinetic differences among the BABD. However, similar end results can be achieved with any of the BABD in the treatment of hypertension[17,57] and in the treatment of angina in patients with ischemic heart disease.[57,58] Thus, if one were to consider individualizing a beta blocker in the management of hypertension or angina, an assessment should be made of the patient's hepatic and renal function, whether or not insulin-dependent diabetes mellitus coexists, the presence of mental depression (in which case a highly lipid-soluble beta blocker might be contraindicated), the history of patient compliance (where once-daily administration of long-acting BABD would be useful), and whether bronchospastic disorders coexist (in which case a cardioselective agent would be valuable). Even though pharmacodynamically these drugs are similar, individualization can be based logically on the various properties related to biotransformation.

REFERENCES

1. Ahlquist, RP: *A study of the adrenotropic receptors.* Am J Physiol 153:586, 1948.
2. Cambridge, D, Davey, MJ, and Massingham, R: *Prazosin, a selective antagonist of postsynaptic α-adrenoreceptors.* Br J Pharmacol 59:514, 1977
3. Haeusler, G: *Cardiovascular regulation by central adrenergic mechanisms and its alteration of hypotensive drugs.* Circ Res 36(Suppl 1):223, 1975.
4. Lefkowitz, RJ: *β Adrenergic receptors: Recognition and regulation.* N Engl J Med 295:323, 1976.
5. Frishman, WH: *Clinical Pharmacology of the β-Adrenoceptor Blocking Drugs.* Appleton-Century-Crofts, New York, 1980.
6. Glaubiger, G and Lefkowitz, RJ: *Elevated beta adrenergic receptor number after chronic propranolol treatment.* Biochem Biophys Res Commun 78:720, 1977.
7. Miller, RR, Olson, HG, Amsterdam, EA, et al: *Propranolol withdrawal rebound phenomenon. Exacerbation of coronary events after abrupt cessation of anti-anginal therapy.* N Engl J Med 293:416, 1975.
8. Leenen, FHH, Coenen, CHM, Zonderland, M, et al: *Effect of cardioselective and non-selective beta-blockade on dynamic exercise in mildly hypertensive men.* Clin Pharmacol Ther 28:12, 1980.
9. Lowenthal, DT, Affrime, MB, Rosenthal, LS, et al: *The neuroendocrine and potassium response to anti-renin anti-hypertensives during exercise.* Clin Exp Hypertens Theory and Practice A4 (9&10):1895, 1982.

10. *The 1980 report of the Joint National Committee on Detection, Evaluation, and Treatment of High Blood Pressure.* Arch Intern Med 140:1280, 1980.

11. BAUER, JH AND BROOKS, CS: *The long-term effect of propranolol therapy on renal function.* Am J Med 66:405, 1979.

12. FALKNER, B, ONESTI, G, LOWENTHAL, DT, ET AL: *The effectiveness of a centrally-acting agent versus diuretic in adolescent hypertension.* Clin Pharmacol Ther 32:577, 1983.

13. FIRSHMAN, WH AND SILVERMAN, R: *Clinical pharmacology of the new beta adrenergic blocking drugs. Part II. Physiologic and metabolic effects.* Am Heart J 97:797, 1979.

14. FRISHMAN, WH AND SILVERMAN, R: *Clinical pharmacology of the new beta adrenergic blocking drugs. Part III. Comparative clinical experience and new therapeutic applications.* Am Heart J 98:119, 1979.

15. KOCH-WESER J: *Metoprolol.* N Engl J Med 301:698, 1979.

16. JACKSON, G, SCHWARTZ, J, KATES, RE, ET AL: *Atenolol: Once daily cardioselective beta blockade for angina pectoris.* Circulation 61:555, 1980.

17. BRODGEN, RN, HEEL, RC, SPEIGHT, TM, ET AL: *Metoprolol: A review of its pharmacological properties and therapeutic efficacy in hypertension.* Drugs 14:321, 1977.

18. LAGER, I, BLOHNÉ, G, SMITH, U, ET AL: *Effect of cardioselective and non-selective beta blockade on the hypoglycemic response in insulin dependent diabetics.* Lancet 1:458, 1979.

19. KOCH, G: *Combined alpha and beta adrenoceptor blockade with oral labetalol in hypertensive patients with reference to hemodynamic effects at rest and during exercise.* Br J Clin Pharmacol 4:729, 1976.

20. KIRKENDALL, WM (ED): *Proceedings of an International Symposium on Pindolol.* Am Heart J 104(Part II):333, 1982.

21. VAUGHAN-WILLIAMS, EM: *Mode of action of beta receptor antagonists on cardiac muscle.* Am J Cardiol 18:399, 1966.

22. COLTART, DJ AND SHAND, DG: *Plasma propranolol levels in the quantitative assessment of beta adrenergic blockade in man.* Br Med J 3:731, 1970.

23. WOOSLEY, RL, KORNHAUSER, D, SMITH, R, ET AL: *Suppression of chronic ventricular arrhythmias with propranolol.* Circulation 60:819, 1979.

24. CRUICKSHANK, JM: *The clinical importance of cardioselectivity and lipophilicity in beta blockers.* Am Heart J 100:160, 1980.

25. MEIER, J: *Pharmocokinetic comparison of pindolol with other beta adrenocepter blocking agents.* Am Heart J 104(Part II):364, 1982.

26. WOOD, AJJ: *Pharmacokinetics and pharmcodynamics of beta blockers.* In MORGANROTH, J AND DREIFUS, L (EDS): *The Clinical Application of Beta Blockers.* Martinus Nijhoff Publishers, The Hague, 1981, p. 41.

27. VESTALL, RE, WOOD, AJJ, BRANCH, RA, ET AL: *Effects of age and cigarette smoking on propranolol disposition.* Clin Pharmacol Ther 26:8, 1979.

28. VESTALL, RE, WOOD, AJJ, SHAND, DG, ET AL: *Reduced beta adrenoceptor sensitivity in the elderly.* Clin Pharmacol Ther 26:181, 1979.

29. WOOD, AJJ, VESTALL, RE, WILKINSON, GR ET AL: *The effects of aging and cigarette smoking on the elimination of antipyrine and indocyaninegreen.* Clin Pharmacol Ther 26:16, 1979.

30. EVANS, GH, NIES, AS, AND SHAND, DG: *The disposition of propranolol. III. Decreased half-life and volume of distribution as a result of plasma binding in man, monkey, dog, and rat.* J Pharmacol Exp Ther 186:114, 1973.

31. NIES, AS, SHAND, DG, AND WILKINSON, GR: *Altered hepatic blood flow and drug disposition.* Clin Pharmacokinet 1:135, 1976.

32. EVANS, GH AND SHAND, DG: *Disposition of propranolol. V. Drug accumulation and steady-state concentrations during chronic oral administration in man.* Clin Pharmacol Ther 14:487, 1973.

33. SHAND, DG, NUKOLLS, EM, AND OATES, JA: *Plasma propranolol levels in adults.* Clin Pharmacol Ther 11:112, 1970.

34. BRIGGS, WA, LOWENTHAL, DT, CIRKSENA, W, ET AL: *Propranolol in hypertensive dialysis patients: Efficacy and compliance.* Clin Pharmacol Ther 18:606, 1975.

35. COTHAM, RH AND SHAND, D: *Spuriously low plasma propranolol concentrations resulting from blood collection methods.* Clin Pharmacol Ther 18:535, 1975.

36. WOOD, M, SHAND, DG, AND WOOD, AJJ: *Altered drug binding due to sampling through heparin locks.* Clin Pharmacol Ther 25:255, 1979.

37. LOWENTHAL, DT, BRIGGS, WA, GIBSON, TP, ET AL: *Pharmacokinetics of oral propranolol in chronic renal disease.* Clin Pharmacol Ther 16:761, 1974.

38. BIANCHETTI, G, GRAZIANI, G, BRANCACCIO, D, ET AL: *Pharmacokinetics and effects of propranolol in terminal uraemic patients and in patients undergoing regular dialysis treatment.* Clin Pharmacokinet 1:373, 1976.

39. Affrime, MB, Ruch, E, Pirano, AJ, et al: *Apparent volume of distribution of propranolol in patients with normal and abnormal renal function.* Clin Res 28:133A, 1980.

40. Lowenthal, DT: *Pharmacokinetics of antiarrhythmics: Propranolol, quinidine, procainamide, lidocaine.* Am J Med 62:532, 1977.

41. Lichter, M, Black, M, and Arias, IM: *The metabolism of antipyrine in patients with chronic renal failure.* J Pharmacol Exp Ther 187:612, 1973.

42. Reidenberg, MM, Odar-Cederlof, I, von Bahr, C, et al: *Protein binding of diphenylhydantoin and desmethylimipramine in plasma from patients with poor renal function.* N Engl J Med 285:264, 1971.

43. Reidenberg, MM, Lowenthal, DT, Briggs, WA, et al: *Pentobarbital elimination in patients with poor renal function.* Clin Pharmacol Ther 20:67, 1976.

44. Walle, T, Conradi, E, Walle, K, et al: *4-Hydroxypropranolol and its glucuronide after single and long-term doses of propranolol.* Clin Pharmacol Ther 27:22, 1980.

45. Schneck, DW, Gibson, TP, Pritchard, JF, et al: *The plasma concentrations of napthoxylactic acid and napthoxyacetic acid in uremic patients receiving chronic propranolol.* Clin Res 27:602A, 1979.

46. Branch, RA, James, J, and Read, AE: *A study of factors influencing drug disposition in chronic liver disease using the model drug (+)-propranolol.* Br J Clin Pharmacol 3:243, 1976.

47. Lowenthal, DT, Pitone, JM, Affrime, MB, et al: *Timolol kinetics in chronic renal insufficiency.* Clin Pharmacol Ther 23:606, 1978.

48. Homeida, M, Jackson, L, and Roberts, CJD: *Decreased first-pass metabolism of labetolol in chronic liver disease.* Br Med J 2:1048, 1978.

49. Ohnhaus, EE, Nuesch, E, Meier, J, et al: *Pharmacokinetics of unlabelled and C^{14}-labelled pindolol in uremia.* Eur J Clin Pharmacol 7:25, 1974.

50. Øie, S and Levy, G: *Relationship between renal function and elimination kinetics of pindolol in man.* Eur J Clin Pharmacol 9:115, 1975.

51. Tjandramaga, TB, Thomas, J, Verbeeck, R, et al: *The effect of end-stage renal failure and hemodialysis on the elimination kinetics of sotalol.* Br J Clin Pharmacol 3:259, 1976.

52. Frishman, W: *Clinical pharmacology of the new beta adrenergic blocking drugs. Part 9. Nadolol—a new long acting beta-adrenoreceptor blocking drug.* Am Heart J 99:124, 1980.

53. Herrere, J, Vukovich, RA, and Griffith, DJ: *Elimination of nadolol by patients with renal impairment.* Br J Clin Pharmacol 7:227S, 1979.

54. Johnsson, G and Rehardh, CG: *Clinical pharmacokinetics of beta-adrenoreceptor blocking drugs.* Clin Pharmacol 1:233, 1976.

55. McAinsh, J, Holmes, BF, Smith, S, et al: *Atenolol kinetics in renal failure.* Clin Pharmacol Ther 28:302, 1980.

56. Flouvat, B, Decaurt, S, Aubert, P, et al: *Pharmacokinetics of atenolol in patients with terminal failure and influence of hemodialysis.* Br J Clin Pharmacol 9:379, 1980.

57. Frisk-Holmberg, M: *β-Adrenoceptor blocking drugs: A comparative evaluation of their present clinical effectiveness and perspectives.* Curr Ther Res 26:1027, 1979.

58. Thadani, U, Davidson, C, Singleton, W, et al: *Comparison of the immediate effects of five β-adrenoreceptor-blocking drugs with different ancillary properties in angina pectoris.* N Engl J Med 300:750, 1979.

Comprehensive Drug Management of Hypertension

Suzanne Oparil, M.D., and Sherry Winternitz, M.D.

GENERAL APPROACH

Although the pathogenesis of essential hypertension remains obscure, reduction of blood pressure by pharmacologic means does delay or prevent such complications as stroke, congestive heart failure, and renal failure. Ideally, therapy should be tailored to correct the specific disturbance responsible for the initiation or maintenance of elevated blood pressure. In practice, however, detailed characterization of hormone patterns and hemodynamics in most patients with essential hypertension is seldom feasible and adds little to the efficacy of drug therapy.

The empiric selection of antihypertensive medication is directed toward a variety of goals. Treatment should be inexpensive, long-acting, effective over the long term, and associated with minimal adverse effects. Therapy should control systolic and diastolic hypertension whether the patient is supine or upright without impairing postural regulation of blood pressure. Poor compliance and therapeutic failure become inevitable with expensive and complicated drug regimens, particularly when they disturb sexual function, mood, or alertness. In general, appropriate use of current drugs, though less than ideal, will permit adequate control of blood pressure in most patients.

Most patients with essential hypertension can be successfully controlled with medical treatment. The guiding principle of antihypertensive treatment in ambulatory patients is to control the blood pressure by use of the simplest regimen (fewest drugs in the lowest doses administered over the most convenient dose schedule) possible. This is usually implemented by a stepped-care program in which therapy is initiated with a small dosage of a single drug, most often a thiazide diuretic; the dosage of that drug is increased until either the blood pressure is controlled or the maximal therapeutic dose is achieved; and additional drugs are added one at a time in increasing dosages until the blood pressure is controlled.[1] An example of such a stepped-care regimen is given in Figure 1. Alternative regimens can be used as required by the needs of patients and the experience and preferences of physicians. In patients who present with moderately severe or severe hypertension, it may be desirable to initiate treatment with more than one agent, because it can be predicted that a diuretic alone will not be adequate to bring the blood pressure into the normal range. It is generally advisable to see the patient once every 1 to 2 weeks during the time that the blood pressure is being lowered and once every 3 to 4 months once the blood pressure is controlled. This interval is thought to be necessary in order to reinforce the need for compliance, to assess the patient for side effects of the medication, and to reassess the blood pressure status in order to titrate the dosage of antihypertensive drugs.

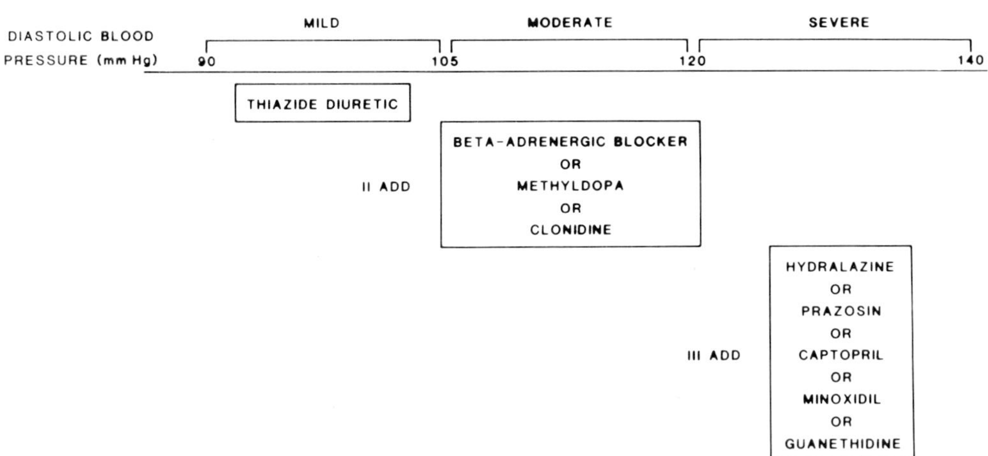

Figure 1. Suggested approach to outpatient treatment of hypertensive patients.

Hypertensive patients frequently require multiple drugs for adequate control. Use of fixed-dose combination tablets provides the convenience of taking several drugs in a single tablet but has several disadvantages. The durations of action of the various components are frequently different and the dosages inappropriate to the patient's needs. Moreover, the fixed-dose ratio precludes the adjustment of dosages of the constituent drugs to suit the requirements of the patient. These advantages and disadvantages must be weighed in deciding whether or not to use fixed-dose combination tablets in antihypertensive treatment. The commonly used fixed-dose combination tablets are listed in Tables 1 and 2 under the entry of their more potent constituent drug.

DIURETICS

Mechanisms of Action Common to Diuretic Agents

Except in the small percentage of cases in which a specific treatable biochemical defect underlies the hypertension, the foundation of medical antihypertensive therapy is the diuretic. Diuretics lower blood pressure and potentiate other antihypertensive drugs. Depletion of extracellular fluid volume with a consequent decrease in cardiac output accounts for their acute antihypertensive effect.[2] Depressed peripheral resistance persists beyond the acute phase and is responsible for their chronic antihypertensive action. The volume-depleting effects of diuretics are central to their potentiation of other antihypertensive agents.[3] Most other antihypertensive drugs predispose to sodium retention, and this effect probably accounts for their decreased efficacy with time.[3,4] Diuretics, on the other hand, continue to be effective as either sole or adjunctive antihypertensive agents as long as they prevent sodium retention.

The commonly used diuretics work by inhibiting sodium reabsorption by the renal tubules. Various agents are selective for specific regions of the nephron. The diuretics that are used as antihypertensive agents belong to three classes: (1) the benzothiadiazines (thiazides), which inhibit sodium reabsorption in the cortical ascending limb of the loop of Henle (cortical diluting segment) and the distal convoluted tubule; (2) the "loop diuretics" (furosemide, ethacrynic acid), which inhibit sodium reabsorption throughout the ascending limb of the loop of Henle; and (3) the potassium-sparing diuretics (spironolactone, triamterene, amiloride), which interfere with ion-exchange processes in the distal convoluted tubules. Table 1 lists the commonly used diuretics with their trade names, dosages, and average duration of action.

Table 1. Commonly used diuretics

Generic Name	Trade Name (Manufacturer)	Daily Adult Dosage	Frequency of Administration	Duration (hours)	Dispensing Unit
BENZOTHIADIAZINE DIURETICS					
Thiazides					
Chlorothiazide	Diuril (MSD)	250–1000 mg	bid	6–12	250 mg 500 mg
Hydrochlorothiazide	Esidrix (CIBA) Hydrodiuril (MSD) Oretic (Abbott)	25–200 mg	qd	12–18	25 mg 50 mg 100 mg
Methyclothiazide	Aquatensen (Mallinckrodt) Enduron (Abbott)	2.5–10.0 mg	qd	24–48	2.5 mg 5 mg
Polythiazide	Renese (Pfizer)	1–4 mg	qd	24–48	1 mg 2 mg 4 mg
Phthalimidines					
Chlorthalidone	Hygroton (USV)	12.5–100 mg	qd	24–72	25 mg 50 mg 100 mg
Metolazone	Zaroxolyn (Pennwalt)	2.5–5 mg	qd	12–24	2.5 mg 5 mg 10 mg
LOOP DIURETICS					
Furosemide	Lasix (Hoechst)	20–1000 mg	bid	3–6	20 mg 40 mg
Ethacrynic acid	Edecrin (MSD)	50–400 mg	bid	3–6	25 mg 50 mg
POTASSIUM-SPARING DIURETICS					
Spironolactone	Aldactone (Searle)	25–100 mg	bid	3–6	25 mg 100 mg
Triamterene	Dyrenium (SKF)	100–200 mg	bid	3–6	50 mg 100 mg
Amiloride	Midamor (MSD)	10–20 mg	qd	24	5 mg
FIXED-DOSE COMBINATION AGENTS					
Thiazide + Potassium-Sparing Diuretic					
Hydrochlorothiazide 25 mg + Spironolactone 25 mg	Aldactazide (Searle)				
Hydrochlorothiazide 25 mg + Triamterene 50 mg	Dyazide (SKF)				
Hydrochlorothiazide 50 mg + Amiloride 5 mg	Moduretic (MSD)				

Thiazide Diuretics

The thiazides are administered orally as sole treatment of mild chronic hypertension and as adjunctive treatment of more severe disease. These agents have flat dose-response curves, so that the effective dosage range is narrow. Larger dosages of drug tend to produce more adverse effects.

Loop Diuretics

The loop diuretics are rapid-acting and extremely potent diuretics.[5,6] They have steep dose-response curves, so that their effective dosage range is broad. When administered to hypertensive patients with normal renal function, the loop diuretics appear to be less effective antihypertensive agents than the thiazides but have similar adverse effects.[7,8] Accordingly, their antihypertensive use should be reserved for (1) patients with renal insufficiency who are refractory to the thiazides, (2) patients with refractory congestive failure or other edematous states, and (3) patients in hypertensive crises.

Potassium-Sparing Diuretics

The potassium-sparing diuretics have weak diuretic and antihypertensive actions. When used in conjunction with other diuretics, they serve to enhance their antihypertensive effects and minimize potassium loss. Spironolactone alone is an effective antihypertensive agent, particularly when used in states of elevated aldosterone production and/or combined with other diuretics,[9,10] but triamterene and amiloride do not have significant antihypertensive properties[11,12]; accordingly, they are used in hypertensive patients only for their potassium-sparing action in conjunction with other diuretics. High-dosage (300 to 400 mg/day) spironolactone therapy has also been shown to be useful in the diagnosis and chronic treatment of primary aldosteronism.[13,14] It is the treatment of choice for primary aldosteronism due to bilateral adrenal hyperplasia and for primary aldosteronism due to adrenal adenoma in patients who are not surgical candidates.[15,16] If spironolactone is not well tolerated, amiloride can be substituted. Patients treated with potassium-sparing diuretics, particularly those with renal insufficiency, should not receive potassium supplementation because of the risk of inducing serious hyperkalemia. Gynecomastia, breast tenderness, menstrual irregularities, and impotence occur frequently in the course of chronic high-dosage spironolactone treatment.[16]

Adverse Effects Common to Diuretic Agents

The most common adverse effects of diuretic therapy relate to volume depletion, decreased renal perfusion, and electrolyte imbalance. Elevations in blood urea nitrogen and creatinine secondary to volume contraction and decreased glomerular filtration occur most often with the loop diuretics but are also seen with the benzothiadiazines and potassium-sparing agents. During the first few days of diuretic treatment, weakness, postural dizziness, fatigue, and muscle cramps are common, probably related to the acute diuretic and potassium-depleting effect. The thiazides and loop diuretics block sodium reabsorption proximal to the distal Na^+-K^+ exchange site and therefore predispose to potassium loss. Chronic diuretic administration further predisposes to hypokalemia via increased renin and aldosterone production secondary to hypovolemia. Hypokalemia develops in approximately 10 percent of patients on chronic thiazide therapy.[17] Moderate hypokalemia does not produce important symptoms or adverse effects on the natural history of hypertensive disease, and therefore does not generally require specific treatment. Modest dietary sodium restriction reduces potassium losses by limiting the amount of sodium available to distal exchange sites and thus tends to minimize the incidence and severity of hypokalemia. Liberal use of foods rich in potassium and of potassium-containing salt substitutes further alleviates the problem. Patients who are taking cardiac glycosides do require potassium replacement, however, because hypokalemia predisposes to digitalis toxicity. Potassium supplementation with KCl or its equivalent to 80 to 120 mEq potassium per day or use of a potassium sparing-diuretic is indicated in this group.

Diuretics also cause the renal loss of magnesium,[18,19] leading to hypomagnesemia in some patients. Magnesium replacement is indicated in those patients who are taking cardiac glycosides because hypomagnesemia also facilitates the development of digitalis toxicity.[20–22] Diuretics inhibit the tubular secretion of uric acid and may induce hyperuricemia and, rarely, gout. The urate retention associated with chronic diuretic treatment results from a combination of direct inhibition of uric acid secretion and diuretic-induced volume contraction.[23] Addition of a uricosuric agent such as probenecid (Benemid) is advised for patients with significant hyperuricemia (plasma uric acid $>$ 10 mg/100 ml), particularly if there is a history of gout. Because diuretics are needed to maintain the efficacy of other antihypertensive agents, it is not generally recommended that they be discontinued in hyperuricemia. Impaired carbohydrate tolerance is a well-known side effect of chronic thiazide treatment and is generally attributed to chronic hypokalemia.[24] Hypercalcemia is a rare side effect of diuretic use in previously normocalcemic patients[25] but occurs so frequently in patients with antecedent hyperparathyroidism or those who are ingesting vitamin D that diuretics should be used with caution in such patients. Hyponatremia sometimes results from diuretic treatment because of impairment of the urinary diluting mechanism.[26] This disorder may become a serious problem in patients who are receiving loop diuretics, particularly if there is underlying renal disease and if dietary sodium is restricted.

SYMPATHOLYTIC DRUGS

Antihypertensive drugs that act as sympatholytic agents affect preganglionic, ganglionic, or postganglionic sites to reduce sympathetic influence and relax arterioles. They exert their principal antihypertensive effect by preventing sympathetic responses to changes in posture, exertion, and plasma volume deficit. Prevention of arterial vasoconstriction by these agents leads to a decrease in total peripheral resistance and reduction in blood pressure. There is also decreased sympathetic activity in the veins, with venous pooling, decreased cardiac output, and orthostatic hypotension. Attenuation of sympathetic activity to the heart decreases cardiac contractility and heart rate with further reductions in cardiac output and blood pressure. Renal plasma flow and glomerular filtration rate are often reduced as a result of the decrease in cardiac output, and sodium retention occurs. Renin secretion, which is mediated in part by adrenergic influences, decreases.

Drugs That Affect the Central Nervous System

Antihypertensive drugs that have their principal effects on sites in the central nervous system reduce preganglionic activity. The most commonly used centrally acting antihypertensive agents, clonidine and alpha-methyldopa, act as alpha$_2$-adrenoceptor agonists.[27] The central receptor involved in their antihypertensive action is of the alpha$_2$ type but is located postsynaptically. Activation of this receptor by either clonidine or alpha-methylnorepinephrine, a metabolite of alpha-methyldopa, engages the depressor pathway in the brain stem and leads to a decrease in norepinephrine release and a reduction in peripheral sympathetic tone. Clonidine and alpha-methyldopa share a similar pattern of peripheral effects, including reductions in preganglionic sympathetic nerve traffic, bradycardia, and decreases in plasma renin activity. The most common side effects are depression, sedation, and bad dreams. Because of the frequency and severity of these side effects, there is an ongoing search for new centrally acting antihypertensive agents that might be better tolerated. Table 2 lists the commonly used centrally acting antihypertensive agents with their trade names, dosages, and average duration of action.

Table 2. Commonly used antihypertensive agents

Generic Name	*Trade Name (Manufacturer)*	*Daily Adult Dosage*	*Frequency of Administration*	*Duration (hours)*	*Dispensing Unit*
	SYMPATHOLYTIC AGENTS				
METHYLDOPA	Aldomet (MSD)	250–2000 mg	bid	3–6	125 mg 250 mg 500 mg
Fixed-dose combination agents: Methyldopa + thiazide					
Methyldopa 250 mg + chlorothiazide 150 mg	Aldoclor 150 (MSD)		bid		
Methyldopa 250 mg + chlorothiazide 250 mg	Aldoclor 250 (MSD)		bid		
Methyldopa 250 mg + hydrochlorothiazide 15 mg	Aldoril 15 (MSD)		bid		
Methylodopa 250 mg + hydrochlorothiazide 25 mg	Aldoril 25 (MSD)		bid		
Methyldopa 500 mg + hydrochlorothiazide 30 mg	Aldoril D30 (MSD)		bid		
Methyldopa 500 mg + hydrochlorothiazide 50 mg	Aldoril D50 (MSD)		bid		
CLONIDINE	Catapres (Boehringer-Ingelheim)	0.1–2.4 mg	bid	6–12	0.1 mg 0.2 mg 0.3 mg
Fixed-dose combination agents: Clonidine + chlorthalidone					
Clonidine hydrochloride 0.1 mg + chlorthalidone 15 mg	Combipres 0.1 (Boehringer-Ingelheim)		bid		
Clonidine hydrochloride 0.2 mg + chlorthalidone 15 mg	Combipres 0.2 (Boehringer-Ingelheim)		bid		
GUANABENZ	Wytensin (Wyeth)	8–64 mg	bid	8–12	4 mg 8 mg
PRAZOSIN	Minipress (Pfizer)	1–20 mg	bid	3–6	1 mg 2 mg 5 mg
Fixed-dose combination agents: Prazosin + thiazide diuretic					
Prazosin hydrochloride 1 mg + polythiazide 0.5 mg	Minizide 1 (Pfizer)		bid		

Prazosin hydrochloride 2 mg + polythiazide 0.5 mg	Minizide 2 (Pfizer)		bid		
Prazosin hydrochloride 5 mg + polythiazide 0.5 mg	Minizide 5 (Pfizer)		bid		
GUANETHIDINE	Ismelin (CIBA)	10–300 mg	qd	24	10 mg 25 mg
Fixed-dose combination agent: Guanethidine + thiazide diuretic					
Guanethidine monosulfate 10 mg + hydrochlorothothiazide 25 mg	Esimil (CIBA)		qd		
BETA-ADRENERGIC BLOCKING AGENTS					
PROPRANOLOL	Inderal (Ayerst)	20–640 mg	bid	6–12	10 mg 20 mg 40 mg 80 mg
Fixed-dose combination agents: Propranolol + thiazide diuretic					
Propranolol hydrochloride 40 mg + hydrochlorothiazide 25 mg	Inderide 40/25 (Ayerst)		bid		
Propranolol hydrochloride 80 mg + hydrochlorothiazide 25 mg	Inderide 80/25 (Ayerst)		bid		
METOPROLOL	Lopressor (CIBA)	100–450 mg	bid	12	50 mg 100 mg
NADOLOL	Corgard (Squibb)	40–640 mg	qd	24	40 mg 80 mg 120 mg 160 mg
ATENOLOL	Tenormin (ICI)	50–100 mg	qd	24	50 mg 100 mg
PINDOLOL	Visken (Sandoz)	7.5–45 mg	qd	24	5 mg 10 mg
TIMOLOL	Blocadren (MSD)	20–40 mg	bid	8–12	10 mg 20 mg
Fixed-dose combination agent: Timolol + thiazide diuretic					
Timolol 10 mg + hydrochlorothiazide 24 mg	Timolide		bid		

Table 2. Commonly used antihypertensive agents (*Continued*)

Generic Name	*Trade Name (Manufacturer)*	*Daily Adult Dosage*	*Frequency of Administration*	*Duration (hours)*	*Dispensing Unit*
	DIRECT VASODILATORS				
HYDRALAZINE	Apresoline (CIBA)	20–300 mg	bid	6–12	10 mg 25 mg 50 mg 100 mg
Fixed-dose combination agents: Hydralazine + thiazide diuretic					
Hydralazine hydrochloride 25 mg + hydrochlorothiazide 25 mg	Apresazide 25/25 (CIBA)		bid		
Hydralazine hydrochloride 50 mg + hydrochlorothiazide 50 mg	Apresazide 50/50 (CIBA)		bid		
Hydralazine hydrochloride 100 mg + hydrochlorothiazide 50 mg	Apresazide 100/50 (CIBA)		bid		
Hydralazine hydrochloride 25 mg + hydrochlorothiazide 15 mg	Apresoline-Esidrix (CIBA)		bid		
MINOXIDIL	Loniten (Upjohn)	5–100 mg	qd	Up to 72	2.5 mg 10 mg
	ANGIOTENSIN-CONVERTING ENZYME INHIBITOR				
CAPTOPRIL	Capoten (Squibb)	37.5–450 mg	tid	6–8	25 mg 50 mg 100 mg

The most common complaints of patients receiving methyldopa or clonidine are drowsiness, nasal congestion, and dry mouth. The incidence of sedation is high, especially during initiation of therapy and when the dosage is increased, but tends to decrease with continued therapy. Some patients are unable to tolerate the drowsiness. Depression is associated with methyldopa therapy in roughly 5 to 10 percent of patients and may necessitate discontinuation of the drug.[28]

Aside from intolerable side effects, other indications for discontinuation of methyldopa therapy include hemolytic anemia, drug-induced fever, and drug-associated hepatitis. A dose-related positive direct antiglobulin (Coombs') test can occur in up to 20 percent of patients taking methyldopa.[29] A positive Coombs' test per se is not an indication for discontinuance but may interfere with blood typing. Rarely these Coombs'-positive patients develop hemolytic anemia that is responsive to drug withdrawal and steroids.[30] Methyldopa-induced fever of up to 104°F[31] has been reported with about a 1 percent incidence.[32] Disturbance of sexual function, including both impotence and failure of ejaculation, also has been reported with methyldopa therapy.[33] Reversible hepatotoxicity, characterized by elevated transaminase and alkaline phosphatase levels, fever, and eosinophilia, may occur in patients receiving alpha-methyldopa.

Potentially serious rebound hypertension can be encountered upon abrupt withdrawal of clonidine.[34] A clinical presentation similar to that of pheochromocytoma (anxiety, headaches, insomnia, vomiting, tachycardia, tremulousness) accompanied by exacerbated hypertension and increased urinary catecholamine excretion has been described.[34–37] Although clonidine is the most notorious offender, other antihypertensive agents, including alpha-methyldopa, guanabenz, beta-adrenergic blocking agents, guanethidine, reserpine, diuretics, saralasin, and several combination drugs, have been shown to produce this "discontinuation syndrome."[38,39] This syndrome can be treated by reintroduction of clonidine or by alpha-adrenergic blockade with an agent such as phentolamine.[40]

Guanabenz is a new centrally acting antihypertensive agent, recently made available for use in this country. Although guanabenz differs chemically from both clonidine and methyldopa in that it is a guanidine derivative, its mechanism of action is similar. It acts as a central $alpha_2$ agonist, thereby producing a decrease in peripheral sympathetic activity.[41] Guanabenz also appears to be a peripheral alpha-adrenergic antagonist, but the contribution of this effect to its antihypertensive action is unclear.[42] During chronic therapy with guanabenz, peripheral vascular resistance is decreased while cardiac output remains unchanged. Plasma renin activity is not affected.[43] Although, unlike clonidine and methyldopa, guanabenz does not cause fluid retention, its effectiveness has been shown to be enhanced by concomitant administration of thiazide diuretics.[43] Sedation, dry mouth, and lethargy are the most common side effects encountered during treatment with guanabenz. Postural hypotension is uncommon.

Beta-Adrenergic Receptor Blocking Agents

Aside from diuretics, beta receptor–blocking agents have become the most commonly used drugs for the management of hypertension. Compared with other adrenergic blocking agents, their use appears to be associated with fewer central nervous system side effects and a much lower incidence of impotence; hence they are better tolerated by most patients. In addition, their usefulness in concomitant disease, particularly ischemic heart disease, makes them the agent of choice in a large number of patients.

The beta receptor–blocking drugs lower blood pressure in hypertensive patients by mechanisms that are incompletely understood. A combination of decreased cardiac output secondary to blockade of myocardial beta-adrenergic receptors, central nervous system effects, and suppression of renin release are thought to be responsible (Fig. 2). Blockage of beta receptors has negative inotropic and chronotropic effects on the heart, resulting in a decrease in cardiac

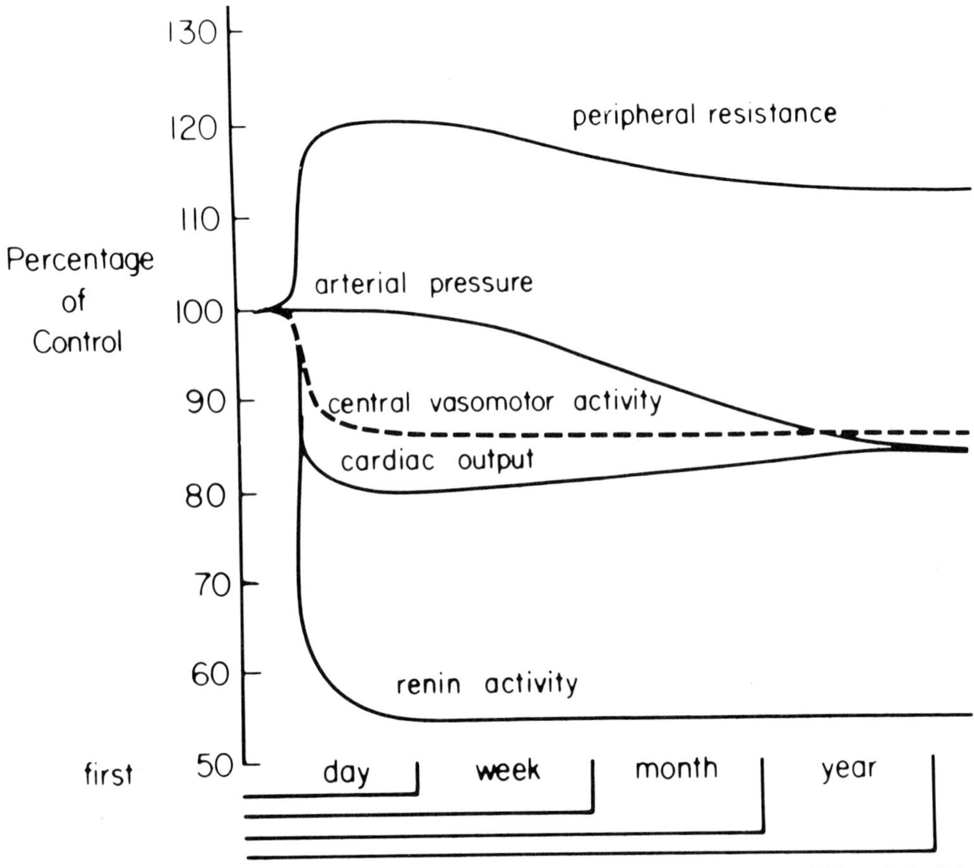

Figure 2. Schematic representation of the multiple actions of beta-blocker therapy over variable periods of time. The solid lines have been measured; the dotted line of central vasomotor activity has not been measured. (From Kaplan, NM: *Clinical Hypertension.* Williams & Wilkins, Baltimore, 1982, p 149, with permission.)

output.[44] These effects contribute to but do not fully explain the antihypertensive action of the beta blockers. It has been shown that increasing the dose of a beta-blocking agent beyond that required to reduce cardiac output has an additional antihypertensive effect in most patients. Furthermore, in some patients, a beta blocker–induced reduction in cardiac output can occur without a change in blood pressure. Beta blockers also alter peripheral vascular resistance. Following initiation of beta-blocker therapy, peripheral resistance is increased owing to unopposed alpha-mediated vasoconstriction; during chronic therapy, peripheral resistance returns to normal and may even be reduced.[45]

Most beta-blocking agents lower plasma renin activity, probably by interfering with intrarenal beta-adrenergic renin-releasing mechanisms.[46,47] Although the decrease in plasma renin activity may account for at least part of the antihypertensive effect of these drugs, most studies have failed to show a correlation between the magnitude of decrease in blood pressure and either pretreatment or post-treatment renin levels.[48] Because neither the hemodynamic nor renin-suppressing properties of the beta-blocking agents can fully explain their antihypertensive effects, it has been proposed that they also lower blood pressure via an effect on the central nervous system. There is now experimental evidence to support this hypothesis, but the mechanism remains poorly understood.[49,50]

Six beta-adrenergic receptor blocking agents are currently available for use in the United States in the management of hypertension. Although none has been shown to have superior

Table 3. Comparison of properties of beta-blocking agents

	Cardioselectivity	*ISA*	*Lipid Solubility*
Propranolol	−	−	+++
Metoprolol	+	−	±
Nadolol	−	−	−
Atenolol	+	−	−
Pindolol	−	+	±
Timolol	−	−	±

antihypertensive efficacy, these agents do have differentiating properties that may have clinical relevance. These include the degree of cardioselectivity, the presence of intrinsic sympathomimetic activity, and the degree of lipid solubility. Membrane-stabilizing activity, in contrast, appears to have no clinical significance. Tables 2 and 3 list the currently available agents and summarize their recommended dosage, duration of action, and pharmacologic properties.

Cardioselectivity refers to the property of certain beta blockers to antagonize $beta_1$ receptors (heart) to a greater extent than $beta_2$ receptors (smooth muscle). Atenolol and metoprolol are cardioselective agents. The potential advantages of using such agents over nonselective beta blockers are that cardioselective agents may have less effect on peripheral beta-adrenergic receptors with less concomitant peripheral vasoconstriction, less tendency to cause hypertensive reactions in states of catecholamine excess, a smaller risk of causing bronchospasm, and less tendency to block glucose release in response to hypoglycemia. They may thus be superior in patients with Raynaud's phenomenon, diabetes mellitus (insulin-dependent), or chronic obstructive pulmonary disease. It should be noted that cardioselectivity is dose-related, and at higher doses all agents act to block both $beta_1$ and $beta_2$ receptors.

Intrinsic sympathomimetic activity (ISA) is the property of having both beta-agonist and beta-antagonist effects. Pindolol is the only available agent with ISA. The potential advantages of agents with ISA are similar to those of cardioselective agents: less bronchospasm and less of a decrease in peripheral blood flow. In addition, agents with ISA cause less bradycardia and may be preferable in patients with low pretreatment heart rates.

The degree of lipid solubility of the beta blockers affects both their duration of action and their central nervous system effects. Agents that are less lipid soluble (and therefore more water soluble), including atenolol and nadolol, escape hepatic metabolism, are primarily excreted by the kidney and have a longer duration of action, and cross the blood-brain barrier less well and are associated with few central nervous system effects. In one study, switching patients from propranolol, the most lipid-soluble beta blocker, to atenolol resulted in a marked reduction in the incidence of central nervous system side effects.[51]

Side effects common to beta-blocking drugs include bronchospasm, congestive heart failure, cold extremities, lethargy, and central nervous system side effects (insomnia, nightmares, and depression). Impotence is rare. Although these problems may occur with any of the agents listed, as discussed previously, they may be minimized by choosing agents that are cardioselective, have ISA, or are relatively lipid insoluble.

Alpha-Adrenergic Receptor Blocking Agents

Use of the nonselective alpha-adrenergic receptor blocking agents phenoxybenzamine and phentolamine in hypertension is limited because of lack of efficacy and numerous adverse effects. Sympathetic vasoconstriction in arteries and veins is attenuated by alpha-adrenergic blocking agents; because the beta-adrenergic receptors are unaffected, baroreceptor-mediated increases in cardiac contractility and heart rate occur. Orthostatic hypotension, nasal congestion, increased gastrointestinal motility, and other effects of attenuation of noncardiac sympathetic stimuli also occur when nonselective alpha blockers are administered. Accordingly, phenoxybenzamine and phentolamine are used almost exclusively for the diagnosis and treatment of pheochromocytoma.

Prazosin

Prazosin lowers blood pressure by selectively blocking postsynaptic alpha-adrenergic receptors, thus causing relaxation of peripheral arterioles and a reduction in total peripheral resistance.[52,53] Unlike conventional alpha-adrenergic receptor blockers, prazosin does not cause tachycardia or renin release.[54–56] Prazosin does not appear to have a central action or to alter the function of adrenergic neurons. It is effective in lowering blood pressure in all grades of hypertension: in less severe cases when used alone and in more severe cases when used in combination with other agents. The combination of prazosin, a beta-adrenergic blocking agent, and a thiazide seems to be particularly effective. Recommended dosage and frequency of administration of prazosin are given in Table 2.

Dizziness and faintness, possibly associated with postural hypotension, are the most commonly reported adverse effects of prazosin. In some patients, severe postural reactions, including syncope, occur with the initial dose or first few doses of prazosin, but this effect can be minimized by beginning treatment with a low dose (0.5 mg) given at bedtime. The "first-dose" postural effects of prazosin appear to be more severe in patients who have been sodium restricted or else sodium depleted by previous diuretic treatment and/or who have been maintained on beta-adrenergic receptor blockers.[57–59]

Combined Alpha- and Beta-Adrenergic Blocking Agents

Recently, agents with combined alpha- and beta-blocking effects have been developed. Of these, labetalol (Trandate) has received the most extensive evaluation and is expected to be available soon for use in this country. Labetalol is a competitive antagonist of both beta and alpha receptors. It is more effective in blocking beta than alpha receptors at a ratio of three to one.[60] Labetalol is less effective than propranolol in blocking beta receptors and, like propranolol, is nonselective. Administration of labetalol results in decreases in peripheral vascular resistance and cardiac output. No consistent effect on plasma renin activity has been observed.[60] Fluid retention occurs during chronic treatment and, therefore labetalol is more effective when used in combination with a diuretic.

During clinical trials, labetalol has been shown to compare favorably with both methyldopa and the combination of a beta blocker and hydralazine for the treatment of mild to moderate hypertension.[61] Its most common adverse effect is postural hypotension, which is more severe shortly after initiation of treatment and with higher doses.[60] Other less frequent side effects include weakness and lethargy, gastrointestinal symptoms such as abdominal pain and nausea, and depression. Although labetalol is reported to have a lesser tendency to cause bronchoconstriction than the pure beta-blocking drugs, its use should be avoided in patients with asthma and chronic obstructive pulmonary disease. Isolated reports of positive antinuclear antibodies and antimitochondrial antibodies during labetalol therapy have appeared; however, their clinical significance remains uncertain.[62] The plasma half-life of labetalol is 7 to 8 hours, and the drug has been shown to be effective when administered on a twice-daily basis. The recommended dose range is 400 to 1600 mg per day, although doses as high as 2400 mg have been used.

Agents That Act at Postganglionic Sites

Guanethidine

Guanethidine lowers blood pressure by interfering with the function of postganglionic sympathetic neurons.[63,64] It depresses neural function by preventing the uptake of norepinephrine into storage granules in a manner similar to that of cocaine. The tricyclic antidepressants and the phenothiazines block the norepinephrine pump and therefore the uptake of guanethidine into the neuron and can cause guanethidine unresponsiveness. Likewise, indirect-acting sympathomimetic amines such as ephedrine and amphetamine can interfere with the entry of guanethidine into nerve endings and can stimulate its release. Guanethidine has a much greater antihypertensive effect in the upright position than in the supine position. Accordingly, treatment should be monitored with blood pressures taken in the sitting or standing position. Additionally, patients taking guanethidine should sleep with the head of the bed elevated to maintain the antihypertensive effect. Cardiac output and heart rate usually fall,[65–67] and glomerular filtration rate and renal plasma flow frequently decrease initially but often return to pretreatment values during prolonged therapy.

The dosage range of clinical usefulness of guanethidine is extremely large (10 to 300 mg per day) (see Table 2). Characteristically, once an effective dose is reached, an extremely steep dose-response curve is exhibited. This phenomenon can be partially explained by variability in gastrointestinal absorption of guanethidine.[68] The starting dosage for most ambulatory patients is 10 mg daily. The dosage is increased by 10 mg every 7 days until the desired effect is reached. Dosage adjustments should be made on the basis of blood pressure recordings obtained with the patient standing. A loading regimen for rapid initial administration of guanethidine has been described that involves administration of an initial dose of 80 mg followed by additional doses every 6 hours for a total of three doses per day.[69] The incremental dose is based on expected excretion rates and is adjusted according to the blood pressure response. Maintenance therapy can then be started by the third or fourth day.

Most adverse effects of guanethidine result from decreased sympathetic activity.[65,70] Orthostatic hypotension occurs in most patients, particularly in the morning. Diarrhea is a common complaint, particularly with larger doses, and can often be relieved by atropine or similar anticholinergic agents. Guanethidine often interferes with male sexual function, usually by causing ejaculatory failure (retrograde ejaculation). Impotence is less common. Guanethidine is contraindicated in patients with pheochromocytoma because it can precipitate hypertensive crisis by releasing large quantities of catecholamines from the tumor.

Reserpine

Reserpine, the most commonly used rauwolfia alkaloid, causes depletion of catecholamines from postganglionic sympathetic nerves and adrenal medulla and of catecholamines and serotonin from brain. The most common and most serious adverse effect of reserpine is drug-induced depression, which may be severe enough to cause suicide.[71–73] Depression occurs so commonly with reserpine in usual antihypertensive doses that the drug should not be used in the routine treatment of hypertension despite its low cost and convenience. Other sympatholytic agents and antihypertensive agents that work by non-neural mechanisms lower blood pressure effectively without producing such generalized effects on the sensorium.

DIRECT VASODILATORS

Vasodilators lower blood pressure by causing relaxation of smooth muscle in the vascular bed. Two types have been recognized: agents that act predominately on arteriolar smooth muscle (precapillary or resistance bed) and those that act on both arterioles and venules (postcapillary or capacitance bed).[74] Agents that act predominantly on the arterial vascular bed, including hydralazine and minoxidil, cause decreases in total peripheral resistance and arterial blood pressure with secondary activation of the carotid and aortic baroreceptors. This activation results in increased sympathetic nervous system activity with tachycardia and increased cardiac contractility and cardiac output, which oppose the reduction in blood pressure. Nitrates and sodium nitroprusside cause vasodilatation in both venous and arterial vascular beds. Accordingly, venous pooling and orthostatic hypotension occur with these agents.

Decreased venous return tends to oppose the baroreceptor-mediated increase in cardiac output. Sodium retention occurs with all nonselective vasodilators due to a relative reduction in renal blood flow and/or to activation of the renin-angiotensin-aldosterone system. Palpitations and angina pectoris may occur with all vasodilators. Headache caused by vasodilatation in the closed calvarium is another frequent adverse effect. Hirsutism is commonly observed with potent vasodilators such as minoxidil.

Hydralazine

When used in combination with sympatholytic agents and diuretics, hydralazine is a very useful drug for patients with moderate or moderately severe hypertension. However, many patients with severe hypertension do not respond to the maximum allowable dosage of hydralazine, and more effective vasodilators are needed. The hyperkinetic cardiovascular state induced by hydralazine causes patients to experience palpitations and, less commonly, causes patients with coronary disease to develop angina pectoris or myocardial infarction. The reflex tachycardia may also precipitate congestive heart failure in patients with underlying left ventricular dysfunction. Nausea and vomiting are common. Prolonged administration of hydralazine in dosages greater than 300 to 400 mg/day may lead to a collagen vascular syndrome with joint pain, fever, and signs and symptoms characteristic of systemic lupus erythematosus.[75] These effects are usually reversible when hydralazine therapy is discontinued, but a long period of time may be required for complete clearing. The adverse effects of hydralazine are more common in slow acetylators and in patients with impaired renal function.[76]

Minoxidil

Minoxidil has a mechanism of action similar to that of hydralazine but is a much more powerful vasodilator. Because vasodilatation is more intense, reflex activation of the sympathetic nervous system and sodium retention are also more pronounced.

Minoxidil is recommended for use only in patients with intractable hypertension, particularly those with renal insufficiency. The combination of minoxidil, a beta-adrenergic receptor blocker, and a diuretic has proven effective in large numbers of patients with severe and refractory essential and renal hypertension.[77–79] The clinical use of minoxidil has been limited by a number of adverse reactions that occur commonly when the drug is administered in therapeutic doses. Hirsutism severe enough to necessitate discontinuation of the drug in female patients has been reported in 80 percent of cases. This side effect usually appears within 3 to 6 weeks after starting therapy and is not associated with virilization or other endocrine abnormalities. Fluid retention usually occurs if a diuretic is not given concomitantly. Edema can generally be treated by increasing the diuretic dose. Unexplained pericardial effusion, occasionally with tamponade, has been reported in a few patients.

Diazoxide and Nitroprusside

Diazoxide and sodium nitroprusside are potent vasodilators that can be administered parenterally for treatment of hypertensive crisis. The clinical use of these agents has been reviewed elsewhere[80,81] and is beyond the scope of this chapter.

ANGIOTENSIN-CONVERTING ENZYME INHIBITORS

Because the renin-angiotensin system is required for the maintenance of some forms of hypertension, angiotensin-converting enzyme inhibitors, which inhibit the production of angiotensin II, are useful as antihypertensive drugs. These agents act as vasodilators and inhibitors of aldosterone production in patients whose peripheral vascular tone and aldosterone production are dependent on inappropriately elevated circulating angiotensin II. Converting enzyme inhibitors lower blood pressure most effectively in sodium-depleted subjects, in whom circulating renin levels are high and in whom the maintenance of vascular tone is dependent on angiotensin II. Therefore, concomitant administration of a diuretic potentiates their antihypertensive action.

The observation that the antihypertensive effect of converting enzyme inhibitors is renin dependent has been used to support the argument that the dominant mechanism by which these agents lower blood pressure in hypertensive patients is blockade of angiotensin II formation. Several other mechanisms, including increases in circulating levels of the vasodilator and natriuretic peptide bradykinin and of the vasodilator 13,14-dihydro-15-keto metabolite of prostaglandin E_2 (PGE_2-M) and diminished vascular reactivity to pressor substances, have been suggested.[82] Further study is needed to establish the relative importance of these antihypertensive effects in various patient groups.

The converting enzyme inhibitors have two distinct advantages over other vasodilator antihypertensive drugs. First, they tend to cause enhanced sodium excretion despite blood pressure reduction, probably because of a combination of renal vasodilation and reduced aldosterone production. For this reason patients tend not to develop tolerance to the chronic antihypertensive action of converting enzyme inhibitors, as they do to other vasodilators. Second, converting enzyme inhibitors do not cause reflex-mediated tachycardia in response to lowered blood pressure. This means that they are better tolerated than other peripheral vasodilators and that their use does not require concomitant administration of beta-adrenergic blockers or other sympatholytic agents for heart rate control.

Captopril

Captopril is the only commercially available orally active converting enzyme inhibitor.[83] It is a derivative of proline (2-D-methyl-3-mercaptopropanoyl-L-proline) that was specifically designed to bind to the active site of angiotensin-converting enzyme. Captopril, administered alone or in combination with a diuretic, is effective in controlling the blood pressure of patients with essential hypertension, renovascular hypertension, or hypertension associated with chronic renal failure.[84] Captopril lowers blood pressure in all hypertensive patients except those with primary aldosteronism, including those with low renin levels, but the magnitude of the reduction is correlated with baseline plasma renin activity. The recommended dosage range and dosing intervals for captopril are listed in Table 2. Captopril and its metabolites are excreted in the urine, and active drug tends to accumulate in the circulation of patients with renal insufficiency who are maintained on high dosages. Accordingly, the dosage and dosing interval of captopril should be adjusted in patients with renal insufficiency.

Despite its demonstrated efficacy and relative freedom from annoying side effects, the clinical usefulness of captopril may be limited because of a number of serious adverse effects that have been related to its free sulfhydryl group.[83] These adverse effects, which resemble those described with penicillamine, another sulfhydryl-containing drug, include proteinuria, membranous glomerulopathy, and agranulocytosis. They can be avoided by careful monitoring of the urinary protein excretion and white blood count of patients on captopril therapy and by not administering captopril to patients with proteinuria, known glomerular pathology, or leukopenia, or those who have diseases or are receiving other medications likely to suppress granulocyte production.

Reversible deterioration in renal function has been reported in patients with pre-existing renal impairment, in those with prerenal azotemia secondary to low cardiac output and severe congestive failure, and in renal allograft recipients.[85] Although renal dysfunction improves in these patients when captopril is discontinued, it is advisable to use extreme caution in administering captopril in these clinical settings. Other more common but less serious adverse effects of captopril include taste disturbances and a syndrome of skin rash, pruritus, fever, erythema, and flushing. These side effects usually occur in the first 2 months of treatment and always disappear after discontinuing or reducing the dosage of drug. Adverse effects tend to be somewhat more common in patients maintained on higher dosage of captopril, particularly those with renal insufficiency in whom blood levels of drug tend to rise because of excretory failure. Many patients with renovascular hypertension are included in that class.

In an effort to eliminate adverse effects, converting enzyme inhibitors that lack a sulfhydryl group are being synthesized. The first of these, MK-421 (N-[(S)-1-(ethoxycarbonyl)-3-phenylpropyl]-L-alanyl-L-proline, Enalpril), has been subjected to extensive clinical testing and appears to be highly effective in lowering blood pressure and remarkably free from adverse effects.[86,87] If the converting enzyme inhibitors prove to be as effective and well tolerated as they appear at present, they could replace the diuretics as first-line drugs to be used in patients with mild to moderate hypertension.

CALCIUM-CHANNEL ANTAGONISTS

The calcium-channel antagonists constitute a new class of antihypertensive agents. By blocking the entry of calcium into smooth muscle cells, these drugs cause vasodilation and hence a decrease in peripheral vascular resistance. They appear to have no effect on venous capacitance, inasmuch as cardiac output may increase and right-sided pressures remain unchanged following their administration.[88] In addition to the effects on the peripheral vasculature, the calcium-channel antagonists have a negative inotropic effect on the heart and produce coronary artery vasodilation. To date, these agents have been used primarily for treatment of angina and supraventricular arrhythmias. Of the agents currently available, nifedipine (Procardia) has been used the most for the treatment of hypertension. It has been shown to be an effective antihypertensive drug both alone and in combination with other agents.[88,89] Side effects due to nifedipine are similar to those seen with other vasodilator agents, the most prominent being flushing and headache. There is, in addition, a mild reflex increase in heart rate that lasts for approximately 1 hour after administration of the drug. If studies confirm the long-term effectiveness of this agent in the management of hypertension, its well-documented antianginal effects may make it one of the agents of choice in the treatment of patients with hypertension and concomitant ischemic heart disease.

REFERENCES

1. Rick, JH and Oparil, S: *Drug treatment of hypertension.* Comprehensive Therapy 3:34, 1977.
2. Tarazi, RC: *Diuretic drugs: Mechanisms of antihypertensive action.* In Onesti, G, Kim, KE, and Moyer, JH (eds): *Hypertension: Mechanisms and Management.* Grune & Stratton, New York, 1973, p 251.
3. Finnerty, FA, Davidov, M, Mroczek, WJ, et al: *Influence of extracellular fluid volume on response to antihypertensive drugs.* Circ Res 27:71, 1970.
4. Dustan, HP, Tarazi, RC, and Bravo, EL: *Dependence of arterial pressure on intravascular volume in treated hypertensive patients.* N Engl J Med 286:861, 1972.
5. Goldberg, M, McCurdy, DK, Foltz, EL, et al: *Effects of ethacrynic acid (a new saluretic agent) on renal diluting and concentrating mechanisms: Evidence for site of action in the loop of Henle.* J Clin Invest 43:201, 1964.
6. Stason, WB, Cannon, PJ, Heinemann, HO, et al: *Furosemide: A clinical evaluation of its diuretic action.* Circulation 34:910, 1966.
7. Anderson, J, Godfrey, BE, Hill, DM, et al: *A comparison of the effects of hydrochlorothiazide and of furosemide in the treatment of hypertensive patients.* Q J Med 40:541, 1971.
8. Healy, JJ, McKenna, TJ, Canning, B, et al: *Body composition changes in hypertensive subjects on long-term oral diuretic therapy.* Br Med J 1:716, 1970.
9. Crane, MG and Harris, JJ: *Effect of spironolactone in hypertensive patients.* Am J Med Sci 260:311, 1970.
10. Johnston, LC and Greible, HG: *Treatment of arterial hypertensive disease with diuretics. V. Spironolactone, an aldosterone antagonist.* Arch Intern Med 119:225, 1967.

11. Cannon, PJ: *Clinical use of diuretics in hypertension.* In Onesti, G, Kim, KE, and Moyer, JH (eds): *Hypertension: Mechanisms and Management.* Grune & Stratton, New York, 1973, p 261.
12. Keim, HJ, Drayer, JIM, Thurston, H, et al: *Trimterene-induced changes in aldosterone and renin values in essential hypertension. Evidence of a role for aldosterone in preventing blood pressure reduction.* Arch Intern Med 136:654, 1976.
13. Brown, JJ, Davies, DL, Lever, AF, et al: *Plasma renin in a case of Conn's syndrome with fibrinoid lesions: Use of spironolactone in treatment.* Br Med J 2:1636, 1964.
14. Ferriss, JB, Beevers, DG, Boddy, K, et al: *The treatment of low-renin ("primary") hyperaldosteronism.* Am Heart J 96:97, 1978.
15. Biglieri, EG, Stockigt, JR, and Schambelan, M: *Adrenal mineralocorticoids causing hypertension.* Am J Med 52:623, 1972.
16. Brown, JJ, Ferriss, JB, and Fraser, R: *Spironolactone in the treatment of hypertension with aldosterone excess.* In Wilson, GM (ed): *Medical Uses of Spironolactone.* Excerpta Medica, American Elsevier, New York, 1971, p 27.
17. Veterans Administration Cooperative Study Group on Antihypertensive Agents: *Double blind control study of antihypertensive agents.* Arch Intern Med 110:230, 1962.
18. Smith, WO, Kyriakopoulos, AA, and Hammarsten, JI: *Magnesium depletion induced by various diuretics.* J Okla State Med Assoc 55:248, 1962.
19. Duarte, CG: *Effects of ethacrynic acid and furosemide on urinary calcium, phosphate and magnesium.* Metabolism 17:867, 1968.
20. Kim, YW, Andrews, CE, and Ruth, WE: *Serum magnesium and cardiac arrhythmias with special reference to digitalis intoxication.* Am J Med Sci 242:87, 1961.
21. Beller, GA, Hood, WB Jr, Smith, TW, et al: *Correlation of serum magnesium levels and cardiac digitalis intoxication.* Am J Cardiol 33:225, 1974.
22. Seller, RH: *The role of magnesium in digitalis toxicity.* Am Heart J 82:551, 1971.
23. DeMartini, FE, Wheaton, EA, Healey, LA, et al: *Effect of chlorothiazide on the renal excretion of uric acid.* Am J Med 32:572, 1962.
24. Conn, JW: *Hypertension, the potassium ion and impaired carbohydrate tolerance.* N Engl J Med 273:1135, 1965.
25. Duarte, CG, Winnacker, JL, Becker, KL, et al: *Thiazide-induced hypercalcemia.* N Engl J Med 284:828, 1971.
26. Brown, JJ, Davies, DL, Lever, AF, et al: *Plasma renin concentration in human hypertension. 1. Relationship between renin, sodium and potassium.* Br Med J 2:144, 1965.
27. Oparil, S: *Therapeutic modalities and advances related to neurogenic mechanisms.* Clin Exp Hypertens A4:579, 1982.
28. Prichard, BNC, Johnston, AW, Hill, ID, et al: *Bethanidine, guanethidine and methyldopa in treatment of hypertension: A within-patient comparison.* Br Med J 1:135, 1968.
29. Carstairs, K, Worlledge, S, Dollery, CT, et al: *Methyldopa and haemolytic anaemia.* Lancet 1:201, 1966.
30. Worlledge, SM, Carstairs, KC, and Dacie, JV: *Autoimmune haemolytic anemia associated with alpha-methyldopa therapy.* Lancet 2:135, 1966.
31. Talgren, LG and Servo, C: *Hyperpyrexia in association with administration of L-alpha methyldopa.* Acta Med Scand 186:223, 1969.
32. Gillespie, L, Oates, JA, Crout, JR, et al: *Clinical and chemical studies with alpha-methyldopa in patients with hypertension.* Circulation 25:281, 1962.
33. Dollery, CT and Bulpitt, CJ: *Alpha-methyldopa in the treatment of hypertension: Long-term experience.* In Onesti, G, Kim, KE, and Moyer, JH (eds): *Hypertension: Mechanisms and Management.* Grune & Stratton, New York, 1973, p 299.
34. Hokfelt, B, Hedeland, H, and Dymling, JF: *Studies on catecholamines, renin and aldosterone following Catapresan®(2-(2,6-dichlor-phenylamine)-2-imidazoline hydrochloride) in hypertensive patients.* Eur J Pharmacol 10:389, 1970.
35. Raftos, J, Bauer, GE, Lewis, RG, et al: *Clonidine in the treatment of severe hypertension.* Med J Aust 1:786, 1973.
36. Hoobler, SW and Sagastume, E: *Clonidine hydrochloride in the treatment of hypertension.* Am J Cardiol 28:67, 1971.
37. Conolly, ME, Briant, RH, George, CF, et al: *A cross-over comparison of clonidine and methyldopa in hypertension.* In *Aspects for the Treatment of Arterial Hypertension. Round Table Discussion: Institute of Cardiovascular Research, University of Milan, November, 1973.* Boehringer-Ingelheim, Florence, 1973, p 185.

38. HOUSTON, MC: *Abrupt cessation of treatment in hypertension: Consideration of clinical features, mechanisms, prevention and management of the discontinuation syndrome.* Am Heart J 102:415, 1981.

39. GOLDBERG, AD, RAFTERY, EB, AND WILKINSON, P: *Blood pressure and heart rate and withdrawal of antihypertensive drugs.* Br Med J 1:1243, 1977.

40. HANSSON, L, HUNYOR, SN, JULIUS, S, ET AL: *Blood pressure crisis following withdrawal of clonidine (Catapres, Catapresan), with special reference to arterial and urinary catecholamine levels, and suggestions for acute management.* Am Heart J 85:605, 1973.

41. BOLME, P, CORRODI, H, AND FUXE, K: *Possible mechanism of the hypotensive action of 2,6 dichlorobenzylidene aminoguanidine: Evidence for central noradrenaline receptor stimulation.* Eur J Pharmacol 20:175, 1973.

42. BAUM, T, SHROPSHIRE, AT, ROWLES, G, ET AL: *General pharmacologic actions of the antihypertensive agent 2,6-dichlorobenzylidene aminoguanidine acetate (WY-8678).* J Pharmacol Exp Ther 171:277, 1970.

43. HOLLAND, OB, FAIRCHILD, C, AND GOMEZ-SANCHEZ, CE: *Effect of guanabenz and hydrochlorothiazide on blood pressure and plasma renin activity.* J Clin Pharmacol 21:133, 1981.

44. TARAZI, RC AND DUSTAN, HP: *Beta adrenergic blockade in hypertension: Practical and theoretical implications of long-term hemodynamic variations.* Am J Cardiol 29:633, 1972.

45. TARAZI, RC: *Antihypertensive effect of beta-blockade: Relation of its hemodynamic component to other mechanisms.* In BRAUNWALD, E (ED): *Beta-Adrenergic Blockade: A New Era in Cardiovascular Medicine: International Congress Series #446.* Excerpta Medica-Elsevier, Amsterdam, 1978, p 210.

46. MICHELAKIS, AM AND MCALLISTER, RG: *The effect of chronic adrenergic receptor blockade on plasma renin activity in man.* J Clin Endrcrinol Metab 34:386, 1972.

47. BRAVO, EL, TARAZI, RC, AND DUSTAN, HP: *On the mechanism of suppressed plasma-renin activity during beta-adrenergic blockade with propranolol.* J Lab Clin Med 83:119, 1974.

48. KAPLAN, NM: *Beta-blockade in the treatment of mild to moderate hypertension.* In BRAUNWALD, E (ED): *Beta-Adrenergic Blockade: A New Era in Cardiovascular Medicine: International Congress Series #446.* Excerpta Medica-Elsevier, Amsterdam, 1978, p 253.

49. TACKETT, RL, WEBB, JG, AND PRIVITERA, PJ: *Cerebroventricular propranolol elevates cerebrospinal fluid norepinephrine and lowers blood pressure.* Science 213:911, 1981.

50. SVENSSON, TH, ALMGREN, O, DAHLOF, C, ET AL: *Alpha- and beta-adrenoreceptor-mediated control of brain noradrenaline neurons and antihypertensive therapy.* Clin Sci 59:479s, 1980.

51. HENNINGSEN, NC AND MATTIASSON, I: *Long-term clinical experience with atenolol—A new selective β-1-blocker with few side-effects from the central nervous system.* Acta Med Scand 205:61, 1979.

52. BROGDEN, RN, HEEL, RC, SPEIGHT, TM, ET AL: *Prazosin: A review of its pharmacological properties and therapeutic efficacy in hypertension.* Drugs 14:163, 1977.

53. MASSINGHAM, R AND HAYDEN, ML: *A comparison of the effects of prazosin and hydralazine on blood pressure, heart rate and plasma renin activity in conscious renal hypertensive dogs.* Eur J Pharmacol 30:121, 1975.

54. CONSTANTINE, JW: *Analysis of the hypotensive action of prazosin.* In *Prazosin—Evaluation of a New Antihypertensive Agent.* International Congress Series 331, 1974, p 16.

55. CAMBRIDGE, D, DAVEY, MJ, AND MASSINGHAM, R: *Prazosin: A selective antagonist of post-synaptic α-adrenoceptors.* Br J Pharmacol 59:514P, 1977.

56. CAMBRIDGE, D, DAVEY, MJ, AND MASSINGHAM, R: *The pharmacology of antihypertensive drugs with special reference to vasodilators, α-adrenergic blocking agents and prazosin.* Med J Aust 2:2, 1977.

57. GRAHAM, RM, THORNELL, IR, GAIN, JM, ET AL: *Prazosin: The first-dose phenomenon.* Br Med J 2:1293, 1976.

58. GRAHAM, RM AND PETTINGER, WA: *Drug therapy: Prazosin.* N Engl J Med 300:232, 1979.

59. STOKES, GS, GRAHAM, RM, GAIN, JM, ET AL: *Influence of dosage and dietary sodium on the first-dose effects of prazosin.* Br Med J 1:1507, 1977.

60. BROGDEN, RN, HEEL, RC, SPEIGHT, TM, ET AL: *Labetalol: A review of its pharmacology and therapeutic use in hypertension.* Drugs 15:251, 1978.

61. BARNETT, AJ, KALOWSKI, S, AND GUEST, C: *Labetalol compared with pindolol plus hydralazine in the treatment of hypertension: A double-blind cross-over study.* Med J Aust 1:105, 1978.

62. WILSON, JD, BOOTH, RJ, BULLOCK, JY, ET AL: *Anti-mitochondrial antibodies associated with labetalol.* Lancet 2:312, 1980.

63. GOLDBERG, LI AND ZIMMERMAN, AM: *Guanethidine and methyldopa as therapeutic agents in hypertension.* Postgrad Med 33:548, 1963.

64. BOURA, ALA AND GREEN, AF: *Adrenergic neuron-blocking agents.* Annu Rev Pharmacol 5:183, 1965.

65. FROHLICH, ED: *Inhibition of adrenergic function in the treatment of hypertension.* Arch Intern Med 133:1033, 1974.

66. DOLLERY, CT, EMSLIE-SMITH, D, AND MILNE, MD: *Clinical and pharmacological studies with guanethidine in the treatment of hypertension.* Lancet 2:381, 1960.

67. Richardson, DW, Wyso, EM, Magee, JH, et al: *Circulatory effects of guanethidine. Clinical, renal and cardiac responses to treatment with novel antihypertensive drug.* Circulation 22:184, 1960.

68. McMartin, C and Simpson, P: *The absorption and metabolism of guanethidine in hypertensive patients requiring different dosages of the drug.* Clin Pharmacol Ther 12:73, 1971.

69. Shand, DG, Nies, AS, McAllister, RG, et al: *A loading-maintenance regimen for more rapid initiation of the effect of guanethidine.* Clin Pharmacol Ther 18:139, 1975.

70. Nies, AS: *Adverse reactions and interactions limiting the use of antihypertensive drugs.* Am J Med 58:495, 1975.

71. Page, LB and Sidd, JJ: *Medical management of primary hypertension.* N Engl J Med 287:960, 1018, 1074, 1972.

72. Qeutsch, RM, Achor, RWP, Litin, EM, et al: *Depressive reactions in hypertensive patients: A comparison of those treated with rauwolfia and those receiving no specific antihypertensive treatment.* Circulation 19:366, 1959.

73. Freis, ED: *Mental depression in hypertensive patients treated for long periods with large doses of reserpine.* N Engl J Med 251:1006, 1954.

74. Chidsey, CA III and Gottlieb, TB: *The pharmacologic basis of antihypertensive therapy: The role of vasodilator drugs.* Prog Cardiovasc Dis 17:99, 1974.

75. Perry, HM: *Late toxicity to hydralazine resembling systemic lupus erythematosus or rheumatoid arthritis.* Am J Med 54:58, 1973.

76. Zacest, R and Koch-Weser, J: *Relation of hydralazine plasma concentration to dosage and hypotensive action.* Clin Pharmacol Ther 13:420, 1972.

77. Wilburn, RL, Blaufuss, A, and Bennett, CM: *Long-term treatment of severe hypertension with minoxidil, propranolol and furosemide.* Circulation 52:706, 1975.

78. Martin, WB, Zins, GR, and Freyburger, WA: *The use of minoxidil, an experimental arteriolar dilator, in 510 patients with refractory hypertension.* Clin Sci Mol Med 48(2):189S, 1975.

79. Dormois, JC, Young, JL, and Nies, AS: *Minoxidil in severe hypertension: Value when conventional drugs have failed.* Am Heart J 90:360, 1975.

80. Koch-Weser, J: *Diazoxide.* N Engl J Med 294:1271, 1976.

81. Palmer, RF and Lasseter, KC: *Sodium nitroprusside.* N Engl J Med 292:294, 1975.

82. Oparil, S: *Angiotensin I converting enzyme inhibitors and analogs of angiotensin II.* In Genest, J, Kuchel, O, Hamet, P, et al (eds): *Hypertension: Physiopathology and Treatment.* McGraw-Hill, New York, in press.

83. Heel, RC, Brogden, RN, Speight, TM, et al: *Captopril: A preliminary review of its pharmacological properties and therapeutic efficacy.* Drugs 20:409, 1980.

84. Brunner, HR, Gavras, H, Waeber, B, et al: *Oral angiotensin-converting enzyme inhibitor in long-term treatment of hypertensive patients.* Ann Intern Med 90:19, 1979.

85. Curtis, JJ, Luke, RG, Whelchel, JD, et al: *Angiotensin converting enzyme inhibition in renal transplant patients with hypertension.* N Engl J Med 308:377, 1983.

86. Patchett, AA, Harris, E, Tristram, EW, et al: *A new class of angiotensin-converting enzyme inhibitors.* Nature 288:280, 1980.

87. Gavras, H, Waeber, B, Gavras, I, et al: *Antihypertensive effect of the new oral angiotensin converting enzyme inhibitor "MK-421."* Lancet 2:543, 1981.

88. Olivari, MT, Bartorelli, C, Polese, A, et al: *Treatment of hypertension with nifedipine, a calcium antagonistic agent.* Circulation 59:1056, 1979.

89. Guazzi, MD, Fiorentini, C, Olivari, MT, et al: *Short- and long-term efficacy of a calcium-antagonistic agent (nifedipine) combined with methyldopa in the treatment of severe hypertension.* Circulation 61:913, 1980.

Clinical Pharmacology of Calcium Antagonists

Philip D. Henry, M.D., and Julio E. Pérez, M.D.

Three calcium antagonists—verapamil, nifedipine, and diltiazem—have recently become available for clinical use in the United States. Although these drugs were introduced in Europe and Japan 10 to 20 years ago, their importance in cardiovascular therapeutics has been recognized only recently. Initially, the calcium antagonists were used in low doses, giving the impression that the drugs were only moderately effective for the treatment of angina pectoris[1] and arterial hypertension.[2] In vitro studies had emphasized the myocardial depressant effects of the drugs,[3] and higher doses were not recommended perhaps because of the fear of precipitating heart failure or producing other untoward effects. Furthermore, in the 1960s, clinical investigators studied primarily the newly introduced beta-adrenergic blockers, and other antianginal drugs were not evaluated in detail.

In recent years, several circumstances have contributed to the renewed interest in calcium antagonists. First, in the 1970s, the treatment of heart failure with agents reducing left ventricular afterload refocused attention on vasodilators in general. Second, coronary artery spasm, a pathogenic mechanism of myocardial ischemia that attracted considerable attention, was reported to be effectively relieved by calcium antagonists.[4] Third, the introduction of a new class of calcium antagonists, the dihydropyridines, stimulated a reappraisal of other calcium antagonists and vasodilators.

In this review, we will briefly discuss the clinical pharmacology of verapamil, nifedipine, and diltiazem—the agents that have received the most clinical attention recently.

GENERAL PHARMACOLOGY

Chemical Structure

Verapamil, nifedipine, and diltiazem are structurally unrelated compounds.[5] Verapamil (M.W.455) is sometimes described as a papaverine derivative, although the similarities of the two compounds are not striking. Nifedipine (M.W.343) is a 1,4-dihydropyridine derivative that is unrelated to drugs used previously in cardiovascular therapeutics. A great number of other dihydropyridine derivatives with calcium antagonistic activity have been synthesized, and some of these compounds have been already evaluated clinically. Diltiazem (M.W.450) is a 1,5-benzothiazepine that is closely related to the neuroleptic agent thiazesim.[6] Verapamil, nifedipine, and diltiazem all possess asymmetric (chiral) centers, and the enantiomers of the drugs exert stereoselective pharmacologic effects on cardiac and smooth muscle.[7] Verapamil and diltiazem have pK_a values of 8.73 and 8.06, respectively, and exist therefore as cations at physiologic pH values.[8] In contrast, dihydropyridines, including nifedipine, are uncharged at physiologic pH values, indicating that a positive charge is not essential for drugs to act as calcium antagonists. Although verapamil, nifedipine, and diltiazem are lipophilic compounds, calcium antagonists need not be highly lipophilic. On the contrary, comparison of various dihydropyridine calcium antagonists reveals that hydrophilic derivatives are as potent as or more potent than the highly lipophilic compounds.[7,8]

Mechanism of Action

It is widely held that verapamil, nifedipine, and diltiazem act by blocking membrane pores that permit the inward flux of calcium.[5,7] Voltage-clamp experiments with isolated myocardium have revealed that the three drugs inhibit the slow inward current that is carried predominantly by calcium ions (Table 1). However, the three drugs produce otherwise dissimilar electrophysiologic effects. In particular, verapamil, but not dihydropyridines, appears to block the delayed potassium outward current (delayed rectifier), and high concentrations of this drug inhibit, in addition, the fast sodium current (local anesthetic effect).[5,7,9] The action of verapamil and diltiazem strongly depends upon cardiac frequency, a phenomenon referred to a frequency- or use-dependence. The action of the drugs increases with the number and duration of membrane depolarizations per unit time. This may reflect, in part, voltage-dependent conformational changes of the drug receptors, membrane depolarization, and hyperpolarization favoring conformations with high and low affinity, respectively.[7]

Recent radioligand experiments have demonstrated that the enantiomers of verapamil and diltiazem influence the binding of dihydropyridines to sarcolemmal fractions from cardiac and smooth muscle.[10,11] The (−) isomer of verapamil produces a biphasic and incomplete displacement of dihydropyridines, whereas the (+) isomer is less active. In contrast, d-cis-diltiazem, but not l-cis-diltiazem, stimulates the binding of dihydropyridines. These interactions have been interpreted as allosteric effects and have been proposed to represent binding of the drugs to different sites of the putative calcium channel.[10] However, verapamil and diltiazem appear to displace multiple agents not currently thought to represent calcium antagonists, raising the question of whether the observed displacements are attributable to nonspecific effects such as changes in lipid-protein interactions.[7]

Pharmacokinetics

The pharmacokinetic properties of verapamil, nifedipine, and diltiazem are summarized in Table 2. The bioavailability of the three compounds is relatively low, mainly because of extensive first-pass extraction in liver. The drugs are extensively metabolized, but most metabolites are inactive. However, some derivatives of verapamil, such as norverapamil, retain some activity. Nifedipine has the shortest half-life of the three drugs, whereas the longer half-lives of verapamil and its derivative may result in drug cumulation during chronic oral therapy.[12]

Table 1. Electrophysiologic effects of Ca antagonists on isolated myocardium[5,7,9,58]

	Dihydropyridine	*Verapamil*	*Diltiazem*
Blockade of slow inward Ca current	+	+	+
Blockade of transient outward K current (Ca activated current)	+	+	+
Blockade of delayed outward K current (delayed rectifier)	−	+	(−?)
Blockade of fast inward Na current (local anesthetic effect)	−	+	+
Frequency and voltage dependence	−	+	+
Blockade of quiescent (oxygenated) myocardium	+	−	?

Table 2. Pharmacokinetics of Ca antagonists[5,12]

	Nifedipine	*Verapamil*	*Diltiazem*
Dose			
Oral	10–40 mg/8 hr	80–160 mg/8 hr	30–120 mg/8 hr
I.V.	5–15 μg/kg	100–200 μg/kg	75–150 μg/kg
Therapeutic plasma concentrations (protein binding, %)	10–75 ng/ml (95%)	50–250 ng/ml (90%)	100–200 ng/ml (80%)
Half-life (T½)	3–5 hr	5-10 hr	4-6 hr
First-pass extraction by liver after oral application	40–60%	75–85%	70–80%
Bioavailability	~50%	~20%	~25%
Hepatic excretion	20	15	60
Renal excretion	80	85	40

Verapamil and diltiazem in therapeutic doses exert direct cardiac effects that consist predominantly of inhibitory actions on the sinus and AV nodes. In contrast, dihydropyridines administered systemically produce negligible direct effects on the heart. It has been suggested that reflex sympathetic discharge counteracts the inhibitory effects of these drugs.[5] However, administration of nifedipine in combination with beta blockers has been generally well tolerated, raising some doubts about the importance of the negative inotropic effects of nifedipine.

Side Effects, Toxicity, and Drug Interactions

Intravenous administration of verapamil is usually well tolerated, and episodes of severe myocardial depression or arterial hypotension have been only rarely observed.[12] Episodes of sinus bradycardia and AV nodal block have been successfully treated with intravenous atropine and isoproterenol, although in some instances transvenous ventricular pacing has been required.[12] Patients with sick sinus syndrome have been reported to be sensitive to intravenous verapamil, and the drug should be used with caution in these patients.[12,13] Liver disease may reduce the hepatic disposal of verapamil and promote the cumulation of active drug.[14] Verapamil appears to be well tolerated by patients with chronic obstructive lung disease and may be useful for the treatment of supraventricular tachyarrhythmias occurring in these patients. Intravenous verapamil administered to patients receiving beta-adrenergic blocking agents may precipitate high-degree AV block.[12] On the other hand, recent studies have demonstrated that the combined administration of oral verapamil and beta blockers in patients with angina is well tolerated.[15,16] Verapamil has been shown to depress the renal clearance of digoxin by as much as 50 percent, an effect associated with dose-dependent increases in plasma digoxin levels.[17] This finding will require further confirmation and evaluation.[18]

Although nifedipine is effective in reducing arterial pressure in hypertensive patients, serious hypotensive episodes seem to occur infrequently.[19] Nifedipine produces nitroglycerin-like side effects including headaches, flushing, dizziness, and pedal edema.[19] The drug has been reported to aggravate angina in some patients, an effect possibly reflecting arterial hypotension and reflex sympathetic discharge.[20] Since nifedipine exerts little direct cardiac depressant effect, it may be safely combined with adrenergic blockers. Nifedipine does not appear to interact with major drugs used in cardiovascular therapeutics, and claimed interactions with digoxin have not been confirmed.[21,22]

Diltiazem is generally well tolerated, although sinus or AV nodal depressions, as encountered with verapamil, have been occasionally observed.[23]

Major side effects of verapamil, nifedipine, and diltiazem are usually attributable to their hypotensive action or depressant effects on the cardiac conducting system. Serious side effects such as allergic reactions, disturbances of the immune system, and blood dyscrasia seem to

Table 3. Vasodilator therapy with Ca antagonists[5,7,58]

	Dihydropyridine	*Verapamil*	*Diltiazem*
Angina			
Rest angina (unstable angina)	+	+	+
Effort angina	+	+	+
Vasospastic angina (Prinzmetal)	+	+	+
Arterial hypertension	+	+	+
Pulmonary hypertension	+		
Congestive heart failure	+		+
Intermittent cerebral ischemia	+		
Vascular headache (migraine)	+		
Cerebral vasospasm	+		
Intermittent claudication	+		
Raynaud's phenomenon	+		
Intestinal ischemia		+	

be extremely rare.[12] Although the agents may potentially inhibit stimulus-secretion coupling of endocrine systems, clinically manifest neuroendocrine disturbances have thus far not been reported. Although calcium antagonists may inhibit insulin secretion in in vitro systems, use of these drugs for many years has failed to reveal a definite diabetogenic action.[22]

THERAPEUTIC USES

Until recently, calcium antagonists have been used primarily as vaso-relaxing agents for the treatment of angiospastic and hypertensive syndromes (Table 3). However, there is increasing evidence that the smooth-muscle relaxing effects of calcium antagonists may have utility in the treatment of spasms involving the respiratory (asthma), gastrointestinal, and

Table 4. Ca antagonists as cell protectants[5,7,58,122–127]

Myocardium
Hypoxia
Ischemia
*Cardiopulmonary bypass
Catecholamine induced cardiac necrosis
*Cardiomyopathy (Syrian hamster; obstructive cardiomyopathy)
Adriamycin cardiomyopathy
Skeletal muscle
*Myopathy (Syrian hamster; clinical myopathies?)
Malignant hyperthermia
Vessels
Vitimin D–induced vascular injury
Hypertensive vascular injury
Experimental atherosclerosis
Kidney
Renal ischemia
Liver
Endotoxic shock
Brain
*Cerebral ischemia
Eyes
Cataract (alloxan-diabetic rat)

*Clinical data available.

genitourinary tracts. In addition, there is some evidence that calcium antagonists may exert protective effects on muscle and non-muscle cells in a variety of syndromes associated with membrane injury and accumulation of intracellular calcium (Table 4).

Effort Angina

Several studies have demonstrated that verapamil in doses of 360 to 480 mg/day is superior to placebo and at least as efficacious as high-dosage beta blockers in patients suffering from stable effort angina. Livesley and coworkers[24] found verapamil (360 mg/day) to be as effective as propranolol (300 mg/day) in a double-blind trial involving 32 patients with exercise-induced angina. More recently, several double-blind, cross-over studies on the effects of verapamil in patients with stable angina have confirmed the antianginal efficacy of verapamil.[25–30] In comparative studies, verapamil was as effective as propranolol or nifedipine in improving exercise tolerance and reducing nitroglycerin consumption.[26,31–34] In one recent double-blind, randomized, cross-over trial, verapamil, 480 mg/day, was more effective than propranolol, 320 mg/day, in reducing the frequency of anginal attacks and the amount of nitroglycerin consumed.[35] Two recent reports suggest that verapamil (up to 480 mg/day) in combination with propranolol (up to 320 mg/day) is efficacious and safe in relieving effort angina.[15,16] The results of these studies appear to contradict earlier reports suggesting that combined therapy with verapamil and beta blockers is hazardous and apt to precipitate bradyarrhythmias and/or heart failure.

Nifedipine has been found to be effective for the treatment of stable exertional angina.[36–39] In comparison with placebo, nifedipine, 60 mg/day, reduced anginal frequency and nitroglycerin consumption, and increased treadmill exercise duration.[36–39] In some studies, nifedipine was found to be comparable or superior in efficacy to therapy with long-acting nitrates or beta blockers such as pindolol[40] or propranolol.[41] In recent years, therapy with nifedipine in combination with beta blockers has been extensively evaluated.[42–44] Current evidence suggests that nifedipine, 30 to 60 mg/day, and propranolol, 240 to 480 mg/day, are more effective than either agent alone in patients with stable angina.[36,45] Nifedipine combined with beta blockers compared with beta blockers alone does not appear to increase the frequency of heart block or heart failure.[45]

Several double-blind, randomized studies have shown that diltiazem is an effective antianginal agent for patients with stable angina.[46–51] Hossack and Bruce[46] demonstrated that diltiazem, 140 to 180 mg/day, produced significant increases in exercise duration, time to onset of angina, and time to development of 1-mm ST segment depression in patients with effort angina subjected to exercise testing. Therapy with combined diltiazem and beta blockers has not been extensively evaluated but should be at least as safe as the combination of beta blockers with verapamil.

The antianginal mechansims of action of calcium antagonists have not been completely elucidated. Claims that the antianginal effects of a drug have been clarified, without having characterized effects on myocardial blood flow and its transmural distribution, cannot be accepted without reservation. Like nitroglycerin, nifedipine may act predominantly by reducing myocardial energy expenditure.[52] However, compared with nitrates, nifedipine may have a greater effect on left ventricular afterload (reduced end-systolic volume and aortic pressure) than on preload (reduced end-diastolic volume or reduced "venous return").[53] Estimations of transmural flow by the xenon method suggest that nifedipine, but not nitroglycerin, increases flow to ischemic zones supplied by a stenosed artery.[54] Calcium antagonists may reduce ischemic diastolic myocardial stiffness, thereby facilitating diastolic myocardial perfusion and left ventricular filling.[55,57] In addition to influencing diastolic function, verapamil (but not nifedipine) may act by reducing cardiac contractility (effect on systolic function). Diltiazem and verapamil (but not nifedipine) may further reduce myocardial energy expenditure by slowing heart rate at rest and during exercise.[58]

Rest or Unstable Angina

Rest or unstable angina is difficult to differentiate from other nonexertional ischemic syndromes, including angiospastic angina and minor subendocardial myocardial infarctions. Furthermore, because of its erratic nature, randomized, double-blind, cross-over studies of this disorder are difficult to conduct. Also, one may be reluctant to omit conventional antianginal regimens for the purpose of evaluating new drugs in patients threatened by episodes of severe myocardial ischemia. Parodi and collaborators[59] have noted that verapamil, 480 mg/day, reduced episodes of chest pain at rest by 79 percent. Mehta and Conti[60] demonstrated that verapamil, 320 to 480 mg/day, decreased the frequency of angina at rest compared with placebo. A large prospective, randomized, double-blind, placebo-controlled trial showed that failure of medical treatment (sudden death, myocardial infarction, or coronary artery bypass surgery within 4 months of initiation of therapy) occurred in 43 of 70 patients receiving placebo, but in only 30 of 68 patients receiving nifedipine, 70 to 80 mg/day, added to therapy with nitrates and propranolol.[61] In other studies, nifedipine was found to be effective in treating unstable angina refractory to nitrates and propranolol.[62,63] In a population of patients with crescendo chest pain at rest, Hugenholtz and associates[64] reported that nifedipine, 60 mg, produced relief in 27 out of 31 patients within 90 minutes. Uncontrolled studies indicate that diltiazem is effective in suppressing ST–T changes occurring during rest angina.[65,66] Therefore, the limited information available appears to support the view that calcium antagonists are effective in treating rest or unstable angina.[67] However, treatment of unstable angina with the different calcium antagonists will require further evaluation.

Variant or Angiospastic Angina

Modern coronary arteriography has confirmed Osler's[68] hypothesis that episodes of angina may result from coronary spasm. However, there is a striking variability in the incidence of documented coronary artery spasm in different centers. Although the high incidence of coronary artery spasm in Japan compared with the United States may reflect true epidemiologic differences, the apparent high incidence of the disease in some North American centers may be the result of patient selection, angiographic techniques, or diagnostic criteria. As pointed out by MacAlpin,[69] coronary spasm may represent a normal constrictor response superimposed on an organic stenosis. Therefore, the occurrence of ischemic symptoms in association with a vasodilator-sensitive coronary narrowing on the arteriogram does not necessarily imply abnormal vasomotion. An uncontrolled study from 11 institutions in Japan involving 243 patients has shown that nifedipine (30 to 60 mg/day), diltiazem (90 to 240 mg/day), and verapamil (120 to 320 mg/day) were effective in reducing or abolishing variant angina in 94, 91, and 86 percent of the patients, respectively.[70] In contrast, beta blockers alone produced relief in only 11 percent of the patients. In a similar open trial involving multiple American centers, nifedipine produced symptomatic relief in 63 percent of the cases.[71] Nifedipine, diltiazem, and verapamil are effective in suppressing ergonovine-induced attacks of chest pain in patients thought to suffer from angiospastic angina.[58,72]

Current evidence supports the initial Japanese observations that calcium antagonists are effective in the treatment of variant angina.[4] However, it remains unclear whether these agents are superior to nitrates or whether some patients might benefit from combinations of two or three calcium antagonists with or without nitrates. Furthermore, the suggestion that beta blockers may aggravate angiospastic angina by abolishing beta-adrenergic vasodilator tone will require further critical scrutiny.

In summary, current information regarding the treatment of anginal syndromes suggests that patients not responding to beta blockers or calcium antagonists alone merit consideration for combined therapy. Nifedipine appears to be less likely to produce electrophysiologic side effects when combined with beta blockers, compared with verapamil or diltiazem.[45]

Effects on Platelets

Recently, the possibility has been considered that platelets play an important role in the pathophysiology of myocardial ischemia, including variant angina.[73–75] Although it has been demonstrated that platelet-derived constrictor substances such as thromboxane are released across the coronary bed during episodes of myocardial ischemia, it has been difficult to establish whether platelet effects are a cause or consequence of myocardial ischemia. Nevertheless, it appears likely that release of thromboxane or serotonin may aggravate or prolong episodes of myocardial underperfusion.[75] Studies in vitro and in vivo suggest that calcium antagonists may exert antiaggregating effects. However, concentrations of verapamil and diltiazem required to inhibit ADP- or epinephrine-induced aggregation are somewhat high ($>10^{-6}$M). Furthermore, there is some question whether the antiaggregating activity reflects a calcium antagonistic effect or an effect on platelet alpha receptors.[7] It has been demonstrated that verapamil and diltiazem may competitively displace yohimbine, a blocking agent with selectivity for alpha platelet receptors. On the other hand, studies demonstrating effects of calcium antagonists on platelets in vivo have unfortunately not included control experiments with noncalcium antagonistic vasodilators. As already mentioned, ischemia as such may produce platelet changes, and correction of ischemia with vasodilators may reduce these changes indirectly via a hemodynamic mechanism.

Arterial Hypertension

Although dihydropyridines were initially thought to be promising antihypertensive agents, calcium antagonists have thus far not been widely used for the treatment of arterial hypertension.[76] The pathophysiologic mechanisms of essential hypertension remain unclear, and the question of whether essential hypertension and other hypertensive syndromes are associated with primary alterations of arterial smooth muscle has been the subject of considerable controversy. It has been suggested that arteries from spontaneously hypertensive rats and from humans with arterial hypertension are excessively sensitive to the constrictor effects of calcium, suggesting that an abnormality of the uptake or extrusion of calcium by smooth muscle may contribute to an excessive constrictor tone.[77,78] If, as has been proposed, calcium leakage across smooth-muscle membranes plays a pathogenic role in hypertension, calcium antagonists might exert a specific antihypertensive effect.[79] However, early clinical trials using calcium antagonists as antihypertensive agents were inconclusive, in part because of inappropriate pharmacologic protocols.[2] Recent trials have demonstrated that calcium antagonists, including verapamil, nifedipine, and diltiazem, are capable of reducing blood pressure in essential hypertension with relatively modest side effects.

In patients with mild essential hypertension, verapamil, 480 mg/day, produced significant decreases in blood pressure without evoking tachycardia, fluid retention, or changes in the plasma concentrations of renin, aldosterone, and catecholamines.[80] In a randomized, double-blind, cross-over trial involving 17 hypertensive patients, verapamil, 360 mg/day, was as effective as pindolol, 15 mg/day, in reducing arterial pressure.[81] In 75 patients given verapamil, 240 to 480 mg/day, tolerance did not develop, and the drug remained effective throughout the 1-year period of observation.[82] In addition, there was no change in serum lipids, including high-density lipoprotein.[82] Study of the diurnal profile of blood pressure in patients receiving verapamil has revealed a consistent reduction of blood pressure throughout the 24-hour cycle, hypotensive effects being most marked during the day.[83] There was no evidence of postural hypotension, and the absolute hypertensive responses to dynamic and isometric exercise were reduced.

Aoki and Guazzi and their coworkers[84–86] were among the first to point out that nifedipine was an effective antihypertensive agent, confirming the early experimental observations by Loev and associates.[76] The efficacy of nifedipine and other dihydropyridines for the treatment of hypertensive emergencies and essential hypertension has been documented in numerous studies.[87–89] As with verapamil, long-term treatment does not appear to be complicated by tolerance or changes in circulating lipids.[87] Unlike verapamil, antihypertensive effects of nifedipine tend to be accompanied by increases in plasma renin activity. The increased plasma renin activity is reduced by combining nifedipine with a beta blocker such as metoprololol.[90] Current evidence suggests that antihypertensive therapy with combined nifedipine and beta blockers is a safe and effective drug regimen. Intravenous nifedipine has been used successfully for the treatment of hypertensive emergencies.[88]

Although diltiazem may reduce arterial pressure in patients with essential hypertension, information on long-term treatment with this drug is still limited.[92]

There is currently a concern about the use of diuretics as first-line antihypertensive agents, inasmuch as the results of various trials have questioned the safety of these drugs in mild hypertension.[93] Diuretic-induced hypokalemia has been reported in 10 to 30 percent of patients on long-term treatment.[94] Recent studies indicate that the hypokalemia may be responsible for an increased mortality probably related to arrhythmias.[93–95] In addition, diuretics may produce glucose intolerance and evoke increases in plasma cholesterol.[93] Similarly, beta blockers may increase long-term atherogenic risks because of their adverse effects on lipids and glucose metabolism.[93] In addition, beta blockers may be contraindicated in patients with chronic lung disease. In view of these considerations, calcium antagonists—agents that appear to produce no changes in serum lipids and may act as mild bronchodilators—appear to have potential advantages over previously used pharmacologic regimens. Although beta blockers may be effective for the treatment of hypertension in young patients with high renin activity, it has been suggested that in older patients with low-renin hypertension calcium antagonists are safer and more effective than beta blockers.[96]

Pulmonary Hypertension

The treatment of pulmonary hypertension remains a major problem in cardiovascular therapeutics. Recently, a number of experimental and clinical studies have suggested that calcium antagonists might be useful in reducing pulmonary vascular resistance and alleviating pulmonary hypertension. Verapamil has been shown to suppress the pulmonary pressor response to acute hypoxia in isolated rat lungs,[97] awake calves,[98] and anesthetized dogs.[99] Nifedipine has been reported to reduce hypoxic pulmonary constriction in isolated pig lungs.[100] In open-chest dogs, nifedipine was more effective than verapamil or diltiazem in reducing hypoxic pulmonary constriction.[99] In a study of 12 patients with pulmonary hypertension, injection of verapamil into the pulmonary artery reduced pulmonary vascular resistance in only 3 out of 12 patients.[101] Other preliminary clinical observations were somewhat more encouraging.[102] However, as with other vasodilators, calcium antagonists appear to lack a selectivity for the pulmonary versus the systemic vascular bed.

Idiopathic Hypertrophic Subaortic Stenosis

Calcium antagonists may reduce the dynamic left ventricular obstruction and provide symptomatic relief in patients suffering from idiopathic hypertrophic subaortic stenosis (IHSS). Intravenous verapamil (0.007 to 0.021 mg/kg/min) has been found to reduce the basal left ventricular outflow tract gradient from 94 down to 49 mm Hg (mean values) in a series of 27 patients.[103] During chronic oral therapy with verapamil (320 to 480 mg/day), a majority of patients appeared to be clinically improved.[104] Other calcium antagonists, including diltiazem[105] and nifedipine,[56] have been observed to exert beneficial effects on IHSS. Although nifedipine may be less effective than verapamil for the treatment of IHSS, it may be useful in combination with beta blockers.[106]

Heart Failure

Reduction of left ventricular ejection impedance with various vasodilators has been shown to be an effective approach to the management of patients with acute and chronic heart failure.[107] Peripheral vasodilation decreases active left ventricular wall stress by reducing ventricular pressure and volume during systole. Important cardiomechanical effects include an improved ejection fraction, an increased cardiac output, and a decreased left ventricular end-diastolic pressure.[108] The last effect decreases pulmonary venous pressure and congestion.[107,108] It has been suggested that vasodilators may possess varying selectivities for the arterial and venous beds. For instance, among the oral agents used to treat cardiac failure, hydralazine and nitrates would act predominantly as arterial and venous dilators, respectively, whereas prazosin would have a balanced arterial/venous effect.[107]

Although calcium antagonists have been used for the treatment of heart failure,[109,114] their advantages or disadvantages compared with other vasodilators remain to be delineated. It is possible that calcium antagonists may be particularly effective in alleviating heart failure associated with decreased diastolic compliance related to myocardial ischemia.[55,57] Because of their relatively potent hypotensive effects, nifedipine and other dihydropyridines might be of particular value in hypertensive heart failure. In patients in whom tachycardia is a major problem, calcium antagonists that reduce ventricular rate (diltiazem, lidoflazine, verapamil) may be more desirable than dihydropyridines or nitrates.[58] However, because of its cardiac depressant effects, verapamil is contraindicated in patients with severe left ventricular disease or disease of the sinus and AV nodes (bradycardia-tachycardia syndrome, atrial fibrillation with slow ventricular response).[12,13] Calcium antagonists have been shown recently to depress certain cardiovascular reflexes, including baroreflex cardiac slowing. Whether these effects are of any importance in the treatment of patients with heart failure and/or hypertension is unknown.[58]

Myocardial Infarction

Numerous physiologic and pharmacologic manipulations have been proposed for the reduction of the extent and severity of ischemic myocardial injury.[5,58] In conscious dogs with acute coronary occlusion, continuous infusion of nifedipine producing minimal or no arterial hypotension may increase collateral flow to moderately ischemic myocardium and decrease permanent ischemic injury. However, perfusion and eventual injury of severely ischemic myocardium do not appear to be influenced by this agent in conscious dogs.[115] In anesthetized dogs, verapamil reduces the extent of myocardial necrosis as quantitated by histologic[116] methods or by planimetry of infarcted zones visualized by an enzymatic method.[117] There is increasing evidence that diltiazem, like verapamil and nifedipine, may have protective effects on the regionally ischemic myocardium of dogs[118] and cats.[119] Administration of calcium antagonists and other vasodilators during acute myocardial infarction may be potentially detrimental, if the treatment precipitates episodes of arterial hypotension.[120] Inasmuch as bolus injections of calcium antagonists tend to lower arterial pressure, particularly in states associated with high sympathetic tone, it would appear preferable to administer the drugs as continuous infusions, carefully monitoring diastolic arterial pressure.[115] Although calcium antagonists may be well tolerated by patients undergoing uncomplicated acute myocardial infarction, controlled clinical studies demonstrating that these agents exert beneficial effects on transmural or non-transmural (subendocardial) infarction are lacking at this time.[53] However, ongoing trials designed to explore this question have thus far yielded encouraging results. As will be discussed below, treatment of ventricular dysrhythmias in acute myocardial infarction has yielded conflicting reports. In summary, the use of calcium antagonists for the treatment of myocardial infarction remains experimental.

Cardiac Preservation

Experimental and clinical studies suggest that nifedipine, diltiazem, and lidoflazine may have protective effects on the heart during hypothermic cardiopulmonary bypass.[121] Unlike cardioplegic maneuvers as such (hypothermia, potassium arrest), calcium antagonists may exert their beneficial action also during the postbypass period.[58] Experimentally, calcium antagonists are effective in preventing myocardial deterioration after temporary withdrawal of calcium ("calcium paradox") or in suppressing reperfusional dysrhythmias.[58] Calcium antagonists may also be effective in treating hypertensive episodes during and after bypass.

Calcium Antagonists as Cell Portectants

Calcium antagonists have been reported to exert protective effects on injured cells in a variety of syndromes involving both muscle and non-muscle cells (see Table 4).[122] In most if not all syndromes, beneficial effects may be attributed to regional and systemic hemodynamic effects.[58] However, the possibility has been considered that calcium antagonists have direct protective effects on injured cells, possibly by preventing the intracellular accumulation of calcium. We have recently demonstrated that dihydropyridines and diltiazem may suppress hypoxic contracture and ATP depletion in isolated rabbit papillary muscles.[123] These experiments demonstrated that calcium antagonists are capable of influencing cardiac cells independent of rhythmic cardiac work or tissue perfusion. Although the action of calcium antagonists on the ischemic heart may in part reflect the energy-saving effects of decreased myocardial work (decreased contractility, decreased impedance to ventricular ejection), it appears likely that the protection is mediated in part by a mechanism not related to contractile work. Recently, Fleckenstein and collaborators[124] have demonstrated that various calcium antagonists may retard the development of cataracts in alloxan-diabetic rats. In addition, there is increasing evidence that calcium antagonists may have beneficial effects on the ischemic brain,[125] liver,[126] and kidney.[127]

Cardiac Arrhythmias

Cardiac muscle is electrically activated by two depolarizing inward currents, a fast sodium inward current and a smaller calcium-dependent slow inward current.[5,7] These currents occur through separate membrane channels referred to as fast and slow channels. Depolarizing currents trigger opposite or repolarizing currents that are unmasked after combined pharmacologic blockade of the fast and slow channels. At least four different outward currents have been described in Purkinje fibers, and there may be considerable variation of these currents in different species. The inward and outward currents are distinguished on the basis of the membrane voltage range in which they activate and inactivate, and on the basis of the effects of agents that selectively block specific channels. Voltage clamps depolarizing working myocardium to a holding potential of approximately −40 mV inactivate the fast channel, and superimposed depolarization steps elicit an inward current occurring through the slow channel. Some cells in myocardium, such as the sinus and AV nodal cells, are normally less polarized than the contractile cells, and activation of these cells appears to be mediated only by the slow current without preceding fast sodium spike.[7] In these cells, the slow current flows both during the upstroke of the action potential and during the later part of the slow diastolic depolarization characteristic of pacemaker activity.[7] Injured contractile cells (myocardial ischemia) may reduce the polarization of working cells, thereby inactivating the fast channel. Like nodal cells, damaged working cells may then depend to a large extent upon the slow channel for activation. The electrophysiology of pacemaker (nodal) cells and injured myocardial cells may in part explain the action of calcium antagonists on arrhythmias in the presence and absence of ischemia.[128,129]

Table 5. Electrophysiologic effects of Ca antagonists in vivo[5,12,58,128–135]

	Dihydropyridine	*Verapamil*	*Diltiazem*
R–R interval	(↓*)	(↑)	(↑)
Sinus node recovery time	0	↑	0
P–R interval	(↓*)	↑	↑
A–H interval	(↓*)	↑	↑
AV nodal effective and functional refractory periods	0	↑	↑
His-Purkinje and ventricular effective refractory periods	0	0	0
Ventricular automacity	0	0	0

↑ = Increase; ↓ = decrease; 0 = no effect
*Probably reflecting reflex sympathetic discharge

Verapamil produces characteristic inhibitory effects on the slow action potential recorded from sinus and AV nodal areas.[7,58,128] First, there is a decreasing rate of spontaneous diastolic depolarization (decrease in the slope of phase 4) and an increase in the membrane threshold potential (initiation of phase 0 from a more positive value)—effects that slow the rate of firing (negative chronotropy). Second, both the rate of rise and the overshoot of the action potential are decreased—effects that slow conduction (negative dromotropy). High concentrations ($>10^{-6}$M) may result in electrical standstill of sinus and AV nodal cells. By prolonging AV nodal conduction and refractoriness, verapamil is effective in reducing the rate of ventricular response to rapid atrial firing. Some of the electrophysiologic effects of verapamil that may contribute to its antiarrhythmic activity are summarized in Table 5.[128,129]

The main indication of verapamil as an antiarrhythmic agent is for the treatment of reciprocating atrioventricular tachycardia with or without an accessory atrioventricular connection (Wolff-Parkinson-White [WPW] syndrome).[45,128,130] According to current concepts, paroxysmal supraventricular arrhythmias may develop when there is a dual, functionally distinct pathway available for AV conduction. The abnormality inviting a re-entrant rhythm is thought to consist of a first pathway with rapid conduction and slow recovery, and a second pathway with reciprocal characteristics—slow conduction and rapid recovery.[58,128] Intravenous verapamil, usually 10 mg or 0.15 mg/kg, appears to abolish AV nodal re-entry by slowing the antegrade pathway without appreciably affecting the retrograde AV nodal pathway.[128,130] However, in some cases, retrograde conduction over the AV node appeared to be greatly prolonged by verapamil.[131] In patients with WPW syndrome, the drug may have little effect on the accessory pathway, but in some instances the antegrade refractory period of the accessory pathway was shortened.[132] The fact that patients with WPW syndrome may respond to verapamil with an accelerated ventricular response during atrial fibrillation is an interesting but poorly understood phenomenon.[132] It has been ascribed to reflex sympathetic discharge, but it would be important to ascertain whether such effects may be related to "non–calcium blocking effects" of verapamil on the accessory pathway.[132,133] It is possible that the efficacy of verapamil and diltiazem[23] in abolishing re-entrant rhythms is a reflection of their frequency- and voltage-dependence.[7] This might explain, in part, why dihydropyridines—agents exhibiting less frequency-dependence—are not effective in abolishing these arrhythmias. Inasmuch as verapamil is effective in the majority of patients with AV nodal re-entry, it has been widely accepted that the drug is the treatment of choice for this disturbance of rhythm. In formal comparisons, verapamil has been found to be more effective than practolol in terminating the arrhythmias, whereas nifedipine was completely ineffective.[45,130] Verapamil may be also effective in abolishing supraventricular tachycardias resulting from sinus nodal re-entry. However, despite similar electrophysiologic features of sinus and AV node re-entry, current evidence suggests that verapamil may be less effective in sinus node re-entry arrhythmias.[128] Chronic oral therapy with verapamil has been reported to prevent paroxysmal supraventricular tachycardias, but some patients are not helped by this treatment.[58,128,134,135] In some cases, it may be necessary to combine oral therapy with beta blockers or digoxin, although such combinations should be used cautiously in view of the possibility of precipitating a high-degree AV block or other dysrhythmias.

Verapamil is somewhat less effective in terminating automatic atrial tachycardias and multifocal atrial tachycardias.[45,128,130] The relative ineffectiveness of verapamil in treating these arrhythmias is not surprising, inasmuch as the automatic mechanisms may not depend predominantly upon slow-channel responses. Verapamil has been reported to convert to sinus rhythm approximately 30 percent of episodes of atrial flutter, and 16 percent of episodes of atrial fibrillation.[128] These figures appear somewhat high, and the vast majority of patients with atrial fibrillation and atrial flutter respond to verapamil only with an increased degree of AV block.[128] However, in the few patients in whom verapamil abolishes atrial fibrillation or flutter, it might be worthwhile to attempt chronic prophylactic treatment with the drug.

The utility of intravenous or oral verapamil in treating ventricular dysrhythmias has not been established.[128] There has been considerable speculation regarding the mechanism of ventricular dysrhythmias in myocardial ischemia.[128,129] Because ischemia may partly depolarize cells and thereby inhibit the fast channels, it has been postulated that arrhythmias during ischemia may depend predominantly on slow responses.[7] However, current experimental evidence suggests that arrhythmias arising from ischemic myocardium are generated by depressed fast responses rather than slow responses.[129] Inasmuch as verapamil indirectly antagonizes adrenergic effects on the heart, some of its efficacy in myocardial ischemia may be ascribed to anti-adrenergic effects. Alternatively, verapamil may act by improving myocardial perfusion, a mechansim that seems established in the dysrhythmias occurring in association with variant angina.[5]

In summary, verapamil and diltiazem, but not dihydropyridines, are effective in terminating supraventricular re-entrant tachyarrhythmias with or without involvement of an accessory pathway. The drugs may be effective in slowing AV conduction during atrial fibrillation and flutter. On the other hand, the utility of these agents in treating other arrhythmias, in particular those occurring during ischemia, is uncertain at this time.

SUMMARY

Verapamil, nifedipine, and diltiazem are effective in the treatment of stable effort angina and angiospastic (variant) angina. In addition, there is evidence that the agents are beneficial in patients diagnosed as having unstable angina. The efficacy of calcium antagonists for the treatment of effort angina appears to be augmented by combining them with beta-adrenergic blockers. Intravenous verapamil, but not nifedipine, is very effective in terminating paroxysmal supraventricular tachycardias caused by re-entrant mechanisms with or without involvement of accessory pathways (WPW syndrome). Verapamil is also effective in slowing the ventricular response to atrial fibrillation or flutter. The use of verapamil for the treatment of ectopic atrial or ventricular dysrhythmias is less well established and will require further evaluation.

REFERENCES

1. Phear, DN: *Verapamil in angina: A double-blind trial.* Br Med J 2:740, 1968.
2. Pedersen, OL: *Does verapamil have a clinically significant antihypertensive effect?* Eur J Clin Pharmacol 13:21, 1978.
3. Fleckenstein, VA; *Die Zuegelung des Myocardstoffwechsels durch Verapamil.* Drug Res 20:1317, 1970.
4. Mabuchi, G, Kishida, H, and Suzuki, K: *Clinical effect of nifedipine on variant form of angina pectoris.* 1st International Nifedipine "Adalat" Symposium, 177–184, 1975.
5. Henry, PD: *Comparative pharmacology of calcium antagonists: Nifedipine, verapamil and diltiazem.* Am J Cardiol 46:1047, 1980.

6. Dreyfuss, J, Swoap, C, Chinn, C, et al: *Excretion and distribution of thiazesim-^{11}C with its biotransformation in vivo and in vitro.* J Pharm Sci 57:1497, 1968.

7. Henry, PD: *Mechanisms of action of calcium antagonists in cardiac and smooth muscle.* In Braunwald, E, Stone, P, and Antman, E (eds): *Calcium Channel Blocking Agents in the Treatment of Cardiovascular Dissorders.* Futura, Mt Kisco, NY (in press).

8. Rodenkirchen, R, Bayer, R, and Mannhold, R: *Specific and non-specific Ca antagonists: A structure-activity analysis of cardiodepressive drugs.* Prog Pharmacol 5:9, 1982.

9. Kass, RS: *Nisoldipine: A new, more selective calcium current blocker in cardiac Purkinje fibers.* J Pharmacol Exp Ther 223:446, 1982.

10. Ferry, DR and Glossmann, H: *Evidence for multiple receptor sites within the putative calcium channel.* Naunyn Schmiedeberg's Arch Pharmacol 41–44, 1982.

11. Murphy, KMM, Gould, RJ, Largent, BL, et al: *A unitary mechanism of calcium antagonist drug action.* Proc Natl Acad Sci 80:860, 1983.

12. McAllister, RG: *Clinical pharmacology of slow channel blocking agents.* Prog Cardiovasc Dis 25:83, 1982.

13. Carrasco, HA, Fuenmayor, PA, Barboza, M, et al: *Effect of verapamil on normal sinoatrial node function and on sick sinus syndrome.* Am Heart J 96:760, 1978.

14. Woodcock, BG and Rietbrock N: *Verapamil bioavailability and dosage in liver disease.* Br J Clin Pharmacol 13:240, 1982.

15. Leon, MB, Rosing, DR, Bonow, RO, et al: *Clinical efficacy of verapamil alone and combined with propranolol in treating patients with chronic stable angina.* Am J Cardiol 48:131, 1981.

16. Subramanian, BV, Bowles, MJ, Davies, AB, et al: *Combined therapy with verapamil and propranolol in chronic stable angina.* Am J Cardiol 49:125, 1982.

17. Klein, HO, Lang, R, Weiss, E, et al: *The influence of verapamil on serum digoxin concentration.* Eur J Pharmacol 3–4:185, 1982.

18. Pedersen, KE, Dorph-Pedersen, A, Hvidt, S, et al: *The long-term effect of verapamil on plasma digoxin concentration and renal digoxin clearance in healthy subjects.* Eur J Clin Pharmacol 22:123, 1982.

19. Ebner, F: *Survey and summary of results obtained during the world-wide clinical investigations of Adalat (nifedipine).* In Lochner, W, Braasch, W, and Kroneberg, G (eds): *2nd International Adalat Symposium.* Springer-Verlag Berlin, New York, 1975.

20. Jariwalla, AG and Anderson, EG: *Production of ischaemic cardiac pain by nifedipine.* Br Med J 1:1181, 1978.

21. Pedersen, KE, Dorph-Pedersen, A, Hvidt, S, et al: *Effect of nifedipine of digoxin kinetics in healthy subjects.* Clin Pharmacol Ther 32:562, 1982.

22. Ebner, F, Leisten, L, Lejeune, PH, et al: *Administration of nifedipine to patients treated with digitalis-glycosides, anti-diabetic agents and beta-blockers.* In Kaltenbach, M and Neufeld, HN (eds): *5th International Adalat Symposium.* Excerpta Medica, Princeton, 1982.

23. Betriu, A, Chaitman, BR, Bourassa, MG, et al: *Beneficial effect of intravenous diltiazem in the acute management of paroxysmal superventricular tachyarrhythmias.* Circulation 67:88, 1983.

24. Livesley, B, Catley, PF, Campbell, RC, et al: *Double-blind evaluation of verapamil, propranolol, and isosorbide dinitrate against a placebo in the treatment of angina pectoris.* Br Med J 1:375, 1973.

25. Subramanian, VB: *Calcium channel blockers in chronic stable angina. A review.* Herz 7:211, 1982.

26. Subramanian, VB, Bowles, MJ, Davies, AB, et al: *Calcium channel blockade as primary therapy for stable angina pectoris. A double-blind placebo-controlled comparison of verapamil and propranolol.* Am J Cardiol 50:1158, 1982.

27. Weiner, DA and Klein, MD: *Verapamil therapy for stable exertional angina pectoris.* Am J Cardiol 50:1164, 1982.

28. Simoons, ML, Taams, M, Lubsen, J, et al: *Treatment of stable angina pectoris with verapamil hydrochloride: A double blind cross-over study.* Eur Heart J 1:269, 1980.

29. Johnson, SM, Mauritson, DR, Corbett, JR, et al: *Double-blind, randomized, placebo-controlled comparison of propranolol and verapamil in the treatment of patients with stable angina pectoris.* Am J Med 71:443, 1981.

30. Pine, MB, Citron, PD, Bailly, DJ, et al: *Verapamil versus placebo in relieving stable angina pectoris.* Circulation 65:17, 1982.

31. Johnson, SM, Mauritson, DR, Willerson, JT, et al: *Comparison of verapamil and nifedipine in the treatment of variant angina pectoris: Preliminary observations in 10 patients.* Am J Cardiol 47:1295, 1981.

32. DePonti, C, Mauri, F, Ciliberto, GR, et al: *Comparative effects of nifedipine, verapamil, isosorbide dinitrate and propranolol on exercise-induced angina pectoris.* Eur J Cardiol 10:47, 1979.

33. Brodsky, SJ, Cutler, SS, Weiner, DA, et al: *Treatment of stable angina of effort with verapamil: A double-blind, placebo-controlled randomized crossover study.* Circulation 66:569, 1982.
34. Sadick, NN, Tan, AT, Fletcher, PJ, et al: *A double-blind randomized trial of propranolol and verapamil in the treatment of effort angina.* Circulation 66:74, 1982.
35. Frishman, WH, Klein, NA, Strom, JA, et al: *Superiority of verapamil to propranolol in stable angina pectoris: A double-blind, randomized crossover trial.* Circulation 65:51, 1982.
36. Lynch, P, Dargie, H, Krikler, S, et al: *Objective assessment of antianginal treatment: A double-blind evaluation of propranolol, nifedipine, and their combination.* Br Med J 281:184, 1980.
37. Mueller, HS and Chahine, RA: *Interim report of multicenter double-blind placebo-controlled studies of nifedipine in chronic stable angina pectoris.* Am J Med 71:645, 1981.
38. Sherman, LG and Liang, CS: *Nifedipine in chronic stable angina: A double-blind placebo-controlled crossover trial.* Am J Cardiol 51:706, 1983.
39. Corbalan, R, Gonzalez, R, Chamorro, G, et al: *Effect of a calcium inhibitor, nifedipine, on exercise tolerance in patients with angina pectoris. A double-blind study.* Chest 79:302, 1981.
40. Cocco, G, Strozzi, C, Chu, D, et al: *Therapeutic effects of pindolol and nifedipine in patients with stable angina pectoris and asymptomatic resting ischemia.* Eur J Cardiol 10:59, 1979.
41. Kenmure, AC and Scruton, JH: *A double-blind controlled trial of the anti-anginal efficacy of nifedipine compared with propranolol.* Br J Clin Pract 33:49, 1979.
42. Ekelund, LG and Oro, L: *Antianginal efficiency of nifedipine with and without a beta-blocker, studied with exercise test. A double-blind, randomized subacute study.* Clin Cardiol 2:203, 1979.
43. Daly, K, Bergman, G, Rothman, M, et al: *Beneficial effect of adding nifedipine to beta-adrenergic blocking therapy in angina pectoris.* Eur Heart J 3:42, 1982.
44. Bassan, M, Weiler-Ravell, D, and Shaley, O: *The additive antianginal action of oral nifedipine in patients receiving propranolol: Magnitude and duration of effect.* Circulation 66:710, 1982.
45. Dargie, H, Rowland, E, and Krikler, D: *Role of calcium antagonists in cardiovascular therapy.* Br Heart J 46:8, 1981.
46. Hossack, KF and Bruce, RA: *Improved exercise performance in persons with stable angina pectoris receiving diltiazem.* Am J Cardiol 47:95, 1981.
47. Pool, PE and Seagren, SC: *Long-term efficacy of diltiazem in chronic stable angina associated with atherosclerosis: Effects on treadmill exercise.* Am J Cardiol 49:573, 1982.
48. Wagniant, P, Ferguson, RJ, and Chaitman, BR: *Increased exercise tolerance and reduced electrocardiographic ischemia with diltiazem in patients with stable angina pectoris.* Circulation 66:23, 1982.
49. Koiwaya, Y, Nakamura, M, Mitsutake, A, et al: *Increased exercise tolerance after oral diltiazem, a calcium antagonist, in angina pectoris.* Am Heart J 101:143, 1981.
50. De Backer, G and Vincke, J: *Double-blind comparison of diltiazem and placebo in the treatment of exercise-inducible chronic stable angina pectoris.* Acta Cardiol 37:245, 1982.
51. Pepine, CJ, Feldman, RL, Whittle, J, et al: *Effect of diltiazem in patients with variant angina: A randomized double-blind trial.* Am Heart J 101:719, 1981.
52. Ludbrook, PA, Tiefenbrunn, AJ, Reed, FR, et al: *Acute hemodynamic responses to sublingual nifedipine: Dependence on left ventricular function.* Circulation 65:489, 1982.
53. Jaffe, AF, Henry, PD, Vacek, JL, et al: *Administration of nifedipine to patients with acute myocardial infarction.* Cardiovasc Med 1:91, 1982.
54. Engel, H-J and Lichtlen, PR: *Beneficial enhancement of coronary blood flow by nifedipine.* Am J Med 17:658, 1981.
55. Beck, OA and Hochrein, H: *Wirkung und Wirkungsdauer von Nifedipin auf den Pulmonalarteriendruck bei dekompensierten Koronarkranken.* Med Klin 73:457, 1978.
56. Waxman, HL: *Verapamil for treatment of supraventricular tachyarrhythmias.* Chest 81:267, 1982.
57. Bonow, RO, Leon, MB, Rosing, DR, et al: *Effects of verapamil and propranolol on left ventricular systolic function and diastolic filling in patients with coronary artery disease: Radionuclide angiographic studies at rest and during exercise.* Circulation 65:1337, 1982.
58. Henry, PD: *Comparative cardiac pharmacology of calcium blockers.* In Flaim, SF and Zelis, R (eds): *Calcium Blockers: Mechanisms of Action and Clinical Applications.* Urban & Schwarzenberg, Baltimore, 1982.
59. Parodi, O, Maseri, A, and Simonetti, I: *Management of unstable angina at rest by verapamil. A double-blind crossover study in coronary care unit.* Br Heart J 41:169, 1979.
60. Mehta, J and Conti, CR: *Verapamil therapy for unstable angina pectoris: Review of double-blind placebo-controlled randomized clinical trials.* Am J Cardiol 50:919, 1982.

61. GERSTENBLITH, G, OUYANG, P, ACHUFF, SC, ET AL: *Nifedipine in unstable angina. A double-blind, randomized trial.* N Engl J Med 306:885, 1982.

62. HAGEMEIJER, F, VAN MECHELEN, R, AND SANTOSO, T: *Benefits from adding nifedipine to the treatment of unstable angina when beta-blockade and isosorbide dinitrate have proved inadequate.* Herz 7:126, 1982.

63. MOSES, JW, WERTEIMER, JH, BODENHEIMER, MM, ET AL: *Efficacy of nifedipine in rest angina refractory to propranolol and nitrates in patients with obstructive coronary artery disease.* Ann Intern Med 94:425, 1981.

64. HUGENHOLTZ, PG, MICHELS, HR, SERRUYS, PW, ET AL: *Nifedipine in the treatment of unstable angina, coronary spasm and myocardial infarction.* Am J Cardiol 47:163, 1981.

65. YASUE, H, OMOTE, S, TAKIZAWA: *Pathogenesis and treatment of angina pectoris at rest as seen from its response to various drugs.* Jpn Circ J 42:1, 1978.

66. NAKAMURA, M AND KOIWAYA, Y: *Beneficial effect of diltiazem, a new antianginal drug, on angina pectoris at rest.* Jpn Heart J 20:613, 1979.

67. HELFANT, RH: *Inpatient treatment of unstable angina: Clinical perspective and sequential management.* Am Heart J 104:697, 1082.

68. OSLER, W: *Angina pectoris.* The Lancet 4517:839, 1910.

69. MACALPIN, RN: *Contribution of dynamic vascular wall thickening to luminal narrowing during coronary arterial constriction.* Circulation 60:296, 1980.

70. KIMURA, E AND KISHIDA, H: *Treatment of variant angina with drugs: A survey of 11 cardiology institutes in Japan.* Circulation 63L:844, 1981.

71. ANTMAN, E, MULLER, JE, GOLDBERG, S, ET AL: *Nifedipine therapy for coronary artery spasm: Experience in 127 patients.* N Engl J Med 302:1269, 1980.

72. WATERS, DD, THEROUX, P, SZIACHCIC, J, ET AL: *Provocative testing with ergonovine to evaluate the efficacy of treatment with nifedipine, diltiazem and verapamil in variant angina.* Am J Cardiol 48:123, 1981.

73. MEHTA, J, MEHTA, P, PEPINE, CJ, ET AL: *Differences in platelet aggregation in coronary artery disease: Effect of propranolol.* Clin Cardiol 1:96, 1978.

74. HIRSH, PD, HILLIS, LD, CAMPBELL, WB, ET AL: *Release of prostaglandins and thromboxane into the coronary circulation in patients with ischemic heart disease.* N Engl J Med 304:685, 1981.

75. ROBERTSON, RM, ROBERTSON, D, ROBERTS, LJ, ET AL: *Thromboxane A_2 in vasotonic angina pectoris.* N Engl J Med 304:998, 1981.

76. LOEV, B, EHRREICH, SJ, AND TEDESCHI, RE: *Dihydropyridines with potent hypotensive activity prepared by the Hantzsch reaction.* J Pharm Pharmacol 24:917, 1972.

77. BÜHLER, FR, AND HULTH'EN, L: *Calcium channel blockers: A pathophysiologically based antihypertensive treatment concept for the future?* Eur J Clin Invest 12:1, 1982.

78. HULTH'EN, UL, BOLLI, P, AMANN, FW, ET AL: *Verapamil-induced vasodilation is enhanced in essential hypertension.* J Cardiovasc Pharmacol 3:313, 1982.

79. NOON, JP, RICE, PJ, AND BALDESSARINI, RJ: *Calcium leakage as a cause of the high resting tension in vascular smooth muscle from the spontaneously hypertensive rat.* Proc Natl Acad Sci 75:1605, 1978.

80. MUIESAN, G, AGABITI-ROSEI, E, ALICANDRI, C, ET AL: *Influence of verapamil on catecholamines, renin and aldosterone in essential hypertensive patients.* In ZANCHETTI, A AND KRIKLER, DM (EDS): *Calcium Antagonism in Cardiovascular Therapy: Experience With Verapamil.* Excerpta Medica, Princeton, 1981.

81. DOYLE, AE, ANAVEKAR, SN, AND OLIVER, LE: *A clinical trial of verapamil in the treatment of hypertension.* In ZANCHETTI, A AND KRIKLER, DM (EDS): *Calcium Antagonism in Cardiovascular Therapy: Experience Wtih Verapamil.* Excerpta Medica, Princeton, 1981.

82. LEWIS, GRJ, STEWART, DJ, LEWIS, BM, ET AL: *The antihypertensive effect of oral verapamil — acute and long-term administrations and its effects on the high-density lipoprotein values in plasma.* In ZANCHETTI, A AND KRIKLER, DM (EDS): *Calcium Antagonism in Cardiovascular Therapy: Experience With Verapamil.* Excerpta Medica, Princeton, 1981.

83. GOULD, BA, MANN, S, KIESO, H, ET AL: *The 24-hour intra-arterial ambulatory profile of blood pressure reduction with verapamil.* In ZANCHETTI, A AND KRIKLER, DM (ED): *Calcium Antagonism in Cardiovascular Therapy: Experience With Verapamil.* Excerpta Medica, Princeton, 1981.

84. AOKI, K, YOSHIDA, T, KATO, S, ET AL: *Hypotensive action and increased plasma renin activity by Ca^{2+} antagonist (nifedipine) in hypertensive patients.* Jpn Heart J 17:497, 1970.

85. GUAZZI, M, OLIVARI, MT, POLESE, A, ET AL: *Nifedipine, a new antihypertensive with rapid action.* Clin Pharmacol Ther 22:528, 1977.

86. GUAZZI, MD, FIORENTINI, C, OLIVARI, MT, ET AL: *Short- and long-term efficacy of a calcium-antagonistic agent (nifedipine) combined with methyldopa in the treatment of severe hypertension.* Circ Res 61:913, 1980.

87. PEDERSEN, OL: *Calcium blockade as a therapeutic principle in arterial hypertension.* Acta Pharmacol Toxicol 49:1, 1981.

88. KUWAJIMA, I, UEDA, K, KAMATA, C, ET AL: *A study on the effects of nifedipine in hypertensive crises and severe hypertension.* Jpn Heart J 19:455, 1978.

89. BAYLEY, S, DOBBS, RJ, AND ROBINSON, BF: *Nifedipine in the treatment of hypertension: Report of a double-blind controlled trial.* Br J Clin Pharmacol 14:509, 1982.

90. COREA, L, ALUNNI, G, BENTIVOGLIO, M, ET AL: *Acute and long-term effects of nifedipine on plasma renin activity and plasma catecholamines in controls and hypertensive patients before and after metoprolol.* Acta Therapeutica 6:177, 1980.

91. COREA, L, MIELE, BENTIVOGLIO, M, ET AL: *Acute and chronic effects of nifedipine on plasma renin activity and plasma adrenaline and noradrenaline in controls and hypertensive patients.* Clin Sci 57:115s, 1979.

92. LEVENSON, J, SIMON, A, ACHIMASTOS, A, ET AL: *Comparative hemodynamic effects of 2 vasodilators: Dihydralazine and diltiazem in permanent essential arterial hypertension.* Arch Mal Coeur 75:167, 1982.

93. AMES, RP: *Negative effects of diuretic drugs on metabolic risk factors for coronary heart disease: Possible alternative drug therapies.* Am J Cardiol 51:632, 1983.

94. KAPLAN, NM: *New approaches to the therapy of mild hypertension.* Am J Cardiol 51:621, 1983.

95. *Multiple Risk Factor Intervention Trial.* JAMA 248:1465, 1982.

96. BÜHLER, FR, HULTH'EN, UL, KIOWSHI, W, ET AL: *The place of the calcium antagonist verapamil in antihypertensive therapy.* J Cardiovasc Pharmacol 4:S350, 1982.

97. MCMURTY, IF, DAVIDSON, BS, REEVES, JT, ET AL: *Inhibition of hypoxic pulmonary vasoconstriction by calcium antagonists in isolated rat lungs.* Circ Res 38:99, 1976.

98. MCMURTY, IF, REEVES, JT, WILL, DH, ET AL: *Reduction of bovine pulmonary hypertension by normoxia, verapamil and hexaprenaline.* Experientia 33:1192, 1977.

99. YOUNG, TE, LUNDQUIST, LJ, CHESLER, E, ET AL: *Comparative effects of nifedipine, verapamil, and diltiazem on experimental pulmonary hypertension.* Am J Cardiol 51:195, 1983.

100. KENNEDY, T AND SUMMER, W: *Inhibition of hypoxic pulmonary vasoconstriction by nifedipine.* Am J Cardiol 50:864, 1982.

101. LANDMARK, K, REFSUM, AM, SIMONSEN, S, ET AL: *Verapamil and pulmonary hypertension.* Acta Med Scand 204:299, 1978.

102. SIMONNEAU, G, ESCOURROU, P, DUROUX, P, ET AL: *Inhibition of hypoxic pulmonary vasoconstriction by nifedipine.* N Engl J Med 304:1582, 1981.

103. ROSING, DR, KENT, KM, BORER, JS, ET AL: *Verapamil therapy: A new approach to the pharmacologic treatment of hypertrophic cardiomyopathy. I. Hemodynamic effects.* Circulation 60:1201, 1979.

104. ROSING, DR, KENT, KM, MARON, BJ, ET AL: *Verapamil therapy: A new approach to the pharmacologic treatment of hypertrophic cardiomyopathy. II. Effects on exercise capacity and symptomatic status.* Circulation 60:1208, 1979.

105. NAGAO, M, YASUE, H, OMOTE, S, ET AL: *Diltiazem-induced decrease of exercise-elevated pulmonary arterial diastolic pressure in hypertrophic cardiomyopathy patients.* Am Heart J 102:789, 1981.

106. LANDMARK, K, SIRE, S, THAULOW, E, ET AL: *Haemodynamic effects of nifedipine and propranolol in patients with hypertrophic obstructive cardiomyopathy.* Br Heart J 48:19, 1982.

107. COHN, JN: *Choice and rationale for vasodilators in the treatment of hypertension or relief of heart failure.* Cardiovasc Reviews and Reports 1:686, 1980.

108. WEBER, KT AND JANICKI, JS: *Afterload and the failing heart.* Pract Cardiol 6:35, 1980.

109. MATSUMOTO, S, ITO, T, SADA, T, ET AL: *Hemodynamic effects of nifedipine in congestive heart failure.* Am J Cardiol 46:476, 1980.

110. BELLOCCI, F, ANSALONE, G, SANTARELLI, P, ET AL: *Oral nifedipine in the long-term management of severe chronic heart failure.* J Cardiovasc Pharmacol 4:847, 1982.

111. FIORETTI, P, BENUSSI, B, SCARDI, S, ET AL: *Afterload reduction with nifedipine in aortic insufficiency.* Am J Cardiol 49:1728, 1982.

112. CANTELLI, I, PAVESI, PC, NACCARELLA, F, ET AL: *Comparison of acute haemodynamic effects of nifedipine and isosorbide dinitrate in patients with heart failure following acute myocardial infarction.* Int J Cardiol 1:151, 1981.

113. ALVES, LE AND ROSE, EP: *Use of nifedipine in older patients and patients with congestive heart failure.* Am J Med 72:462, 1982.

114. KINOSHITA, M, KUSUKAWA, R, SHIMONO, Y, ET AL: *The effect of diltiazem hydrochloride upon sodium diuresis and renal function in chronic congestive heart failure.* Drug Res 29:676, 1979.

115. HENRY, PD, SHUCHLEIB, R, BORDA, L, ET AL: *Effects of nifedipine on myocardial perfusion and ischemic injury in dogs.* Circ Res 43:372, 1978.

116. Reimer, KA, Lowe, JE, and Jennings, RB: *Effects of the calcium antagonist verapamil on necrosis following temporary coronary artery occlusion in dogs.* Circulation 55:581, 1977.

117. Maroko, PR: *Experimental infarction studies.* Clin Invest Med 3:139, 1980.

118. Nakamura, M, Kikuchi, Y, Senda, Y, et al: *Myocardial blood flow following experimental coronary occlusion. Effects of diltiazem.* Chest 78:205, 1980.

119. Bush, LR, Li, YP, Shlafer, M, et al: *Protective effects of diltiazem during myocardial ischemia in isolated cat hearts.* J Pharmacol Exp Ther 218:653, 1981.

120. Selwyn, AP, Welman, E, Fox, K, et al: *The effects of nifedipine on acute experimental ischemia and infarction in dogs.* Circ Res 44:16, 1979.

121. Clark, RE, Christlieb, IY, Spratt, JA, et al: *Myocardial preservation with nifedipine: A comparative study at normothermia.* Ann Thorac Surg 31:3, 1981.

122. Henry, PD: *Calcium Antagonists as Cell Protectants.* Exerpta Medica (in press).

123. Henry, PD and Wahl, AM: *Diltiazem and nitrendipine suppress hypoxic contracture in quiescent ventricular myocardium.* Eur J Cardiol (in press).

124. Fleckenstein, A, v.Witzleben, H, Frey, M, et al: *Prevention of cataracts of alloxan-diabetic rats by long-term treatment with verapamil.* Pflügers Arch Ges Physiol [Suppl] 391:12, 1981.

125. Raichle, M: *Pathophysiology of brain ischemia.* Ann Neurol 13:2, 1983.

126. Sayeed, MM and Doroba, A: *Effects of diltiazem in the early phase of endotoxin shock in rats.* Circul Shock 9:193, 1982.

127. Ishigami, M, Stowe, N, Smith, C, et al: *Protective effect of Ca^{++} entry blocker in dog kidneys subjected to 120 min warm ischemia.* Fed Proc 42:843, 1983.

128. Zipes, DP and Gilmour, RF: *Management of arrhythmias with "calcium antagonists."* J Vasc Dis 540, 1982.

129. Gilmour, RF and Zipes, DP: *Electrophysiological response of vascularized hamster cardiac transplants to ischemia.* Circ Res 50:599, 1982.

130. Rowland, E, Evans, T, and Krikler, D: *Effect of nifedipine on atrioventricular conduction as compared with verapamil.* Br Heart J 42:124, 1979.

131. Klein, GJ, Gulamhusein, S, Prystowsky, EN, et al: *Comparison of the electrophysiologic effects of intravenous and oral verapamil in patients with paroxysmal sypraventricular tachycardia.* Am J Cardiol 49:117, 1982.

132. Gulamhusein, S, Ko, P, Carruthers, SC, et al: *Acceleration of the ventricular response during atrial fibrillation in the Wolff-Parkinson-White syndrome after verapamil.* Circulation 65:348, 1982.

133. Harper, RW, Whitford, E, Middlebrook, K, et al: *Effects of verapamil on the electrophysiologic properties of the accessory pathway in patients with the Wolff-Parkinson-White syndrome.* Am J Cardiol 50:1323, 1982.

134. Mauritson, DR, Winniford, MD, Walker, WS, et al: *Oral verapamil for paroxysmal supraventricular tachycardia: A long-term, double-blind randomized trial.* Ann Intern Med 96:409, 1982.

135. Tonkin, AM and Shorne, L: *The prophylaxis of AV nodal re-entry tachycardia.* Clin Exp Pharmacol Physiol 6:135, 1982.

Parenteral Nitroglycerin: Clinical Usefulness and Limitations

John T. Flaherty, M.D.

For nearly a century, sublingual nitroglycerin has been the cornerstone of therapy for angina pectoris. Sustained-action oral forms and cutaneous ointment have been used prophylactically to prevent anginal attacks and more recently have been used for the treatment of chronic congestive heart failure. For the past 8 years, my associates and I have been studying the hemodynamic and anti-ischemic effects of intravenous nitroglycerin in patients with acute myocardial infarction.[1-5] In the surgical intensive care unit, we have also compared intravenous nitroglycerin with sodium nitroprusside in a randomized crossover study for the management of acute hypertension developing after coronary artery bypass surgery.[6] On October 1, 1981, intravenous nitroglycerin was released by the Federal Food and Drug Administration for general clinical use.

Nitroglycerin acts primarily by relaxing vascular smooth muscle. The exact mechanism of action is poorly understood but may involve disulfide bond formation at a smooth-muscle nitrate receptor or, alternatively, may release prostaglandins from endogenous stores. Although dilation of venous smooth muscle predominates at lower doses, nitroglycerin at higher doses produces dilation of both venous and arterial smooth muscle in a dose-dependent fashion. Venodilation results in peripheral venous pooling and thereby reduction in left ventricular filling pressure. Arterial dilation results in reduction of peripheral vascular resistance and thereby increases stroke volume, especially in failing ventricles. Dilation of the large extramural coronary arteries has been demonstrated. In addition, and perhaps more importantly, nitroglycerin has been shown to dilate intercoronary collateral channels and to redistribute myocardial blood flow to deeper subendocardial layers.

Nitroglycerin is distributed widely in the body and is rapidly metabolized in the liver by the enzyme glutathione–organic nitrate reductase. As a result, intravenous nitroglycerin has a short half-life, estimated at 2 to 3 minutes, with hemodynamic alterations reversing quickly after discontinuation of an intravenous infusion. Serum levels of nitroglycerin can be measured by gas-liquid chromatography (in ng/ml) and have been shown previously to correlate with hemodynamic changes following transcutaneous and sublingual administration. Nitroglycerin is bound approximately 60 percent to plasma proteins. Tolerance to nitroglycerin can be demonstrated in vitro; however, tolerance to nitrates seems less important clinically with persistent hemodynamic effects demonstrable after 3 months of treatment with nitroglycerin ointment. Withdrawal symptoms from nitrates have been reported in munitions workers but have not been reported when patients receiving chronic therapy with long-acting nitroglycerin preparations are abruptly withdrawn from the drug.

CLINICAL USEFULNESS

Unstable Angina

The intravenous route of administration has the practical advantage of allowing maintenance of steady blood levels of nitroglycerin. This characteristic would make its use for the management of unstable angina pectoris appear especially attractive.[8–10] Mikolich and coworkers reported that in 40 of 45 patients (89 percent) nitroglycerin dosage could be titrated to maintain a pain-free state.[10] Only two patients (4 percent) developed hypotension that required reduction of the infusion rate. Intravenous nitroglycerin has also been reported to successfully treat attacks of Prinzmetal's angina, presumably by reversing coronary vasospasm. [11] An important mechanism for the beneficial effects of intravenous nitroglycerin in unstable angina may be prevention of such coronary vasospasm in the presence as well as the absence of signficant fixed coronary disease.

Infusion can be started at 5 to 10 μg/min and the rate increased progressively at 3- to 5-minute intervals until a given hemodynamic end point, such as a 10 percent lowering of mean arterial pressure, is obtained. This particular hemodynamic end point, while arbitrary, was shown in previous clinical trials in patients with acute myocardial infarction to be safe and to be associated with a low incidence of side effects.[3,14] Since the therapeutic goal in patients with unstable angina is the prevention of further episodes of chest pain, upward titration of the infusion rate should follow each episode of ischemic chest pain unless excessive lowering of blood pressure is encountered. Side effects, such as headache or nausea and vomiting not responsive to usual symptomatic treatment, can also limit the maximal infusion rate tolerated by an individual patient.

Acute Myocardial Infarction

The greatest clinical experience with intravenous nitroglycerin has been obtained in patients with acute myocardial infarction. Lowering blood pressure and thereby coronary perfusion pressure would be especially critical in those patients who are demonstrating electrocardiographic changes of acute ischemia. Thus, precordial ST segment mapping was used to monitor the effects of nitroglycerin infusion on the severity of regional ischemia in patients with anterior infarctions.[1,2,4] It was found that lowering mean arterial pressure by 10 to 35 percent was associated with an improvement in the sum of precordial ST segment voltages in all patients.

The hemodynamic effects of intravenous nitroglycerin appear to vary according to presence or absence of left ventricular failure[2] (Fig. 1). Patients with normal stroke volume and normal left ventricular filling pressure demonstrate an almost pure preload-lowering effect. Because nitroglycerin is a potent venodilator, a fall in left ventricular filling pressure would be expected. Nitroglycerin also increases the diastolic compliance of the regionally ischemic left ventricle. The resulting downward shift of the diastolic pressure-volume relationship would result in a lower end-diastolic pressure for any given diastolic volume. Both these mechanisms act to lower left ventricular preload. Patients with normal left ventricular function will demonstrate a fall in cardiac output during nitroglycerin infusion as their left ventricular filling pressure moves down the Starling curve. Since these patients have a normal baseline cardiac output, such a reduction is usually well tolerated. However, it should be noted that patients with low left ventricular filling pressure and/or patients with right ventricular infarction can be especially sensitive to the hypotensive effects of nitroglycerin.

The magnitude of the increase in stroke volume obtained by vasodilator therapy has been shown to depend upon the presence of, or severity of, left ventricular failure[12] (Fig. 2). Patients with normal left ventricular function will show little or no increase in stroke volume when systemic vascular resistance is lowered. On the other hand, patients with severe left

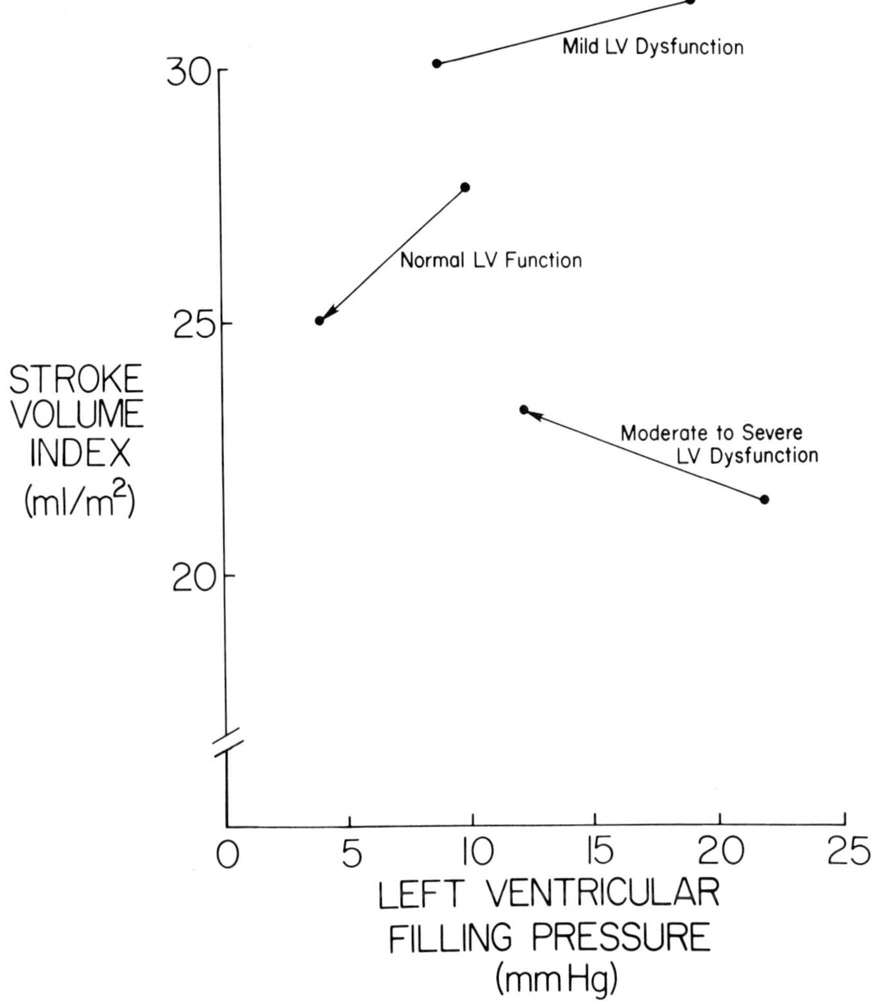

Figure 1. Responses of stroke volume index to infusion of intravenous nitroglycerin in patients with acute myocardial infarction according to their hemodynamic subgroup (i.e., normal left ventricular [LV] function, mild LV dysfunction, and moderate to severe LV dysfunction). See text for details.

ventricular failure demonstrate marked improvement in stroke volume when systemic vascular resistance is lowered. Our own hemodynamic data in patients with acute myocardial infarction and mild left ventricular dysfunction (i.e., normal stroke volume with elevated left ventricular filling pressure) demonstrated combined preload- and afterload-lowering effects, with preload-lowering effect predominating. Patients with more severe left ventricular dysfunction (see the lower right quadrant of Fig. 1) demonstrated more balanced afterload- and preload-lowering effects with stroke volume increasing as left ventricular filling pressure was reduced. Thus, patients with more severe degrees of left ventricular failure appear to obtain the most significant hemodynamic benefits from intravenous nitroglycerin therapy.

In contrast, the anti-ischemic effects of short-term acute administration of intravenous nitroglycerin appeared equal in all hemodynamic subgroups.[2] In our recently completed randomized clinical trial of intravenous nitroglycerin in acute myocardial infarction,[3,14] myocardial perfusion and left ventricular function were significantly improved most often when nitro-

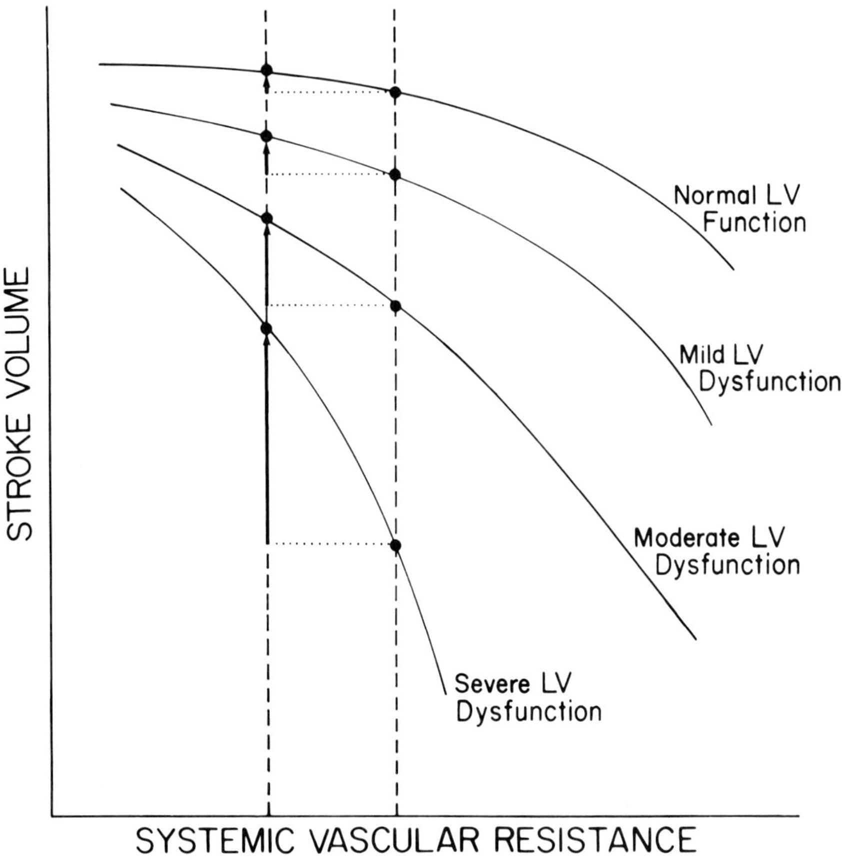

Figure 2. Differential effects of afterload reduction on stroke volume according to hemodynamic subgroup. Curves shown are for patients with normal left ventricular (LV) function as well as patients with mild, moderate, and severe degrees of LV dysfunction. Vertical dashed lines indicate pretreatment (right) and post-treatment (left) levels of systemic vascular resistance (SVR). Vertical arrows indicate the magnitude of the increase in stroke volume index that would be expected from this given reduction in SVR in each hemodynamic subgroup.

glycerin treatment was initiated less than 10 hours after the onset of chest pain. Both perfusion defect score, assessed quantitatively from thallium-201 images, and left ventricular ejection fraction, assessed by gated blood pool scintigraphy, showed significant improvement more often when patients had a 48-hour infusion of nitroglycerin initiated early after symptom onset. The incidence of in-hospital complications of acute infarction, including infarct extension, new congestive heart failure, or early cardiac death, was likewise reduced in frequency by early nitroglycerin therapy. However, larger clinical trials will be necessary before this therapy can be considered routine.

Acute Left Ventricular Failure

The beneficial effects of acute administration of intravenous nitroglycerin to patients with left ventricular pump failure complicating acute myocardial infarction have been discussed above. Theoretically, similar beneficial effects might be expected in patients with acute mitral regurgitation or acute ventricular septal rupture complicating acute infarction. Lowering impedance to left ventricular ejection would reduce both the regurgitant fraction and the magnitude of the left-to-right shunt, respectively.

In the past, nitroprusside has been considered the parenteral drug of choice for lowering afterload in the setting of acute left ventricular failure with or without complicating mechanical lesions. Nitroglycerin might offer several advantages over nitroprusside, because the vasodilating effects of these two agents on intercoronary collateral flow have been shown by several investigators to differ markedly.[13,15,16] In both clinical and animal model studies, nitroglycerin was shown to dilate intercoronary collateral vessels and improve regional ischemia, whereas nitroprusside decreased collateral flow and worsened ischemia. Furthermore, in the lower dosage range, significant preload-lowering and anti-ischemic effects can be obtained with nitroglycerin without significantly reducing mean arterial pressure, thereby facilitating its use in borderline hypotensive patients. In the future, intravenous nitroglycerin may also prove effective for the treatment of pulmonary edema, and may be preferred in patients with significant coronary disease.

Perioperative Applications

Having demonstrated potent afterload-lowering effects in patients with acute myocardial infarction, my colleagues and I tested the ability of intravenous nitroglycerin to lower arterial pressure in postoperative coronary artery bypass surgery patients. During the first 3 hours post–cardiopulmonary bypass, approximately two thirds of these patients develop sudden and persistent increases in arterial pressure associated with an increase in peripheral vascular resistance and a decrease in cardiac output.[17] Though the mechanisms responsible for these hypertensive episodes remain uncertain, we have hypothesized that persistent beta blockade, in the face of markedly elevated plasma catecholamines, would allow unopposed alpha stimulation and thereby result in intense vasoconstriction. Vasodilator therapy would reverse this potentially injurious rise in oxygen demands and also reduce the risk of increased surgical bleeding. Using a randomized crossover study design, nitroglycerin and nitroprusside were shown to lower both arterial pressure and peripheral vascular resistance equally in 85 percent of patients, at comparable infusion rates (μg/min).[6] Intravenous nitroglycerin appeared to result in more potent vasodilating effects in the pulmonary circulation with a greater lowering of mean pulmonary artery pressure being obtained, especially in patients with initially elevated pulmonary artery pressures. Nitroglycerin also resulted in a decrease, in contrast to nitroprusside which resulted in an increase, in intrapulmonary shunting. Kaplan and associates have also reported the use of intravenous nitroglycerin in the management of intraoperative hypertension in patients undergoing coronary artery bypass.[18] In this clinical setting, we recently demonstrated the induction of segmental left ventricular wall motion abnormalities during endotracheal intubation. Segmental akinesis most often developed before or in the absence of electrocardiographic changes. Prophylactic use of a vasodilator such as nitroglycerin during induction of anesthesia could prevent this potentially disastrous induction of regional ischemia in these unstable patients.

Induction of controlled hypotension during certain orthopedic, plastic, or neurosurgical procedures is another clinical indication for intravenous nitroglycerin. The arterial dilating ability of nitroglycerin can be used to precisely and reversibly lower arterial blood pressure and thereby minimize surgical bleeding.

LIMITATIONS

In previous sections, I have reviewed the current clinical indications for intravenous nitroglycerin therapy as well as several potential future applications. To balance such a discussion, however, I think it is important to discuss the limitations, present the adverse reactions and contraindications, and describe the loss of drug through standard intravenous infusion sets.

For the management of unstable angina in a coronary care unit, administration of intravenous nitroglycerin appears to offer advantages over sublingual, oral, or transcutaneous routes. However, it must be pointed out that patients will be quite sensitive to any failure of infusion pumps to deliver drug at a constant rate or failure of the nursing staff to manage such an infusion. Whereas angina may result from failure of delivery, arterial hypotension can result from accidental delivery of excessive drug. Intravenous nitroglycerin will not control pain episodes in all patients with unstable angina. Addition of calcium-channel blockers with or without beta-adrenergic blockers would be a logical next step. Intra-aortic balloon counterpulsation and/or emergency bypass surgery may be required for the remaining patients who fail to respond to maximal medical therapy. It remains to be demonstrated whether the recently introduced transcutaneous nitroglycerin delivery systems, which advertise once-daily dosing, will provide a means of delivering nitroglycerin in doses sufficient to control unstable angina. If effective, the transdermal route of administration would decrease the need for frequent blood pressure monitoring, the need for costly infusion pumps, and perhaps the frequency of accidental interruptions or excesses in drug delivery.

For the treatment of left ventricular failure complicating acute myocardial infarction, intravenous nitroglycerin may not produce sufficient afterload lowering in all patients. Such patients may require the addition or substitution of intravenous sodium nitroprusside in order to maximally increase forward cardiac output. Similarly, the addition of oral hydralazine or prazosin may be required to obtain the desired afterload lowering when sufficient afterload lowering is not obtained by nitroglycerin infusion rates in excess of 300 μg/min.

A similar limitation exists for nitroglycerin usage in the postoperative setting. Approximately 15 percent of patients were found in our study to be relatively "nitroglycerin resistant." In these patients, doses of 1100 μg/min were infused in an attempt to match the arterial pressure lowering obtained with sodium nitroprusside. In one case, equal blood pressure lowering was obtained; in another case, only 50 percent of the desired lowering was obtained; and in the last case, no significant arterial pressure lowering was obtained. In such patients, nitroprusside would appear to remain the parenteral drug of choice for controlling blood pressure.

Adverse Reactions

Potential adverse reactions to intravenous nitroglycerin therapy include hypotension, sinus tachycardia, sinus bradycardia, headache, and nausea or vomiting. In our clinical experience, drug-induced hypotension is quickly reversed by discontinuing or reducing the rate of infusion. We have only rarely encountered a significant increase in heart rate with the intravenous route of administration but have, in approximately 4 percent of patients, noted sinus bradycardia and associated hypotension. Discontinuing the infusion is usually all that is required. However, if necessary, leg elevation with or without a small dose of atropine (0.5 mg) rapidly reverses both the bradycardia and hypotension. Headache and nausea or vomiting appear to be dose-related and can usually be reversed by reducing the rate of infusion. Methemoglobinemia and uncoupling of oxidative phosphorylation are theoretically possible side effects that have not as yet been reported clinically. Increased intrapulmonary shunting would appear to be less severe with nitroglycerin than with nitroprusside therapy.

Sinus tachycardia or sinus bradycardia might be expected if the blood pressure is rapidly or overzealously lowered.[19] Reflex effects can be minimized by slow incrementing of the infusion rate, thus slowly lowering arterial pressure. Blood pressure usually can be monitored noninvasively using an ultrasonic cuff. In patients with borderline blood pressure and severe left ventricular failure, optimization of preload and afterload lowering becomes even more critical. Placement of a balloon flotation catheter in the pulmonary artery allows assessment of both the pulmonary capillary wedge pressure and the cardiac output, and therefore allows more precise adjustment of both left ventricular filling pressure and peripheral vascular resistance.

Contraindications

Intravenous nitroglycerin should not be administered to patients with (1) hypotension (< 90/60 mm Hg) or hypovolemia, (2) increased intracranial pressure, (3) constrictive pericarditis or pericardial tamponade where an adequate filling pressure is critical, (4) inadequate cerebral perfusion, or (5) known hypersensitivity or idiosyncratic reactions to nitroglycerin or other organic nitrate preparations.

Absorption of Drug by Standard Infusion Sets

Because nitroglycerin is rapidly absorbed into plastic bags, it should be mixed only in glass bottles. Furthermore, 20 to 80 percent of the nitroglycerin will be absorbed during the passage through standard polyvinylchloride (PVC) intravenous administration sets.[7] This absorption through the tubing is neither constant nor saturable, and therefore no simple calculation will predict the amount of nitroglycerin actually delivered to the patient. In any case, the infusion rate should not be chosen according to the nitroglycerin dose administered but instead should be titrated to the hemodynamic response of the individual patient. The problem of loss of drug into and through the PVC tubing is eliminated by using special commercially available infusion sets that are relatively impermeable to nitroglycerin. Because all clinical experience reported in the literature used standard PVC tubing, the final nitroglycerin infusion rates required to obtain the same hemodynamic end point using the new tubing could well be considerably lower than published rates. Bolus dosing causes sudden and relatively uncontrolled hemodynamic changes and therefore is generally not recommended.

SUMMARY

It would appear that nitroglycerin, which has been the time-honored therapy for angina pectoris, has a much broader therapeutic scope. Since the Food and Drug Administration has only recently released intravenous nitroglycerin for general clinical use, other clinical applications may develop in the future. Intravenous nitroglycerin appears to provide predictable and rapid lowering of left ventricular filling pressure and mean arterial pressure in patients with ischemic heart disease. The ability to increase cardiac output appears to be greatest in those patients with severe left ventricular failure. However, anti-ischemic effects are evident in all hemodynamic subgroups. Compared with sodium nitroprusside, nitroglycerin appears to have more favorable effects on intercoronary collateral flow, pulmonary artery pressure, and intrapulmonary shunting. In the perioperative setting, nitroglycerin appears to be as effective an afterload-lowering agent as nitroprusside in the majority of patients. In view of its more favorable effects on coronary collateral resistance, nitroglycerin may be preferable to nitroprusside for many such afterload-lowering applications, especially in patients with significant obstructive coronary disease. With greater clinical use, intravenous nitroglycerin will undoubtedly prove to be a valuable new tool for the management of patients with ischemic heart disease.

REFERENCES

1. Flaherty, JT, Reid, PR, Kelly, DT, et al: *Intravenous nitroglycerin in acute myocardial infarction.* Circulation 51:132, 1975.
2. Flaherty, JT, Come, PC, Baird, MG, et al: *Effects of intravenous nitroglycerin on left ventricular function and ST segment changes in acute myocardial infarction.* Br Heart J 38:612, 1976.
3. Flaherty, JT, Becker, LC, Bulkley, BH, et al: *A randomized prospective trial of intravenous nitroglycerin in patients with acute myocardial infarction.* Circulation (in press).
4. Come, PC, Flaherty, JT, Baird, MG, et al: *Reversal by phenylephrine of the beneficial effects of intravenous nitroglycerin in patients with acute myocardial infarction.* N Engl J Med 293:1003, 1975.

5. COME, PC, FLAHERTY, JT, BECKER, LC, ET AL: *Combined administration of nitroglycerin and propranolol to patients with acute myocardial infarction.* Chest 80:416, 1981.

6. FLAHERTY, JT, MAGEE, PA, GARDNER, TL, ET AL: *Comparison of intravenous nitroglycerin and sodium nitroprusside for the treatment of acute hypertension developing after coronary artery bypass surgery.* Circulation 65:1072, 1982.

7. BAASKE, DM, AMANN, AH, WAGENKNECHT, DM, ET AL: *Nitroglycerin compatibility with intravenous fluid filters, containers, and administration sets.* Am J Hosp Pharm 37:201, 1980.

8. DAUWE, F, AFFAKI, G, WATERS, DD, ET AL: *Intravenous nitroglycerin in refractory unstable angina.* Am J Cardiol 43:416, 1979.

9. LEINBACH, RL AND GOLD, HK: *Intermittent and continuous nitroglycerin infusions for control of myocardial ischemia.* Circulation 56(Suppl III):194, 1977.

10. MIKOLICH, JR, NICOLOFF, NB, ROBINSON, PH, ET AL: *Relief of refractory angina with continuous intravenous infusion of nitroglycerin.* Chest 77:375, 1980.

11. ANTMAN, E, GUNTHER, S, AND BARRY, W: *Beneficial effects of intravenous nitroglycerin in a case of Prinzmetal angina.* Br Heart J 43:88, 1980.

12. COHN, JN AND FRANCIOSA, JA: *Vasodilator therapy of cardiac failure.* N Engl J Med 297:27, 254, 1977.

13. CAPURRO, NL, KENT, KM, AND EPSTEIN, SE: *Comparison of nitroglycerin-, nitroprusside-, and phentolamine-induced changes in coronary collateral function in dogs.* J Clin Invest 60:295, 1977.

14. FLAHERTY, JT, BULKLEY, BH, WEISFELDT, ML, ET AL: *Importance of early administration of intravenous nitroglycerin to preserve ischemic myocardium.* Am J Cardiol 47:490, 1981.

15. CHIARIELLO, M, GOLD, HK, LEINBACH, RC, ET AL: *Comparison between the effects of nitroprusside and nitroglycerin on ischemic injury during acute myocardial infarction.* Circulation 54:766, 1976.

16. MANN, T, COHN, PF, HOMAN, BL, ET AL: *Effect of nitroprusside on regional myocardial blood flow in coronary artery disease. Results in 25 patients and comparison with nitroglycerin.* Circulation 57:732, 1978.

17. WHELTON, PK, FLAHERTY, JT, MACALLISTER, NP, ET AL: *Hypertension following coronary artery bypass surgery: The role of preoperative propranolol therapy.* Hypertension 2:291, 1980.

18. KAPLAN, JA, DUNBAR, RW, AND JONES, EL: *Nitroglycerin infusion during coronary artery surgery.* Anesthesiology 45:14, 1976.

19. COME, PC AND PITT, B: *Nitroglycerin induced severe hypotension and bradycardia in patients with acute myocardial infarction.* Circulation 54:624, 1976.

Acute Myocardial Infarction: Pharmacologic Treatment in the Coronary Care Unit

J. O'Neal Humphries, M.D.

Optimal resources for the care of patients with acute myocardial infarction were recently updated by the Coronary Heart Disease Study Group of the Inter-Society Commission for Heart Disease Resources.[1] All patients with an acute myocardial infarction or patients suspected to have an acute infarction should be placed as soon as possible in a hospital unit with the resources described in this latter report.

In the coronary care unit (CCU), the management of patients with an uncomplicated infarction is so distinctly different from the management of patients with complications of the infarction that this discussion must necessarily be restricted to a discussion of the routine care of patients without serious complications. Discussion of the management of some of the complications of acute infarction is presented elsewhere in this book. The patient with an uncomplicated infarction would fit into Class I or II as described by Killip and Kimball.[2]

UNCOMPLICATED ACUTE MYOCARDIAL INFARCTION

Even patients without hemodynamic complications of the acute infarction are at very high risk of abruptly developing serious, life-threatening complications such as ventricular tachycardia and fibrillation, hypotension and shock, pulmonary edema, thromboembolism, and recurrent ischemic pain. Thus, the primary aims of treatment during this acute phase are (1) to reduce to a minimum the risk of developing the complications, (2) to immediately detect the onset of any complication and promptly institute the appropriate therapy for that complication, and (3) to reduce the work of the left ventricle while maintaining coronary flow and myocardial oxygen delivery.

ANXIETY

Anxiety and fear are common but undesirable during acute infarction because they tend to provoke tachycardia, hyperventilation, and cardiac arrhythmias. Efforts to reduce anxiety are necessary but often forgotten in the heat of battle. Preventive methods include a quiet, pleasant environment where the patient can rest and have some privacy while still benefiting from the reassurance that he or she is being closely cared for by competent professionals. A benzodiazepine such as diazepam, 2 to 5 mg, may be given orally three to four times daily to help relieve anxiety.

All unnecessary testing and procedures should be avoided. The purpose of all necessary procedures and drugs should be explained to the patient and family before the procedure. The indications for the drugs and procedures may be so obvious and routine to health professionals that they forget the lack of understanding by the general public. All one has to do to appreciate the general lack of understanding of medical care by the general public is to watch a motion picture or television show about medicine.

Sleep deprivation is very common in many coronary care units. Physician orders to obtain vital signs and laboratory studies throughout the night contribute to this factor. In the uncomplicated infarction, the major risk is the abrupt onset of a life-threatening arrhythmia, and this disorder can be monitored without entering the patient's room. In these patients, a 4:00 AM temperature is of little value. Perhaps a 4:00 AM blood pressure may detect an unexpected fall or rise that needs prompt attention, but this occurrence seems unlikely if the patient is sleeping soundly. The breathing pattern can be observed without waking the patient in order to detect the development of pulmonary edema. Auscultation of the lungs and heart can be postponed until the patient awakens in the morning. A sedative such as flurazepam, 15 to 30 mg, or chloral hydrate, 30 to 60 mg, may be given orally at the anticipated time of sleep. Room lights should be dimmed and the door to the room closed to keep out the noise of the unit, especially the noise that might be generated during the care of a desperately ill patient in a nearby room.

MORPHINE

Pain early in the course of acute infarction contributes to the anxiety of acute infarction and usually represents continuing myocardial ischemia. Pain can usually be relieved promptly by morphine sulfate, 4 to 8 mg, given intravenously. Repeat doses may be necessary. As much as 100 to 200 mg of morphine may be required. Care should be taken promptly to detect any adverse effects of morphine, such as respiratory depression, bradycardia, hypotension, and nausea. Respiratory depression can be treated with naloxone hydrochloride (Narcan) administered intravenously, 0.4 mg, at 5-minute intervals, but such therapy is rarely necessary. Nausea may be treated with small doses of a phenothiazine, such as trimethobenzamide hydrochloride (Tigan). Hypotension and bradycardia are the result of the vagomimetic effects of morphine and are particularly likely to occur in patients with acute inferior infarctions. However, atropine, 0.5 to 1.0 mg, may be given with the morphine in these latter patients, especially if the heart rate is relatively slow or blood pressure relatively low. If the heart rate is very slow (below 40 beats per min) or blood pressure very low (below 80 mm Hg systolic), then morphine should not be given.

In addition to the analgesic effect, morphine relieves anxiety and promotes euphoria, the value of which has been emphasized earlier, and it also causes both arterial and venous dilatation. This vasodilatory effect, in general, reduces the work of the myocardium. Reduction of the work of the myocardium in the acute phase of a myocardial infarction is highly desirable, as will be discussed later in this chapter.

Other analgesics such as meperidine have no advantage over morphine.

If morphine is ineffective in relieving the pain, there are a variety of alternative approaches to the control of ischemic heart pain, including the use of other vasodilators, the intra-aortic balloon pump, and coronary bypass surgery.

OXYGEN

Oxygen is usually administered at a rate of 2 to 4 L/min by mask or nasal prongs during the first 1 to 2 days of an acute uncomplicated infarction. If care is taken to keep the mask or prongs in place, an inspired oxygen content of about 30 to 40 percent can be maintained. The latter may be useful in correcting a mild hypoxemia that is often present because of impaired left ventricular function, even in the uncomplicated infarction.

In the absence of hypoxemia, however, the administration of oxygen does not increase the delivery of oxygen to the body tissues (including the myocardium) and thus is of little value.

Also, oxygen may cause arteriolar constriction and actually increase the work of the left ventricle. In the absence of hypoxemia and signs of left ventricular failure such as gallop rhythm or pulmonary rales, it would be reasonable not to administer oxygen, especially if the mask or nasal prongs are irritating to the patient.

LIDOCAINE

Lidocaine administered intravenously is an effective and relatively safe antiarrhythmic agent. There are three recommended methods of administering lidocaine during an acute infarction. Each method has its proponents, and each has merits to justify its choice.[3] The three methods are (1) give lidocaine to all patients with an acute infarction or strongly suspected of having an acute infarction who are seen within the first 24 hours after onset of symptoms; (2) give lidocaine just to those patients who exhibit warning ventricular arrhythmias; or (3) give lidocaine just to those patients who experience one or more episodes of ventricular tachycardia or fibrillation. These options are discussed below.

Ventricular fibrillation (VF) has been observed to develop in the setting of acute myocardial infarction in approximately 6 to 12 percent of cases. About one half of these patients develop VF in the absence of heart failure or shock. Such an episode is termed primary ventricular fibrillation (PVF) and is most likely to occur within the first hours after onset of symptoms. If these patients are promptly and successfully treated, their prognosis is relatively good and not much different from that of patients with similar infarctions who have not experienced PVF. Ventricular fibrillation that develops in the patient with severe left ventricular failure, manifest clinically as congestive heart failure or shock or both, is termed secondary ventricular fibrillation. Though the arrhythmia may be treated, the prognosis is not good in the latter situation because of the extensive damage to the left ventricle causing the heart failure and shock.

In properly staffed and monitored coronary care units (CCUs), the onset of PVF is promptly noted and treated. The patients who recover from PVF can be treated with intravenous lidocaine initially and with an oral antiarrhythmic agent subsequently in an effort to reduce the risk of recurrent VF. This approach avoids the unnecessary administration of antiarrhythmic agents to the 88 to 94 percent of patients who are not destined to develop VF. This method obviously reduces the incidence of side effects to the drugs, and also it probably reduces the cost of care.[4]

The concept of treating only those patients with warning arrhythmias is based on the assumptions that warning arrhythmias will precede the onset of PVF in the majority of patients and that these warning arrhythmias will be promptly detected so that lidocaine therapy can be instituted. Both of these assumptions have been challenged. There are a substantial number of patients who develop PVF who do not have warning arrhythmias[5–8]; and in many who do have warning arrhythmias prior to PVF, the interval between the onset of the warning arrhythmias and the onset of the PVF is so short that it is not practical to administer adequate amounts of lidocaine. Moreover, it is recognized that in most CCUs, many instances of warning arrhythmias are overlooked; this circumstance was established by comparing conventional monitoring with computer-assisted monitoring.[9,10]

The rationale for the routine administration of lidocaine as early as possible in the course of documented or highly suspected myocardial infarction is based on the following arguments: (1) Primary ventricular fibrillation usually happens in the first several hours after the onset of symptoms, and it occurs in 3 to 6 percent of cases. (2) PVF is often not preceded by warning arrhythmias, or else the warning arrhythmias are not noted. There are studies[6–8] to suggest that PVF occurs just as frequently in patients without warning arrhythmias as it does in patients with such arrhythmias; assuming the latter to be true, there would be no reason to arbitrarily elect to give lidocaine only to those patients with warning arrhythmias if the purpose of giving the lidocaine is to prevent PVF. (3) Ventricular fibrillation, even if promptly detected and treated, is associated with temporary reduction in coronary (and cerebral) blood flow.[11] (4) When lidocaine is administered properly, its side effects are minimal and reversible.[3]

Whether administration of lidocaine is to be given to all patients, just to those with warning arrhythmias, or just those with ventricular tachycardia or fibrillation, it is essential to give the drug properly. It is important to obtain a therapeutic blood level (1.5 to 6.0 μg/ml) as quickly as possible and to maintain this blood level as long as the high risk period persists or until another effective antiarrhythmic drug has been introduced. A loading dose of 75 to 100 mg is administered intravenously as a bolus over a several-minute period. Simultaneously, a continuous infusion of 50 μg/kg body weight/min (3 mg/min in a 60-kg person) is begun. After the first bolus, two to three more 50-mg boluses should be administered every 5 minutes. Alternatively, after the first bolus, it is reasonable to maintain the continuous infusion rate at 200 μg/kg body weight/min (12 mg/min) for 15 to 20 minutes and then to reduce the rate to 50 μg/kg/min. After steady state has been achieved in 3 to 5 hours, it might be wise to reduce the rate to 40 μg/kg/min; this method should maintain therapeutic blood levels and avoid toxicity.

The infusion rate must be adjusted to maintain therapeutic plasma levels. Premature ventricular complexes (PVCs) usually are reduced or eliminated, but their persistence does not necessarily justify adding or changing to another antiarrhythmic agent inasmuch as the lidocaine may reduce the risk of PVF without eliminating all PVCs.

If lidocaine toxicity develops, the dose should be reduced or another management approach chosen. Toxicity is recognized by tremulousness, drowsiness, seizures, and coma.

Lidocaine is primarily metabolized in the liver. Thus, if hepatic blood flow is reduced, as in congestive heart failure or shock, or if there is liver disease, it is important to reduce the dose of lidocaine administered.[3,12] For example, Harrison and Berte[3] suggest administering the same initial bolus over a longer period of time, a reduction in subsequent doses by about 50 percent, and frequent measurements of plasma concentrations.

In the absence of complications, the lidocaine infusion is continued for 48 hours and then stopped. This approach is based on the high risk of PVF in the first several hours of infarction and on the low risk after 48 hours.

If serious ventricular arrhythmias develop despite the aforementioned program, one might choose to increase the dosage of lidocaine by giving another 50-mg bolus and increasing the infusion rate, or one might elect to add (or substitute) another antiarrhythmic agent. Serious ventricular arrhythmias include frequent uniform or multiform PVCs, two or more PVCs in a row, and PVCs with very short coupling intervals (so-called R-on-T PVCs).[13] The greatest experience in the United States has been with the addition of procainamide. Initially, the procainamide is given as intravenous bolus doses of 50 mg every 5 minutes until an effect has been achieved or a total dose of 1000 mg has been given. The bolus doses are followed by a continuous infusion at a rate of 20 to 80 μg/kg/min. Most patients who continue to have serious arrhythmias despite the proper use of lidocaine will require the long-term administration of an oral antiarrhythmic agent.

The persistence or recurrence of serious ventricular arrhythmias despite the use of lidocaine and procainamide requires the consideration of whether any of the treatments may be provoking the arrhythmias. Obviously, care should be taken to ascertain that other factors that might provoke arrhythmias have been searched for and corrected as well as possible; such factors would include hypokalemia, acidosis or alkalosis, hypoxia, hypotension, and so on.

In the presence of sinus tachycardia or systemic arterial hypertension, consideration of the use of a beta-adrenergic blocking agent would be justifed if serious ventricular arrhythmias persist despite lidocaine administration.

If serious ventricular arrhythmias complicate sinus bradycardia and/or atrioventricular heart block, then the approach would not be to increase the lidocaine, add another antiarrhythmic drug, or add a beta-adrenergic blocking agent, but rather to eliminate the bradycardia by the use of atropine and/or an artificial pacemaker.

ANTICOAGULANTS

The popularity in the 1960s of routine anticoagulation for patients with uncomplicated myocardial infarction has diminished. This reduced popularity is probably related to the many reports that anticoagulation did not decrease the risk of infarct extension or recurrence and that anticoagulation could cause serious hemorrhagic complications.

Nevertheless, there are numerous studies[14–16] showing that thromboembolic complications, both venous thrombosis and systemic embolization, can be reduced by the administration of so-called "minidose" heparin and that the risk-benefit ratio is favorable if patients with recent gastrointestinal bleeding or known hemorrhagic disorders were not entered into the study. Thus in the absence of a contraindication, it seems justifiable to administer 5000 units of heparin subcutaneously every 8 hours until the patient is fully ambulatory. Middle-of-the-night dosing should be avoided, and the medication should be discontinued if there is serious local pain or bleeding. Early ambulation and the use of elastic stockings on the lower legs probably play a more important role than anticoagulants in reducing the risk of thromboembolic complications in the patient with an uncomplicated infarction.

If pulmonary embolism or systemic embolism complicates acute infarction, then full heparin anticoagulation is indicated to reduce the risk of recurrence, and, in selected cases, thrombolytic therapy should be considered.

THROMBOLYTIC THERAPY

Should all patients seen early in the course of an acute myocardial infarction receive systemic or regional thrombolytic therapy? Studies to answer this question have been underway for over a decade,[17] and a recent review of all randomized studies[18] has favored the use of these agents in selected patients. The authors of this review suggest that intravenous streptokinase therapy reduces mortality over the subsequent few weeks after infarction by about 20 percent and that the complication rate of thrombolytic therapy is acceptable. In many medical centers, thrombolytic agents are being administered directly into the coronary arteries if the patient is seen within the first few hours after the onset of symptoms.[19] Which patients should be treated with thrombolytic agents and which route of administration should be used are unclear at this time.

NITRATES

Nitroglycerin has many desirable effects for the patient with an acute infarction, including reduction in the work of the left ventricle, increase in collateral coronary flow to the subendocardial area of the myocardium, dilatation of the epicardial coronary arteries, reduction in pulmonary venous pressure and pulmonary congestion, and reduction in the size of an ischemic myocardium as assessed by thallium-201 perfusion scans and left ventricular contraction patterns.[20] Thus, it is tempting to suggest that nitroglycerin should be given to all patients who have experienced an acute myocardial infarction. However, nitroglycerin also has hazards if given to the wrong person in the wrong amount. It is a potent vasodilator (venous dilation greater than arterial), and it may cause profound hypotension in the patient who is hypovolemic or in the patient who is already hypotensive. In the patient with a normal stroke volume and low left ventricular filling pressure, nitroglycerin reduces both parameters and may cause serious hypotension. During the first few hours of infarction, the stroke volume and systemic blood pressure may be increased above normal (for that individual), probably due to release of catecholamines; but both tend to return to normal or even low levels as anxiety and other stimuli subside. If these patients were to receive nitroglycerin during the hypertensive phase, then disastrous hypotension could follow during the subsiding phase. If decreased cardiac output and hypotension result from the use of nitroglycerin, the patient's legs should be raised and the nitroglycerin reduced in dose or discontinued. If bradycardia accompanies the hypotension, atropine should be administered also.[21]

Nitroglycerin would appear to be indicated in the patient with acute infarction who has evidence of left ventricular failure (either on clinical grounds or on measurements with a Swan-Ganz balloon flotation catheter) in the absence of overt shock, and it would be particularly indicated in those patients with persisting or recurring ischemic heart pain.

Therapeutic blood levels and effective hemodynamic changes in the systemic and coronary vascular beds can be obtained by administering nitroglycerin sublingually, transcutaneously, or intravenously. The most precise control of hemodynamic response can be obtained by the intravenous route. The dosage is started at 5 μg/min and then adjusted every 3 to 5 minutes until the mean arterial pressure is reduced about 10 percent below the control mean arterial pressure.[20] The fall in mean arterial pressure is primarily due to the arterial dilating effect of the nitroglycerin. This dosage also will cause marked venodilatation and reduction in left ventricular filling and pulmonary venous pressure (and pulmonary congestion, if present).

Nitroglycerin is readily and continuously absorbed into plastic at an unpredictable rate. Thus, the drug should be prepared only in glass bottles and administered through special intravenous tubing in order to minimize loss.[20]

Intravenous nitroglycerin has a very short half-life, estimated at 2 to 3 minutes. Therefore, if hypotension and decreased cardiac output develop owing to the nitroglycerin, these effects usually reverse in a matter of minutes after the infusion is discontinued. However, if the hypotension and fall in cardiac output are not immediately detected by proper monitoring, disaster may result.

The intense hemodynamic monitoring required for the use of intravenous nitroglycerin is not warranted in most patients with uncomplicated infarction. In other words, the potential benefit of intravenous nitroglycerin to the patient without complications is outweighed by the potential bother and hazards of unnecessary instrumentation (or every-3-minute cuff blood pressure determination).

The dosage of nitroglycerin administered sublingually or transcutaneously to achieve the maximal hemodynamic effects described above is much well less defined, but it does correlate with serum levels measured by gas-liquid chromatography. Small doses, designed to result in some venodilatation and little or no arterial dilatation, might reduce ventricular volume and pressure and thus benefit the ischemic myocardium. The apparent response of ischemic heart pain to sublingual or transcutaneous nitroglycerin would favor this argument. However, no studies are available to indicate that the routine administration of small doses of nitroglycerin (or other nitrates) reduces myocardial damage, prevents complications, or reduces mortality in patients with uncomplicated infarction.

Currently, it cannot be recommended that nitroglycerin (or other nitrates) be given by any route to all patients with uncomplicated myocardial infarction. But nitrates may be of value in those patients who have evidence of mild left ventricular failure or those who have persistent or recurrent ischemic pain, and they are of particular value in patients with ischemic mitral regurgitation or ruptured ventricular septum. Careful observation and adjustment of dosage are necessary to avoid hypotension. Intravenous nitroglycerin probably should be reserved for those patients with frank pulmonary congestion and/or unresponsive ischemic heart pain in whom hemodynamic monitoring would be appropriate anyway.

BETA-ADRENERGIC BLOCKING AGENTS

For patients who have survived the acute phase of an infarction without serious complications, the administration of beta-adrenergic blocking agents beginning 4 to 10 days after the onset of symptoms appears to reduce the risk of death (including sudden death and other causes of cardiac death) during the subsequent 12 or more months, if care is taken to avoid giving the drug to patients who might be expected to develop adverse effects to the beta blockade (for example, those with bronchospastic asthma, bradycardia, AV block, or left ventricular failure).[22]

The value of administering beta blockers during the first hours of acute infarction is much more controversial. During the first 24 to 48 hours of infarction, deterioration of left ventricular function can develop so rapidly and so unexpectedly that the presence of beta blockade might be hazardous. However, one double-blind randomized study from Sweden where the administration of the beta blocker (or placebo) was begun as soon as possible after the patients arrived in the hospital did demonstrate a 36 percent reduction in mortality within 90 days in those treated with the beta blocker.[23] These investigators believe that lives were saved by giving the beta blockers immediately, and they base this conclusion on the fact that ventricular tachycardia and fibrillation requiring treatment occurred much more frequently in the placebo group than in the treatment group and on the additional fact that the treatment group had a 15 percent reduction in enzyme-estimated infarct size. In this latter study, 15 mg of metoprolol was given intravenously over 6 minutes and, if hypotension, bradycardia, or AV block did not develop, was followed in 15 minutes by an oral dose of 50 mg and then 50 mg orally every 6 hours for 48 hours and thereafter 100 mg orally every 12 hours. The results of this study are in contrast to those of numerous other studies in which no difference in mortality was demonstrated between beta-blocker-treated and placebo-treated groups of acute infarct patients if the treatment was begun as soon as possible after the onset of symptoms.[24–26] Studies are underway in which the mortality in patients receiving beta blockers immediately is to be compared with the mortality in patients not receiving beta blockers until several days after the onset of symptoms.

If beta blockers are to be used early in the course of infarction or, for that matter, even late in the course of infarction, great care must be taken to immediately detect adverse effects so that the dose can be reduced or the drug discontinued. In the Swedish study,[23] hypotension (blood pressure <90 mm Hg) and bradycardia (heart rate <40 beats per min) developed much more frequently in the beta-blocker-treated group than in the placebo-treated group, but angina and arrhythmias developed much less frequently.

Even if beta blockers are given only to those patients with elevated blood pressure and heart rate, these precautions are important because the hypertension and sinus tachycardia of the early infarction period may be due to high sympathetic activity that usually resolves spontaneously within hours.

CALCIUM-CHANNEL BLOCKING AGENTS

Calcium-channel blocking agents are potent dilators of arteries, including the coronary arteries. There is evidence that vasospasm may play a role in the provocation of some infarctions and some postinfarction angina syndromes.[27–29] Thus, it is reasonable to consider administering a calcium-channel antagonist to all patients with an uncomplicated myocardial infarction. However, studies designed to establish the value and hazards of these agents in this setting are not yet available.

SUMMARY

It is reasonable to consider treating the patient with an uncomplicated infarction with as many as 10 drugs: a benzodiazepine, a sedative, oxygen, morphine, lidocaine, a nitrate, an anticoagulant, a thrombolytic agent, a beta blocker, and possibly a calcium-channel antagonist. Obviously, experienced judgment must be used in selecting the appropriate agents for each patient. A properly staffed and equipped coronary care unit continues to be the most important preventative for unnecessary deaths during the acute phase of myocardial infarction.

REFERENCES

1. Yu, PN, Conti, CR, Jones, P, et al: *Optimal resources for the care of patients with acute myocardial infarction and chronic coronary heart disease.* Circulation 65:654B, 1982.

2. Killip, T and Kimball, JT: *Treatment of myocardial infarction in a coronary care unit: A two-year experience with 250 patients.* Am J Cardiol 20:457, 1967.
3. Harrison, DC and Berte, LW: *Should prophylactic antiarrhythmic drug therapy be used in acute myocardial infarction?* JAMA 247:2019, 1982.
4. Carruth, JE and Silverman, ME: *Ventricular fibrillation complicating acute myocardial infarction: Reasons against the routine use of lidocaine.* Am Heart J 104:545, 1982.
5. Dhurandher, RW, MacMillan, RL, and Brown, KWG: *Primary ventricular fibrillation complicating acute myocardial infarction.* Am J Cardiol 27:347, 1971.
6. El-Sheriff, N, Myerburg, RJ, and Scherlag, BJ: *Electrographic antecedents of primary ventricular fibrillation: Value of the R-on-T phenomenon in myocardial infarction.* Br Heart J 38:415, 1976.
7. Lawrie, DM, Higgins, MR, and Godman, JJ: *Ventricular fibrillation complicating acute myocardial infarction.* Lancet 2:523, 1968.
8. Lie, KI, Wellens, HJ, and VanCapelle, FJ: *Lidocaine in the prevention of primary ventricular fibrillation.* N Engl J Med 291:1324, 1974.
9. Romhelt, DW, Bloomfield, SS, and Chout, C: *Unreliability of conventional electrocardiographic monitoring for arrhythmia detection in coronary care units.* Am J Cardiol 31:457, 1973.
10. Vetter, NJ and Julian, DG: *Comparison of arrhythmia computer and conventional monitoring in coronary-care unit.* Lancet 1:1151, 1975.
11. Conley, MJ, McNeer, JF, and Lee, CL: *Cardiac arrest complicating acute myocardial infarction: Predictability and prognosis.* Am J Cardiol 39:7, 1977.
12. Zito, R and Reid, PR: *Lidocaine kinetics predicted by indocyanine green clearance.* N Engl J Med 278:1160, 1978.
13. Campbell, RWF, Murray, A, and Julian, DC: *Ventricular arrhythmias in first 12 hours of acute myocardial infarction.* Br Heart J 46:351, 1981.
14. Cooperative Study Group: *Anticoagulants in acute myocardial infarction.* JAMA 225:724, 1973.
15. Wray, R, Maurer, B, and Shillingford, J: *Prophylactic anticoagulant therapy in the prevention of calf-vein thrombosis after myocardial infarction.* N Engl J Med 292:146, 1975.
16. Wessler, S: *Prevention of venous thromboembolism by low-dose heparin.* Mod Concepts Cardiovasc Dis 45:105, 1976.
17. European Working Party: *Streptokinase in recent myocardial infarction: A controlled multi-centre trial.* Br Med J 3:325, 1971.
18. Stampfer, MJ, Goldhaber, SZ, Yusuf, S, et al: *Effect of intravenous streptokinase on acute myocardial infarction: Pooled results from randomized trials.* N Engl J Med 307:1180, 1982.
19. Ganz, W and Geft, I: *What is the role of thrombolytic therapy in acute myocardial infarction?* Cardiovasc Clin 13(1):163, 1983.
20. Flaherty, JT: *Intravenous nitroglycerin.* Johns Hopkins Med J 151:36, 1982.
21. Come, PC and Pitt, B: *Nitroglycerin-induced severe hypotension and bradycardia in patients with acute myocardial infarction.* Circulation 54:624, 1976.
22. May, GS, Eberlein, KA, Furberg, CD, et al: *Secondary prevention after myocardial infarction: A review of long-term trials.* Prog Cardiovasc Dis 24:331, 1982.
23. Hjalmarson, A, Herlitz, J, Malek, I, et al: *Effect on mortality of metoprolol in acute myocardial infarction: A double-blind randomized trial.* Lancet 2:823, 1981.
24. Balcon, R, Jewitt, DE, Davies, JPH, et al: *A controlled trial of propranolol in acute myocardial infarction.* Lancet 2:917, 1966.
25. Clawsen, J, Felsby, M, Schonau-Jorgensen, F, et al: *Absence of prophylactic effect of propranolol in myocardial infarction.* Lancet 2:920, 1966.
26. Wilcox, RG, Rowley, JM, Hampton, JR, et al: *Randomized placebo-controlled trial comparing oxprenolol with disopyramide phosphate in immediate treatment of suspected myocardial infarction.* Lancet 2:765, 1980.
27. Maseri, A, L'Abbate, A, Baroldi, G, et al: *Coronary vasospasm as a possible cause of myocardial infarction.* N Engl J Med 299:1271, 1978.
28. Oliva, PR and Breckinridge, JC: *Arteriographic evidence of coronary arterial spasm in acute myocardial infarction.* Circulation 56:366, 1977.
29. Schuster, EH and Bulkley, BH: *Early post-infarction angina: Ischemia at a distance and ischemia in the infarct zone.* N Engl J Med 305:1101, 1981.

Pharmacologic Management of the Myocardial Infarction Patient After Discharge From the Hospital

Howard S. Rosman, M.D., and Sidney Goldstein, M.D.

Therapeutic interventions in the post–myocardial infarction patient have been legion. The physician is frequently faced with a patient who is likely to progress to significant morbidity and mortality, often suddenly. The anxiety and uncertainty permeating the physician-patient relationship can occasionally lead to desperate and dangerous interventions, with associated risks exceeding those of the underlying disease itself.

Following myocardial infarction, most people are placed on numerous medications.[1] Drugs may be given to these patients to treat symptoms or signs related to myocardial infarction (MI), to treat risk factors associated with coronary atherosclerosis, or to prevent progression of the pathophysiologic process that led to the MI. These three categories of interventions encompass our present understanding of the pathophysiology of myocardial ischemia. However, our knowledge is limited. In fact, physicians must confess ignorance concerning the process leading to myocardial infarction. Because of the numerous variables occurring in arteriosclerotic heart disease, the only proof of the effectiveness of a specific drug is that which we can amass from careful, preferably randomized, prospective studies. After decades of therapeutic intervention in post–myocardial infarction patients, only beta blockers have been shown to be effective in prolonging life in survivors of myocardial infarction. No other drug has been satisfactorily shown to be of benefit. The clinical pharmacology of most of the drugs used in post–myocardial infarction patients are discussed in individual chapters in this book. This chapter, therefore, will concentrate on the indications for individual drugs in the post–myocardial infarction patient. We will review some of the prognostic factors after MI and the results of therapeutic drug trials. We will stress the options available in drug therapy and place particular emphasis on the side effects and adverse interactions of these agents, recognizing that marginal benefit from a drug does not justify its use if side effects or complications are great. Finally, we will attempt to place cardiac drugs within the overall perspective of total care of the patient after myocardial infarction.

PROGNOSTIC FACTORS

In order to plan a rational therapy for a patient surviving a myocardial infarction, the physician must be aware of pertinent prognostic and risk factors for subsequent infarction or cardiac death. It is important to focus on the fact that the 1-year mortality following discharge from the hospital after an acute myocardial infarction is between 5 and 10 percent. There are, however, subgroups at low 1-year mortality risk, that is, less than 5 percent, and those with extremely high risk approaching 20 percent.[2] Studies predicting mortality after MI collect information either in a routine manner or by using special techniques. Routine information includes history, physical examination, electrocardiogram, chest x-ray, and often arrhythmia monitoring in a coronary care unit. There are numerous retrospective and prospective surveys of large populations that use these parameters. Other studies are prospective with smaller populations and use more sophisticated tests such as dynamic electrocardiograms, exercise tests with and without nuclear tracers, invasive hemodynamic measures, and coronary angiography in order to develop prognostic indicators.

There is a remarkable consistency in the findings among this vast literature.[2] The Peel prognostic index lists six pertinent variables: age greater than 65, prior history of angina, hypotension, basilar rales, exertional dyspnea, and electrocardiographic changes with Q waves or abnormal ST segments and T waves.[3] The Norris prognostic index, following patients up to 6 years post–myocardial infarction, indicates that the degree of myocardial damage sustained is the one best indicator of subsequent survival.[4,5] The Coronary Drug Project analyzed 40 entry characteristics in 3000 men post–myocardial infarction and found that variables reflecting myocardial damage and loss of ventricular function correlate most closely with subsequent mortality.

Data gleaned from more sophisticated tests confirm these earlier studies. One-, 10-, and 24-hour continuous electrocardiographic monitoring in more than 2000 male survivors of myocardial infarction show that complex ventricular ectopy predicts subsequent death. This ectopy is strongly associated with congestive heart failure.[7–9] Exercise testing, 2 to 6 weeks after infarction, can predict subsequent unstable angina and death. Patients with diffuse ST segment changes, greatly reduced exercise capacity, and fall in exercise blood pressure are at particular risk. All of these parameters are indicative of large areas of dysfunctioning myocardium.[10,11] Coronary angiography and electrophysiologic studies demonstrate independent prognostic importance of left ventricular contractility, degree of occlusion of coronary arteries supplying the noninfarcted myocardium, and ventricular ectopy.[12–14] Yet many of these features are interrelated and are not easily separated.

In summary, once a myocardial infarction occurs, prognosis is most closely associated with age, amount of necrotic myocardium, amount of jeopardized viable myocardium, and degree of ventricular arrhythmia. Secondary preventive measures can affect only the latter two prognostic factors.[15]

CLINICAL TRIALS

As we have already emphasized, after MI, a patient's prognosis is closely associated with the amount of functioning left ventricle. The mode of subsequent cardiac death is usually another infarction or sudden death due presumably to ventricular fibrillation. Cardiac drug therapy is designed to prevent reinfarction and sudden death. Unfortunately, the etiology and pathophysiology of MI and sudden death are not well understood.[16] Therefore, clinical drug trials have attempted to alter what we currently perceive as the mechanisms of myocardial infarction, that is, further intravascular lipid deposition, platelet aggregation, thrombosis, spasm, and excessive myocardial oxygen demand. In addition, trials have been directed at the treatment of complications of myocardial infarction, notably congestive heart failure, angina pectoris, and ventricular arrhythmia.[17,18] A superb report by May and associates reviews the significant secondary prevention trials.[17]

Prevention of Intravascular Lipid Deposition

It is well established that elevated plasma cholesterol is associated with increased coronary atherosclerosis. It is less certain that it is a risk factor for recurrent infarction.[17] The relationship among lipoprotein receptors, cholesterol, and the development of atherosclerosis is being explored. The complex interactions with platelets, arterial smooth muscle cells, and vascular endothelium are imperfectly defined.[19,20]

Several trials have succeeded in reducing plasma cholesterol between 6.5 and 20 percent with various lipid-lowering agents. Earlier studies using estrogen compounds[21–23] were discontinued when serious cardiovascular complications of pulmonary embolism, thrombophlebitis, and increased myocardial infarction occurred. In addition, many male patients were unable to tolerate the treatment because of decreased libido and enlarging, tender breasts.

Nicotinic acid has been used alone and in combination with clofibrate.[23–25] Although the incidence of nonfatal recurrent myocardial infarction appears to be less frequent, patients on the agent show no difference in mortality. Intolerable side effects including rhythm abnormalities and gastrointestinal distress also occur.

Other therapeutic interventions actually increased total mortality without significantly affecting cardiac mortality. Dextrothyroxine has been shown to increase cardiac mortality and recurrent myocardial infarction.[26] Clofibrate may reduce myocardial reinfarction and coronary death, but total mortality is virtually identical to that seen in placebo groups in three studies.[24,25,27] A greater incidence of gallstones, thromboembolism, angina, peripheral claudication, and gastrointestinal carcinoma was observed.

In summary, it appears that the various lipid-lowering agents show no benefit in reducing mortality after myocardial infarction.

Inhibition of Platelet Aggregation

Platelet hyperfunction is observed in most patients with coronary heart disease. This platelet overactivity can cause vasoconstriction and vascular damage. It is not clear, however, whether it is a primary factor or occurs secondary to the damage inflicted on the endothelium by the atherosclerotic process.[28]

Three recent large multicenter trials have evaluated the efficacy of platelet-active agents prescribed subsequent to myocardial infarction.[29–31] The largest trial, the Aspirin Myocardial Infarction Study (AMIS), enrolled 4500 patients in whom aspirin at a dosage of 1 gm/day was compared with placebo. Compliance was excellent in this double-blind study; followup was continued for a minimum of 3 years. Mortality was 10.8 percent in the aspirin group and 9.7 percent in the placebo group. Three times as many aspirin patients had gastrointestinal complications, and twice as many developed symptomatic gout.[29]

All the other trials testing platelet-active drugs, including the Persantine-Aspirin Reinfarction Study (PARIS)[30] and the Anturane Re-infarction Trial (ART),[31] showed a trend toward decreased cardiac mortality, but in none was the difference significant statistically. Furthermore, the observation that these agents are effective in the first 6 months post–myocardial infarction was made subsequent to the inspection of end points. Controversy over the design of the Anturane study continues,[32] and it is likely that new trials with different design and more patients will be necessary to establish its efficacy.

Prevention of Thrombosis

The hypothesis that coronary thrombosis is often the final event causing myocardial infarction is supported by DeWood's recent observations at coronary arteriography during acute infarction.[33] Numerous trials of anticoagulation therapy performed in the late 1950s and 1960s had serious flaws in design and conduct.[17] More recently, randomized and blinded trials with these drugs have been carried out. The control group took placebo in two trials[34,35] and aspirin in a third.[36] In none of the latter studies was there a significant difference in overall mortality. In the German trial,[34] patients were entered 4 to 6 weeks post–myocardial infarction, whereas in the Dutch study,[35] all patients were randomized at 6 months to 6 years after the event. As anticipated, thromboembolic events are less and hemorrhagic problems more frequent in patients receiving anticoagulants.

Prevention of Coronary Artery Spasm

Spasm of the coronary arteries as a contributor to angina or myocardial infarction has intermittently been in vogue. Osler believed spasm was important, Prinzmetal reaffirmed the belief,[37] and recently Maseri demonstrated its occurrence during myocardial ischemia.[38] Rarely, patients without coronary atherosclerosis may have enough spasm to cause infarction or death. More commonly, however, spasm occurs in a vessel already partially obstructed by atheroma and thrombus. The spasm appears to be related to the release of thromboxane A_2, a potent arterial vasoconstrictor, by activated platelets.

There are no published randomized trials of the efficacy of calcium-channel blockers in preventing death after myocardial infarction. Recently, however, Gerstenblith and colleagues[39] studied 138 patients with unstable angina despite therapy with nitrates and beta blocker who were given either nifedipine or placebo and observed for 4 months. Though symptoms improved with nifedipine, myocardial infarction and mortality were distressingly and equally high in both groups.

Beta-Adrenergic Blockade

It is believed that beta blockers reduce angina by diminishing myocardial oxygen requirements. It has also been postulated that alterations in autonomic tone play a role in sudden death.[40] The sympatholytic effect of beta blockers is antihypertensive, antiarrhythmic, and perhaps suppressive of platelet aggregation. Because all of these diverse effects may be beneficial in preventing myocardial infarction and sudden death, it is not surprising that there have been 10 large randomized trials reported since 1974. The drugs studied include alprenolol, practolol, propranolol,[41–43] atenolol,[42] timolol,[44] and metoprolol.[45] The only drugs demonstrated to have unequivocal benefit in prolonging life post–myocardial infarction are beta blockers. In this discussion, we will pay particular attention to the Beta Blocker Heart Attack Trial (BHAT).

The BHAT was a randomized, double-blind, multicenter trial comparing propranolol with placebo in 3837 post-infarction patients. The patients were enrolled within 3 weeks of infarction and received either placebo or 120 mg daily of propranolol for 1 month, and thereafter propranolol was increased to 180 to 240 mg daily. The intervention group had a 26 percent lower mortality after 24 months (9.5 percent mortality in placebo group versus 7.0 percent in propranolol group). The benefit occurred independent of age, sex, or location of infarction. Side effects from propranolol were infrequent but included depression, hypotension, and gastrointestinal complaints. The results were sufficiently conclusive to terminate the study 9 months early.

The other nine studies enrolled a total of approximately 8000 patients. Eight of the nine studies showed a favorable trend toward decreased cardiac mortality in the beta-blocker group, with four studies reaching statistical significance. Also of note is the fact that the three largest studies all showed a significant benefit from intervention.[43,44,46] These studies prove that beta blockers prolong life after myocardial infarction.

The cardiac agents discussed thus far in this section are used in hopes of preventing recurrence of myocardial infarction. They either counter the known pathophysiologic phenomena associated with myocardial ischemia or prevent the abnormalities that occur at the endothelial blood cell interface, that is, intravascular lipid deposition, platelet aggregation, thrombosis, and spasm. Other cardiac agents, discussed below, are employed to treat the two most ominous prognosticators associated with myocardial infarction, that is, congestive heart failure and "malignant" ventricular arrhythmias. For these latter conditions, patients receive cardiac drugs primarily for amelioration of symptoms and secondarily to prolong life.

Treatment of Congestive Heart Failure

Therapy for congestive heart failure (CHF) includes agents like digoxin that increase inotropy; those that reduce afterload, such as hydralazine, captopril, and prazosin; and those that reduce preload, including diuretics and nitrates. Thus far, there have been no large randomized trials studying change in mortality post-infarction with these drugs.

Digoxin is of unquestioned benefit in controlling atrial fibrillation. Recent studies indicate that its inotropic benefit is sustained for months in patients with CHF.[47] Hemodynamic monitoring shows significant deterioration of cardiac index after cessation of digoxin.[48] It, therefore, seems reasonable to assume that digoxin is indicated in post–myocardial infarction patients with CHF. However, it has not been shown to prolong life, and one retrospective study suggests that it increases the mortality post–myocardial infarction.[49]

Hydralazine, prazosin, and captopril reduce symptoms of CHF and improve cardiac output acutely.[50–52] There is controversy as to whether these effects are sustained.[53] Studies examining whether these agents alter prognosis are underway.

Treatment of Ventricular Arrhythmia

The major mechanism of death in most survivors of a myocardial infarction is electrical, usually ventricular fibrillation. This terminal arrhythmia may be caused by acute myocardial ischemia, which all of the drug interventions discussed thus far attempt to avert. Antiarrhythmic agents are employed to prolong life by increasing electrical stability and suppressing ventricular arrhythmias and premature beats.[17]

Five double-blind, randomized studies have studied the effect on post-MI mortality of various antiarrhythmic agents including phenytoin,[54] tocainide,[55,56] mexiletine,[57] and aprindine.[58] The only study demanding ventricular arrhythmia as an entry criterion was the aprindine study. All others registered virtually unselected post–myocardial infarction patients. In addition, the studies did not attempt to match patients with comparable ventricular function. Three of the five studies showed higher mortality in the treated group[17]; and only in the aprindine study was the mortality lower in the intervention group. However, none of the mortality figures reached statistical significance. Phenytoin and mexiletine can cause distressing tremor and ataxia. Blood dyscrasias have been described with tocainide. Although ventricular ectopy can be reduced by these agents, there is nothing to suggest that life can be prolonged. Patients who survive a sudden death experience or who show repetitive ventricular ectopy on dynamic electrocardiography or electrophysiologic stimulation may represent a subset in whom this therapy could be lifesaving. Prospective studies are underway to better understand these puzzling problems.

DRUG THERAPY

Familiarity with important prognostic factors enables the physician to recognize a subset of high-risk patients in whom interventions might be attempted. Knowledge of the results of pharmacologic trials compels the physician to be cautious in administering drugs. Only beta blockers have been proven to prolong life after myocardial infarction, and the mechanism of their benefit is uncertain.

Decision Making

It is logical to treat symptoms in the post-MI patient. Even if it is unproven that drug therapy for angina pectoris or CHF prolongs life, it relieves suffering. Beta blockers should be prescribed routinely if there is no contraindication. We do not believe there are sufficient data to recommend the routine use of aspirin, dipyridamole, sulfinpyrazone, anticoagulants, or lipid-lowering agents.

It is reasonable to treat patients who demonstrate frequent or complex ventricular ectopy at the time of hospital discharge post-MI.[59] The immediate goal is to eliminate complex ectopy and reduce frequency by at least 85 percent. Although the long-term goal is to reduce the incidence of sudden death,[60] there are no data to substantiate this hope.

Clinicians cannot always wait for rigorous proof from uncontested large randomized trials prior to embarking on therapies. Decisions often must be made based on ever-expanding knowledge. Numerous logical regimens can be selected.[61] Wenger and associates assessed physician practice in the management of patients post-MI in 1970 and again in 1980.[1] The results, not unexpectedly, indicate an enormous variety of therapeutic regimens.

Side Effects

If the anticipated benefit to a patient of a drug is marginal and serious side effects or complications occur, the drug must be discontinued. The need for each drug must be repeatedly reassessed. For example, patients may take an antiarrhythmic agent for years though their ventricular ectopy was confined to the peri–myocardial infarction period. Whether or not they should take that drug, or any drug, forever is not known.

The careful physician will not await symptoms before considering potential adverse effects of medication. Side effects should be anticipated at the time of consideration and introduction of a new agent to a patient's regimen. Whenever the status of a patient deteriorates—whether via unpleasant symptoms, physical changes, or laboratory perturbations—the physician must exclude an adverse drug reaction as the cause. Points to be considered include whether there is an appropriate time interval between the occurrence of a given problem and the introduction of a drug, whether that reaction has been described with that drug, and whether the clinical state or other nondrug therapies can reasonably explain the adverse reaction. If a drug reaction is likely, the drug should be withdrawn as a diagnostic and therapeutic experiment. If the symptoms abate, a rechallenge with the agent can be considered.[62]

Table 1. Common and dangerous side effects of cardiac drugs[63–65]

Drug	*Side Effects*
Digoxin	Anorexia, visual disturbances, extrasystoles, gynecomastia
Quinidine	Cinchonism, diarrhea, increased ectopy, ventricular tachycardia
Procainamide	Drug-induced lupus, diarrhea
Disopyramide	Anticholinergic effects, CHF
Amiodarone	Corneal microdeposits, pulmonary fibrosis
β-Blockers	Bronchospasm, CHF, depression, hypoglycemia
Verapamil	Hypotension, AV block, bradycardia
Coumadin	Hemorrhage with overdose
Clofibrate	Increased gallstones, GI complaints, ? increased neoplasms
Cholestyramine	Constipation, malabsorption of vitamins K and D and iron
Hydralazine	Diarrhea, fluid retention, tachycardia, drug-induced lupus
Prazosin	First-dose orthostasis, somnolence, tachycardia
Methyldopa	Sedation, depression, hepatitis, hemolytic anemia, drug fever
Furosemide	Chemical abnormalities (Na, K, Mg, uric acid), ototoxicity
Thiazides	Chemical abnormalities (Na, K, Mg, uric acid)
Spironolactone	Hyperkalemia, gynecomastia, encephalopathy

This chapter is not the forum for an exhaustive analysis of side effects from cardiac drugs, but Table 1 lists some common and dangerous clinical problems.[63–65]

Drug Interactions

As with medication side effects, the practitioner must anticipate adverse drug interactions. A careful history regarding other prescribed and over-the-counter medications must be taken. Foods interact with various drugs, as might preservatives or pesticide residue.[66] The potential for side effects and drug interactions is virtually infinite. New drugs should be prescribed with caution. Their known pharmacologic effects should be reviewed by the physician and then looked for in the recipient. Unexpected effects should be scrutinized.

Computerized drug interaction screening systems[67] and reference texts can be of benefit but cannot replace clinical thoroughness and reasonable skepticism. For example, the synergism between quinidine and digoxin was recognized only recently. This combination was used for decades prior to the recognition that it caused occasional digitalis toxicity and death. It was not until 1979 that a group of British practitioners noted that two of their patients developed digitalis toxicity after quinidine was prescribed for ectopy.[68] This clinical impression was confirmed by plasma digoxin levels; it could never have been confirmed by a computer search.

Table 2. Cardiac drugs: selected adverse interactions*[64–66]

Cardiac Drugs	*Interacting Drug*	*Effect(s)*
Digoxin	Antacids	↓ Digitalis effect
	Diuretics	↑ Digitalis toxicity (when K^+ ↓)
	Quinidine	↑ Digitalis effect
	Sympathomimetics	↑ Ectopy
Quinidine	Anticoagulants	↑ Prothrombin time
	Digoxin	↑ Digitalis effect
	Barbiturates, phenytoin	↓ Quinidine effect
Propranolol	Clonidine	Paradoxic hypertension
	Cimetidine	↑ Propranolol effect[71]
	Hypoglycemics, oral	↓ Glucose
	Indomethacin	↓ Blood pressure reduction
	Lidocaine	↑ Lidocaine effect
	Theophylline	↑ Theophylline effect
Verapamil	Methylxanthines (caffeine)	↓ Verapamil effect
	Digoxin	↑ Digoxin levels[72]
	Propranolol	↓ Inotropy, chronotropy[73]
Cholestyramine	Thyroid hormones	↓ Thyroid effect
Methyldopa	Haloperidol	↑ Haloperidol toxicity
	Lithium	↑ Lithium toxicity
	Hypoglycemics, oral	↓ Glucose
Furosemide	Cephalosporins (esp. cephaloridine)	↑ Nephrotoxicity
	Chloral hydrate	↓ Blood pressure
	Digoxin	↑ Digitalis toxicity (when K^+↓)
	Indomethacin	↓ Blood pressure reduction ↓ Diuresis
	Lithium	↑ Lithium toxicity
	Phenytoin	↓ Diuresis

*Effects with anticoagulants, anesthetic agents not included.

When cimetidine was shown to potentiate propranolol effects by reducing hepatic blood flow, Melmon and Nierenberg predicted lidocaine might be similarly potentiated.[69] That interaction was described a year later.[70] Melmon and Nierenberg emphasized that therapy cannot be conducted by cookbook approach, but only by the reasonable application of therapeutic principles by prepared clinical observers.[69] Table 2 lists both classic and recently discovered drug interactions. It must be re-emphasized that this table is woefully incomplete.

NONDRUG THERAPIES IN THE POST-MI PATIENT

Although drugs play an important role in the care of the post-MI patient, their place in the overall scheme should be placed in clinical context. Some patients need no drugs after an infarct. All of them, however, need emotional and psychologic support. Hancock states that preventing psychologically induced invalidism may be the physician's greatest contribution to the patient.[74] Prudent diet and physical activity may never be proven to prolong life, but there is little doubt that the patient may gain crucial psychologic benefit.

Stubborn insistence upon drug treatment may endanger the life of a patient with critical coronary artery stenosis, where coronary angiography followed by coronary artery surgery or percutaneous transluminal angioplasty may be the only beneficial therapy.

CONCLUSION

> "The history of medicine has never been a particularly attractive subject in medical education, and one reason for this is that it is so unrelievedly deplorable a story. For century after century, all the way into the remote millenia of its origins, medicine got along by sheer guesswork and the crudest sort of empiricism . . . it was in retrospect, the most frivolous and irresponsible kind of human experimentation, based on nothing but trial and error, and usually resulting in precisely that sequence. Bleeding, purging, cupping, the administration or infusion of every known plant, every conceivable diet including total fasting, most of these based on the weirdest imaginings about the cause of disease, concocted out of nothing but thin air. This was the heritage of medicine until a little over a century ago."[75]

Lewis Thomas is more sanguine about the medicine of this century because of the development of the scientific method. Reproducible, meticulous examination of patients combined with epidemiologic studies of large populations helps us to understand better the natural history of disease. Randomized clinical trials enable us to determine whether our therapeutic attempts benefit the patient. Careful scrutiny of the individual after a new drug is introduced can minimize serious side effects and adverse interactions. By combining these techniques, we are able to plan a rational pharmacologic treatment plan for the myocardial infarction patient following discharge from the hospital.

REFERENCES

1. WENGER, MK, HELLERSTEIN, HK, BLACKBURN, H, ET AL: *Physician practice in the management of patients with uncomplicated myocardial infarction: Changes in the past decade.* Circulation 65:421, 1982.
2. MOSS, AS: *Factors influencing prognosis after myocardial infarction.* In HARVEY, WP (ED): *Current Problems in Cardiology.* IV, Year Book Medical Publishers, Chicago, 1979.
3. PEEL, A, SEMPLE, T, WAYNE, I, ET AL: *A coronary prognostic index for grading the severity of infarction.* Br Heart J 24:745, 1962.
4. NORRIS, R, CAUGHEY, D, MERCER, C, ET AL: *Coronary index for predicting survival after recovery from acute myocardial infarction.* Lancet 2:485, 1970.
5. NORRIS, R, CAUGHEY, D, MERCER, C, ET AL: *Prognosis after myocardial infarction, 6 year follow-up.* Br Heart J 36:786, 1974.

6. SCHLANT, R, FORMAN, S, STAMLER, J, ET AL: *The natural history of coronary heart disease: Prognostic factors after recovery from myocardial infarction in 2,789 men.* Circulation 66:401, 1982.

7. RUBERMAN, W, WEINBLATT, E, GOLDBERG, J, ET AL: *Ventricular premature complexes in sudden death after myocardial infarction.* Circulation 64:297, 1981.

8. RUBERMAN, W, WEINBLATT, E, FRANK, C, ET AL: *Repeated 1 hour electrocardiographic monitoring of survivors of myocardial infarction at 6 month intervals: Arrhythmia detection in relation to prognosis.* Am J Cardiol 47:1197, 1981.

9. KLEIGHER, R, MILLER, J, THANAVARO, S, ET AL: *Relationship between clinical features of acute myocardial infarction and ventricular runs 2 weeks to 1 year after infarction.* Circulation 63:64, 1981.

10. STARLING, M, CRAWFORD, M, KENNEDY, G, ET AL: *Exercise testing early after myocardial infarction: Predictive values for subsequent unstable angina and death.* Am J Cardiol 46:909, 1980.

11. MILLER, D AND BOHRER, J: *Exercise testing early after myocardial infarction.* Am J Med 72:427, 1982.

12. SANZ, G, CASTAÑER, A, BETRIU, A, ET AL: *Determinants of prognosis in survivors of myocardial infarction.* N Engl J Med 306:1065, 1982.

13. GREENE, H, REID, B, AND SCHAEFFER, A: *The repetitive ventricular response in man: A predictor of sudden death.* N Engl J Med 299:729, 1978.

14. PLATIA, E, GRUNWALD, L, MELLITS, E, ET AL: *Clinical and arteriographic variables predictive of survival in coronary artery disease.* Am J Cardiol 46:543, 1980.

15. SLOMAN, J, PENINGTON, C, SUTTON, L, ET AL: *Management of late phase of acute myocardial infarction.* In YU, P (ED): *Progress in Cardiology, 9.* Lea & Febiger, Philadelphia, 1980.

16. BRAUNWALD, E: *The present state and future of academic cardiology.* Circulation 66:487, 1982.

17. MAY, GS, EBERLEIN, K, FURBERG, C, ET AL: *Secondary prevention after myocardial infarction: A review of long-term trials.* Prog Cardiovasc Dis 24:331, 1982.

18. ROSMAN, H AND GOLDSTEIN, S: *Preventing a second myocardial infarction.* Cardiovasc Med 7:961, 1982.

19. BROWN, M, KOVANEN, P, AND GOLDSTEIN, J: *Regulation of plasma cholesterol by lipoprotein receptors.* Science 212:628, 1981.

20. OLIVER, M: *Serum cholesterol: The knave of hearts and the joker.* Lancet 2:1090, 1981.

21. STAMLER, J, PICK, R, KATZ, LN, ET AL: *Effectiveness of estrogens for therapy of myocardial infarction in middle-aged men.* JAMA 183:106, 1963.

22. THE CORONARY DRUG PROJECT RESEARCH GROUP: *Findings leading to discontinuation of the 2.5 mgm/day estrogen group.* JAMA 226:652, 1973.

23. DETRE, KM AND SHAW, L: *Long-term changes of serum cholesterol with cholesterol-altering drugs in patients with coronary heart disease: Veterans Administration Drug Lipid Cooperative Study.* Circulation 50:998, 1974.

24. THE CORONARY DRUG PROJECT RESEARCH GROUP: *Clofibrate and niacin in coronary heart disease.* JAMA 231:360, 1975.

25. CARLSON, LA, DANIELSON, M, EKBERG, I, ET AL: *Reduction of myocardial infarction by the combined treatment with clofibrate and nicotinic acid.* Atherosclerosis 28:81, 1977.

26. THE CORONARY DRUG PROJECT RESEARCH GROUP: *Findings leading to further modifications with protocol with respect to dextrothyroxine.* JAMA 208:996, 1972.

27. *Report by a Research Committee of the Scottish Society of Physicians: Ischemic heart disease: A secondary prevention trial using clofibrate.* Br Med J 4:775, 1971.

28. MEHTA, J AND MEHTA, T: *Role of blood platelets and prostaglandins in coronary artery disease.* Am J Cardiol 48:336, 1981.

29. THE ASPIRIN MYOCARDIAL INFARCTION STUDY RESEARCH GROUP: *A randomized controlled trial of aspirin in persons recovered from myocardial infarction.* JAMA 243:661, 1980.

30. THE PERSANTINE ASPIRIN RE-INFARCTION STUDY RESEARCH GROUP: *Persantine and aspirin in coronary heart disease.* Circulation 62:49, 1980.

31. THE ANTURANE RE-INFARCTION TRIAL RESEARCH GROUP: *Sulfinpyrazone in the prevention of sudden death after myocardial infarction.* N Engl J Med 302:250, 1980.

32. HOOD, WB: *More on sulfinpyrazone after myocardial infarction.* N Engl J Med 306:988, 1982.

33. DEWOOD, MA, SPORES, J, NOTSKY, R, ET AL: *Prevalence of total coronary occlusion during the early hours of transmural myocardial infarction.* N Engl J Med 303:897, 1980.

34. BREDIN, K, LOEW, D, LECHER, K, ET AL: *Secondary prevention of myocardial infarction. Comparison of acetylsalicylic acid, phenprocoumon and placebo. A multicentered two-year prospective study.* Thromb Haemostas 40:225, 1979.

35. The Sixty-Plus Re-Infarction Study Research Group: *A double blind trial to assess long-term anticoagulation therapy in elderly patients after myocardial infarction.* Lancet 2:989, 1980.

36. EPSIM Research Group: *A controlled comparison of aspirin and oral anticoagulants in the prevention of death after myocardial infarction.* N Engl J Med 307:701, 1982.

37. Prinzmetal, M, Kennamer, R, Merliss, R, et al: *A variant form of angina pectoris.* Am J Med 27:375, 1959.

38. Maseri, A, L'Abbate, A, Baroldi, G, et al: *Coronary vasospasm as a possible cause of myocardial infarction: A conclusion derived from the study of "re-infarction" angina.* N Engl J Med 299:1271, 1978.

39. Gerstenblith, G, Ouyang, T, Achuff, SC, et al: *Nifedipine in unstable angina.* N Engl J Med 306:885, 1982.

40. Zipes, D, Heger, J, and Prystowsky, E: *Sudden cardiac death.* Am J Med 70:1151, 1981.

41. Baber, NS, Wainwright-Evans, D, Howitt, G, et al: *Multicenter post infarction trial in 49 hospitals in the United Kingdom, Italy and Yugoslavia.* Br Heart J 44:96, 1980.

42. Wilcox, RG, Roland, JM, Banks, DC, et al: *A randomized trial comparing propranolol with atenolol in immediate treatment of suspected myocardial infarction.* Br Med J 1:885, 1980.

43. *The beta-blocker heart attack trial.* JAMA 246:273, 1981.

44. The Norwegian Multicenter Study Group: *Timolol induced reduction in mortality and re-infarction in patients surviving acute myocardial infarction.* N Engl J Med 304:801, 1981.

45. Elmfeldt, D, Herlitz, J, Holmberg, S, et al: *Effect on mortality of metoprolol in acute myocardial infarction: A double blind randomized trial.* Lancet 2:823, 1981.

46. Multicenter International Study: *Improvement in prognosis of myocardial infarction by long-term beta adrenergic receptor blockade using practolol.* Br Med J 3:735, 1975.

47. Arnold, S, Byrd, R, Meister, W, et al: *Long-term digitalis therapy improves left ventricular function in heart failure.* N Engl J Med 303:11443, 1980.

48. Chia-Sen Lee, D, Johnson, R, Bingham, J, et al: *Heart failure in outpatients. A randomized trial of digoxin versus placebo.* N Engl J Med 306:699, 1982.

49. Moss, A, Davis, H, Conard, D, et al: *Digitalis associated cardiac mortality after myocardial infarction.* Circulation 64:1150, 1981.

50. Franciosa, JA, Pierpont, G, and Cohn, JN: *Hemodynamic improvement after oral hydralazine in left ventricular failure.* Ann Intern Med 86:388, 1977.

51. Awan, NA, Miller, RR, DeMaria, AN, et al: *Efficacy of ambulatory systemic vasodilator therapy with oral prazosin in chronic refractory heart failure.* Circulation 56:346, 1977.

52. Ader, R, Chatterjee, K, Ports, T, et al: *Immediate and sustained hemodynamic and clinical improvement in chronic heart failure by an oral angiotensin-converting enzyme inhibitor.* Circulation 61:931, 1980.

53. Packer, MD, Meller, J, Gorlin, R, et al: *Hemodynamic and clinical tachyphylaxis to prazosin-mediated afterload reduction in severe chronic congestive heart failure.* Circulation 59:531, 1979.

54. Collaborative Group: *Phenytoin after recovery from myocardial infarction: Controlled trial in 568 patients.* Lancet 2:1055, 1971.

55. Ryden, L, Arnman, K, Conradson, TB, et al: *Prophylaxis of ventricular tachyarrhythmias with intravenous and oral tocainide in patients with and recovering from acute myocardial infarction.* Am Heart J 100:1006, 1980.

56. Bastian, BC, McFarland, P, McLauchlan, J, et al: *A prospective randomized trial of tocainide in patients following myocardial infarction.* Am Heart J 100:1017, 1980.

57. Chamberlain, DA, Jewitt, D, Julian, D, et al: *Oral mexiletine in high risk patients after myocardial infarction.* Lancet 2:1324, 1980.

58. Vandurme, J, Hagemeijer, F, Bogaert, M, et al: *Chronic antidysrhythmic treatment after myocardial infarction. Design of the Gent-Rotterdam Aprindine Study.* In Boissel, J and Klimt, CR (eds): *Multicenter Control Trial: Principles and Problems.* INSERM, Paris, 1977, p 43.

59. Ruberman, W, Weinblatt, AB, Goldberg, JD, et al: *Ventricular premature complexes in sudden death after myocardial infarction.* Circulation 64:297, 1981.

60. Webb, CR, Ritter, G, and Goldstein, S: *Sudden cardiac death due to coronary artery disease: Prediction and prevention.* Cardiovascular Reviews & Reports 2:695, 1981.

61. Braunwald, E: *Which drugs for MI? A family physician's guide.* Modern Medicine, September 1982, p 60.

62. Karch, F and Lasagna, L: *Toward the operational identification of adverse drug reactions.* Clin Pharmacol Ther 21:247, 1977.

63. Gilman, AG, Goodman, L, and Gilman, A: *The Pharmacologic Basis of Therapeutics,* ed. 6. Macmillan, New York, 1980.

64. DUKES, MNG: *Meyler's Side Effects of Drugs,* ed 9. Excerpta Medica, Amsterdam, 1980.
65. *United States Pharmacopeia Dispensing Information 1980.* The United States Pharmacopeial Convention Inc., Rockville, Md, 1980.
66. *Adverse interactions of drugs.* Med Lett Drugs Ther 23:17, 1981.
67. GREENLAW, C: *Evaluation of the computerized interaction screening system.* Am J Hosp Pharm 38:517, 1981.
68. HOLT, D, HAYLOR, A, EDMONDS, M, ET AL: *Clinically significant interaction between digoxin and quinidine.* Br Med J 2:1401, 1979.
69. MELMON, K AND NIERENBERG, D: *Drug interactions in the prepared observer.* N Engl J Med 304:723, 1981.
70. KNAPP, A: *Lidocaine-cimetidine interaction can be toxic.* JAMA 247:3174, 1982.
71. FEELY, J, WILKINSON, G, AND WOOD, A: *Reduction of liver blood flow and propranolol metabolism by cimetidine.* N Engl J Med 304:692, 1981.
72. KLEIN, H, LANG, R, WEISS, E, ET AL: *The influence of verapamil on serum digoxin concentration.* Circulation 65:998, 1982.
73. PACKER, M, MELLER, J, MEDINA, N, ET AL: *Hemodynamic consequences of combined β-adrenergic and slow calcium channel blockade in man.* Circulation 65:660, 1982.
74. HANCOCK, EW: *Acute myocardial infarction.* Scientific American Medicine 1:X-21, 1982.
75. THOMAS, L: *Medical lessons from history.* In *The Medusa and the Snail.* Viking Press, New York, 1979, p 159.

Comprehensive Drug Management of Angina Pectoris

Carl J. Pepine, M.D., Robert L. Feldman, M.D., and C. Richard Conti, M.D.

Angina pectoris is the symptom associated with transient myocardial ischemia. Transient myocardial ischemia ensues when restricted coronary artery blood flow eventually limits myocardial oxygen delivery relative to myocardial oxygen demands. The clinical characteristics of myocardial ischemia are well known and are beyond the scope of this review. Certain features of angina, however, provide the clinician with important clues regarding the pathophysiologic basis for transient myocardial ischemia. The clinical evaluation also provides the opportunity to exclude possible non–coronary artery causes of myocardial ischemia, such as aortic valve disease or cardiomyopathy. This chapter will be limited to a review of drug management of patients with angina pectoris caused by coronary artery disease. Before addressing these approaches, it is helpful to briefly review some important pathophysiologic mechanisms relative to myocardial ischemia and the angina syndrome.

PATHOPHYSIOLOGY OF ANGINA SYNDROMES

The pathophysiologic basis for transient myocardial ischemia and angina resides in at least three mechanisms.[1] Probably the most common mechanism responsible for angina pectoris is a *transient increase in myocardial oxygen demand* ($M\dot{V}O_2$) in a patient with restricted coronary blood flow. The increase in oxygen requirement eventually exceeds the capacity of diseased coronary arteries to supply sufficient oxygen to maintain aerobic myocardial metabolism. As cellular hypoxia ensues, myocardial function deteriorates, and aerobic myocardial metabolism generates a variety of metabolic byproducts that perpetuate this dysfunction. Changes in both mechanical and biochemical left ventricular function occur. Mechanical changes are reflected in left ventricular pressure and wall motion, whereas biochemical changes are generally reflected in the electrocardiographic ST segment or T wave. These changes not only are readily detectable when sought, but provide objective evidence that transient ischemia is present. After a variable period, the patient perceives the sensation described as angina pectoris. It should be emphasized that angina pectoris is not a uniform accompaniment of myocardial ischemia, and when present, it is often variably perceived by individual patients. For these reasons, the usefulness of angina alone as a marker of myocardial ischemia and guide to subsequent drug therapy is limited. Thus, when possible, the clinician should seek to identify objective manifestations of ischemia as a guide for drug therapy.

A second mechanism, operative in a smaller proportion of patients with angina, is *transient reduction in myocardial oxygen supply* through an abrupt decrease in coronary blood flow. This mechanism usually occurs as a result of spasm of a large epicardial artery. But recent evidence suggests that it could also occur as a result of arteriolar constriction in the coronary

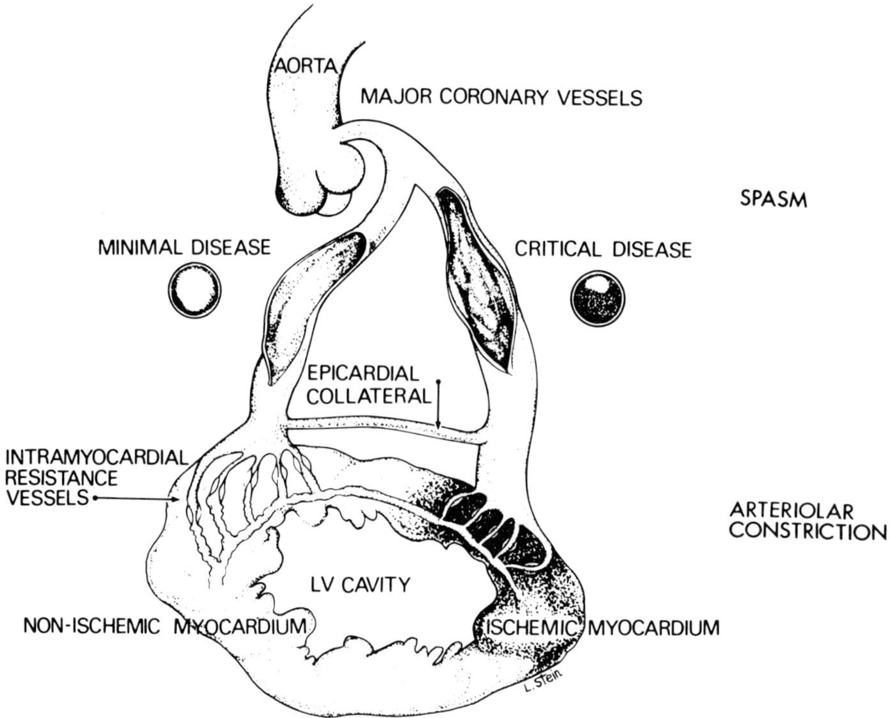

Figure 1. Diagrammatic representation of anatomic and dynamic factors involved in myocardial ischemia. In this schematic, flow to left ventricular myocardium occurs through two large epicardial arteries. One has minimal and the other has physiologically important (critical) atherosclerotic narrowing. Transient ischemia can result from the interaction of both anatomic and dynamic factors. Increasing oxygen demand would cause ischemia in the region supplied by the critically narrowed artery. Dynamic factors such as spasm involving either the minimally or critically diseased vessel, arteriolar constriction at more distal sites, and platelet aggregation can also produce ischemia. Under certain conditions even normal vasoreactivity could result in obstruction of vessels with critical or noncritical disease. (From Pepine, CJ and Conti, CR: *Calcium blockers in coronary heart disease. Part I.* Mod Concepts Cardiovasc Dis 50(11):61, 1981, with permission.)

bed distal to large-vessel artery obstruction.[2] In the latter instance, both intramyocardial and epicardial collateral networks could be involved. More recently, others have also suggested that reduction in coronary artery flow could occur at sites of large-vessel atheromatous plaques in coronary arteries with normal vasomotion.[3]

Third, there is a group of patients in whom *both mechanisms* operate, simultaneously or at different times, to result in myocardial ischemia and angina pectoris. These anatomic and physiologic factors are of prime importance in understanding the drug approach to transient ischemia. They are illustrated in Figure 1.

Patient History and Drug Management of Angina

The most important clues to the pathophysiologic mechanism responsible for ischemia can be obtained from the patient's history. These clues are important in the selection of appropriate drug therapy. For example, *angina occurring either at rest or at relatively low-level activity* is an important clue to possible transient reduction in myocardial oxygen supply such as occurs with coronary artery spasm. In such patients, clinical evaluation also provides important clues through assessment of simple hemodynamic determinants of myocardial oxygen demand, such as heart rate and blood pressure. Heart rate and blood pressure regularly show no important increase either preceding or at the onset of angina in patients with coronary artery spasm.

Another subset of patients will have symptoms occurring predominantly with effort or other forms of stress. *Angina precipitated by exercise* suggests that the basis for transient ischemia resides in an increase in myocardial oxygen demand. The increases in blood pressure, heart rate, and myocardial contractility that occur with exercise raise cardiac oxygen requirements to a level exceeding the ability of a diseased coronary circulation to deliver adequate oxygen. Thus, in the patient with regularly predictable effort angina, it is likely that myocardial ischemia is related to the increase of myocardial oxygen requirements provided through stress.

Finally, a subset of patients have symptoms suggesting myocardial ischemia *both at rest and with exercise.* Some within this group may exhibit widely variable effort tolerance. In this subset, the possibility of *both a decrease in myocardial oxygen supply* and *increase in myocardial oxygen demand,* as a basis for transient ischemia, should be considered. Where patients with "inappropriate arteriolar constriction" fit into this scheme has not yet been determined.

THEORETICAL SITES FOR PHARMACOLOGIC INTERVENTION

Theoretically, there are two major mechanisms that could be approached by pharmacologic means to prevent angina. One would be to prevent reduction in coronary blood flow and, hence, oxygen delivery. Ideally, to prevent a decrease in oxygen delivery, the precise mechanism responsible for reduction in blood flow must be identified. Unfortunately, this is not readily accomplished in many individuals. Alternatively, one could block coronary vasoconstrictor responses. Nonspecific blockade of coronary vasoconstrictor responses would have the potential for preventing coronary artery spasm. In theory, the drug should block only the coronary constrictor responsible for the patient's myocardial ischemia. Unfortunately, this approach is not yet possible.

The second theoretical approach would be to prevent increases in myocardial oxygen requirement. The necessity here is that coronary vasoconstrictor responses to this blockade of increased myocardial oxygen requirement be left intact, to prevent the potential for "coronary steal." Without appropriate coronary vasoconstriction in response to reduced $M\dot{V}O_2$, it is possible that blood flow may be "stolen" or shifted away from regions distal to coronary obstruction toward other regions. Fortunately, this mechanism is relatively easy to approach through a variety of sites. It is also important to avoid the potential for spasm as noted above. Mechanisms responsible for increases in myocardial oxygen demand are well defined and easily altered by vasodilators or catecholamine blockers.

DRUG INTERVENTION

The major classes of pharmacologic agents used in management of transient myocardial ischemia are vasodilators and beta-adrenergic blocking drugs.

Vasodilators

Nitrates

The cornerstone of drug management of angina pectoris continues to be organic nitrates. The action of these compounds include dilatation of both arterial and postcapillary venous beds. As a result of these changes, there is prompt decline in left ventricular systolic and diastolic pressures, ejection time and size.[4] These changes result in a reduction in myocardial oxygen demand. There are some compensatory reflex changes, however, that may tend to offset reduction in myocardial oxygen demand. These reflex changes include increases in heart rate and cardiac contractility. Nitrates also have a direct influence on the coronary circulation. They are potent dilators of the large epicardial coronary arteries.[5] For this reason, nitrates are useful when given to patients with coronary artery spasm.[6] In addition, nitrates dilate coronary arteries narrowed by atherosclerosis, and they also dilate coronary artery collateral channels. Evidence has been presented to indicate that blood flow to ischemic regions increases after administration of nitrates.[7]

The relative amount of dilatation occurring in the systemic venous and arterial beds seems to be dependent upon the rate, site, and dose by which nitroglycerin is administered. For example, when a relatively small dose ($\leq 100\ \mu g$) is administered directly into a coronary artery, intense large-vessel coronary dilatation occurs almost immediately. This dilatation appears more marked in mid and distal coronary arteries, possibly because the coronary artery wall is thinner and more highly innervated by alpha-adrenergic receptors in these regions. Little systemic effect is observed, and major benefit would accrue to patients who have angina as a result of coronary artery spasm. In patients with coronary artery spasm, this intracoronary route of administration provides almost immediate relief of obstruction and prompt increases of coronary blood flow.[6] When nitrates are administered into the systemic circulation rapidly and in large doses, as occurs with amyl nitrite inhalation or with nitrates injected into a systemic vein, intense systemic arterial dilatation predominates.[8] The latter effect results in a sudden decline in arterial blood pressure, which in turn evokes intense reflex-mediated responses. These responses include increased heart rate and constriction of some vascular beds. These sympathetically mediated responses tend to limit the hypotensive response, which is usually relatively brief. Total coronary blood flow under these circumstances declines because oxygen requirements and coronary perfusion pressure both decline. When nitrates are given slowly into the systemic circulation, as occurs with slow intravenous infusion or sublingual or topical administration, there is predominant dilatation of the systemic venous bed and only minimal to moderate arteriolar dilatation. Thus, changes in arterial perfusion pressure are minimal. Reflex-mediated changes in heart rate, myocardial contractility, and vasoconstrictive responses are minimal. The major effect is a reduction in venous return, that is, preload. Within the coronary circulation, ischemic regions supplied by arteries with important narrowings show an increase or no change in blood flow.[7] These beneficial effects of nitrates tend to make these agents extremely useful in patients with ischemic heart disease.

Clinical use of nitrates should, in general, begin with the lowest possible dose to achieve prompt relief of myocardial ischemia. Usually, it is wise to begin with 0.15 or 0.3 mg *sublingually*. Patients should be educated to use nitrates prophylactically prior to strenuous efforts that are known to regularly provoke symptoms. Patients need to be reassured that nitrates are neither an analgesic agent nor habit forming. Rather, they are extremely beneficial cardioactive drugs, and the patient should not attempt to do without them during an ischemic attack. Preferably, patients should take nitrates at the earliest time that symptoms develop. Prolonged or severe bouts may require additional doses.

Parenteral nitrate preparations can be administered by several routes. Intracoronary administration is used to relieve spasm immediately during coronary angiography; generally, 50 to 100 μg is administered by bolus injection directly into a coronary artery.[6,9] For intravenous use, to relieve acute myocardial ischemia, one may also begin with bolus injection of approximately 100 μg. Alternatively, one may start an intravenous infusion beginning at 50 μg/min and adjust the rate according to the patient's symptoms and blood pressure response. For continuous administration, the rate is titrated to the patient's hemodynamic response. The response is often widely variable—depending upon the patient's disease, cardiac function, loading conditions, previous nitrate history, and concurrent administration of agents that block the reflex-mediated responses (beta blockers) or exaggerate the vasodilator responses (calcium-channel blockers)—and therefore the dosage must be individualized. It is important to emphasize that when a nitrate is administered parenterally, plastic and rubber containers, tubing, syringes, and so forth must be avoided, because "absorption" in plastic occurs. This characteristic makes the amount delivered widely variable and often unpredictable. Glass syringes and infusion bottles, stainless steel needles and stopcocks, or polyethylene infusion sets will eliminate this problem.

Topical use is generally begun with 1 to 2 inches of 2 percent paste or ointment (depending upon the patient's preference) at 3- to 4-hour intervals. The amount is adjusted according to the patient's symptoms. In patients requiring large doses, the drug can be covered with an occlusive dressing to achieve high blood levels and avoid soiling clothes. Recently, three novel topical preparations have been introduced. Two preparations take advantage of the fact that nitrates can be absorbed through a plastic material. In one preparation, nitrate absorbed to a polymer gel is applied to the skin by an adhesive bandage patch. It is claimed that the active agent diffuses through this patch at a relatively constant rate into the systemic circulation. Moreover, this patch has been claimed to be active for 24 hours or longer. Another topical form uses nitrate absorbed to a small plastic wafer that is placed on the buccal region, just above the gum line. These wafers are comfortable and can be worn throughout the day without difficulty; the manufacturer recommends 6- to 8-hour changes. More recently, nitrates have been prepared in the form of an aerosol spray. The advantage of the spray is that the solution is quite stable when stored in its pressurized atomizer and has an extremely long shelf and storage life, as opposed to the relatively short storage life of the usual sublingual tablets. In addition, the spray is metered so that one application delivers approximately 200 μg to the tongue and buccal region. In theory, since the nitrate is already in solution, this preparation would act more readily than the tablets, which must be dissolved before being absorbed.

There are numerous nitrate preparations that, although chemically different, appear to act like glyceryl trinitrate. Many of these nitrates are available for sublingual or parenteral use. The preparations selected appears to be a matter of individual preference. Certain preparations also may offer a somewhat longer duration of action than sublingual glyceryl trinitrate.

Molsidomine

Molsidomine is a new non-nitrate vasodilator under trial for patients with effort-induced angina. This agent appears to have pharmacologic actions similar to those of nitrates but has an extremely long duration of action. Both venous and arterial dilatation occur, and the action is reported to last 5 to 8 hours after oral, sublingual, or intravenous administration.[10,11] A 2-mg dose administered intravenously prevented angina and ischemia-related left ventricular dysfunction during exercise stress in one recently reported trial.[10] The long-term effectiveness and safety of this agent need to be evaluated before additional recommendations can be made.

Calcium-Channel Antagonists

The use of this group of drugs to treat myocardial ischemia is particularly exciting. These agents are dealt with in more detail elsewhere in this book. The pharmacokinetics of currently available first-generation calcium-channel antagonists are summarized in Table 1. Since the chemical structures of these agents vary, the clinician should be familiar with each of the three drugs. These calcium antagonists also vary in their side effects, which are summarized in Table 2. The relative potency of these agents on various cardiovascular functions is summarized in Table 3. Because these agents have different chemical structures, a strategy will have to be developed by prescribers relative to choice of a particular drug for a given patient with angina. For example, a patient with angina who also has atrioventricular block or bradyarrhythmias should probably be managed with nifedipine rather than diltiazem or vera-

Table 1. Pharmacokinetics of calcium-channel blockers

	Nifedipine	*Verapamil*	*Diltiazem*
Dose			
Oral	10–40 mg q 8 h*	80–160 mg q 8 h	30–90 mg q 8 h
IV (μg/kg)	5–15	150	75–150
Onset of action	20 min	30 min	15 min
Peak effect	1–2 h	4–5 h	30 min
Excretion			
Renal (%)	∽80	∽70	∽35
Fecal (%)	15	15	65

*Also used sublingually.

pamil. In contrast, the angina patient who has supraventricular tachycardia should be treated with diltiazem or verapamil. The patient who has systemic hypertension or heart failure in addition to angina would be more likely to benefit from nifedipine or, perhaps, diltiazem. Verapamil must be avoided in the patient with heart failure. If the patient has a condition requiring that hypotension be avoided, such as left main coronary stenosis or carotid artery stenosis, the agent least likely to cause an important decrease in blood pressure would be diltiazem.

Since these compounds are likely to be given in combination with other drugs, additional considerations are warranted before their use. Many patients with ischemic heart disease are already receiving nitrates in some form. It is important to recognize that nitrates cause vasodilatation through a different mechanism than that of the calcium-channel antagonist. Thus, nitrates would be expected to intensify the decrease in blood pressure or reflex increase in heart rate occurring with nifedipine. Modification of the dosage of either nitrate or nifedipine is warranted in this instance. Combination of a nitrate and diltiazem should not cause this difficulty. In addition, in patients who have effort angina, beta blockers are likely to be considered in the therapeutic plan as outlined below. The combination of a beta blocker with nifedipine is highly desirable because nifedipine counteracts many undesirable actions of beta blockers, such as aggravation of peripheral vascular or airway disease. Nifedipine's reflex increase in heart rate tends to counteract the bradycardiac effect of beta blockers. Within the coronary circulation, both diltiazem and nifedipine will cause coronary arterial dilatation and counteract the coronary constrictor effects of beta blockers. However, it is wise to avoid combination of verapamil and beta blockers when possible, because of combined depression of cardiac contractility and AV node conduction. Since nifedipine appears to increase digoxin

Table 2. Side effects of calcium-channel antagonists

Side Effects	*Nifedipine*	*Verapamil*	*Diltiazem*
Cardiovascular			
Dizziness/headache	++++	+++	++
Hypotension/postural syncope	+++	+	0
AV block	0	++	0
Heart failure	0	+	0
Other			
Constipation/abdominal pressure	++	+++	+
Edema	+	0	0
Patients with side effects	∽17%	∽9%	∽4%
Drug discontinued	5%	1%	—

Table 3. Cardiovascular effects of calcium-channel blockers

	Nifedipine	*Verapamil*	*Diltiazem*
Vascular			
Coronary resistance	↓↓↓↓	↓↓	↓↓
Systemic resistance	↓↓↓↓	↓↓↓	↓↓
Electrophysiologic			
Heart rate	↑↑↑	0/↓EX	0
A–H interval	0	↑↑	↑
Left ventricular			
Cardiac output	↑↑	↑/↓	↑/0
LVEDP	↓	↓/0	↓/0

↓ = decrease; ↑ = increase; 0 = unchanged; EX = exercise.

levels by approximately 45 percent and verapamil causes as much as a 70 percent increase in free digoxin, both nifedipine and verapamil must be used with caution in digoxin recipients. The effect of diltiazem with digoxin levels has not been reported in detail, although there is anecdotal evidence to suggest that the combination is well tolerated. Benzodiazepines (e.g., diazepam [Valium] and chlordiazepoxide hydrochloride [Librium]) are some of the more frequently prescribed drugs in cardiovascular disorders. Their use in combination with nifedipine or verapamil appears safe. However, diltiazem shares a common chemical structure with benzodiazepines, and the possibility of interaction should be considered. Cimetidine, one of the most commonly used drugs in the world, is taken by many patients with cardiovascular disease or chest pain. Cimetidine causes a marked decrease in hepatic blood flow and microsomal metabolism. Since all first-generation calcium-channel blockers are metabolized in the liver, it may be necessary to decrease their dose when they are given in combination with cimetidine. Additionally, the major pathway for excretion of diltiazem is hepatobiliary and ultimately via the feces, whereas nifedipine and verapamil are excreted primarily by the kidney. Thus, diltiazem is preferred in the patient with renal insufficiency. Disopyramide is likely to be used in combination in some patients with angina who have dysrhythmias. Use of this combination in patients receiving nifedipine appears acceptable, but the combination of disopyramide and verapamil should be avoided, since verapamil could aggravate the cardiac depression that occurs with disopyramide. The use of diltiazem in combination with disopyramide may be acceptable but has not been studied in large numbers of patients.

The side effects encountered with these agents are another consideration (see Table 2). In our experience, nifedipine is commonly associated with side effects (15 to 20 percent of patients) related to an extension of its pharmacologic action, that is, intense vasodilatation (dizziness, flushing, erythema). In addition, a large number of patients receiving verapamil, particularly older patients, have constipation that at times can be severe. These side effects have not been a problem in our experience with diltiazem. Thus, diltiazem seems to be the agent of choice when the possibility of side effects must be minimized. It is also likely that in certain circumstances, combinations of the three first-generation calcium-channel antagonists might control manifestations of ischemic heart disease. The latter approach is particularly applicable in patients who experience unacceptable control of the manifestations of myocardial ischemia or intolerable side effects at higher doses of one agent given alone. Combination of two calcium-channel antagonists may effectively control angina and minimize side effects encountered with large doses of one agent. In our opinion, the combination of diltiazem and nifedipine appears most rational because it takes advantage of different sites of action within the calcium–calmodulin–light chain kinase system that controls vascular smooth-muscle contraction and relaxation. In addition, this combination tends to add some AV node slowing effect to the nifedipine. Combination of diltiazem and verapamil should be avoided because of potential to aggravate atrioventricular block.

Beta-Adrenergic Blocking Agents

Drugs capable of blocking beta-adrenergic receptors are very useful adjuncts in the drug approach to angina pectoris. These agents can be divided into those that (1) nonselectively act at both myocardial (β_1) and vascular (β_2) receptors; (2) selectively block the myocardial (β_1) receptors; and (3) have intrinsic sympathomimetic activity (ISA).

Nonselective Beta Blockers

At the time of this writing, the nonselective beta blocker propranolol appears to be the most useful agent in this class for management of angina. Propranolol, in adequate doses, reduces frequency of angina in most patients. The dose must be individualized, however, and is not readily predictable from either the plasma level or heart rate. Daily doses ranging from 160 mg to more than 1000 mg are not uncommon. The decrease in sympathetically mediated augmentation of cardiac contractility and heart rate, which necessarily accompanies effort, reduces myocardial oxygen requirements for any given activity.[12] To some extent, the systolic blood pressure rise that occurs with exercise is reduced and oxygen requirements lowered. These agents, however, prolong the duration of systolic ejection and may increase ventricular end-diastolic size. In theory, the latter effects partially oppose other actions of beta blockers that reduce myocardial oxygen requirements. Overall, the net benefit observed relative to prevention of angina and prolongation of exercise time with propranolol indicates that effects tending to reduce oxygen consumption outweigh any possible increase in oxygen requirement imposed by increases in ventricular size and duration of ejection.

Important adverse effects include cardiac depression, atrioventricular conduction defects, bradycardia, increased peripheral vascular resistance with aggravation of claudication, and increased airway resistance with aggravation of bronchospasm. Considerable controversy centers about vasodilator control of the coronary circulation and use of beta blockers in patients with suspected coronary spasm. Coronary dilatation depends upon both beta$_1$- and beta$_2$-adrenergic receptors.[13] Theoretically, a nonspecific beta blocker, such as propranolol, blunts coronary vasodilator responses, while alpha-adrenergic constrictor responses remain unopposed. Both epicardial coronary vessel constriction[14] and increase in coronary vascular resistance[15] occur after propranolol administration. However, proper testing has not yet been done to determine whether these changes in coronary caliber act to increase myocardial ischemia. Anecdotally, propranolol has been found to be occasionally effective, ineffective, or even harmful in some patients with coronary spasm.[16]

Other nonselective beta blockers include nadolol (Corgard), timolol (Blocadren), sotalol (Sotacor), and carteolol (Abb. 43326). Though they possess increased potency, increased bioavailability, and longer half-life, these newer agents all appear to reduce angina frequency in a manner similar to that of propranolol.

Selective Beta Blockers

Cardioselective beta blockers are, in theory, less likely to produce bronchoconstriction and to increase peripheral vascular resistance. Thus, atenolol (Tenormin) and metoprolol (Lopressor) may be used in management of angina in patients with symptoms due to bronchoconstriction or peripheral vascular disease. However, despite relative cardioselectivity, these agents can induce bronchospasm in susceptible individuals and should be used cautiously. It has not been determined whether these agents offer an advantage within the coronary circulation for the angina patient with both spasm and atherosclerotic narrowings.

Some newer beta-blocking agents also possess intrinsic sympathomimetic activity. These agents activate the beta receptor while blocking responses to sympathetic stimulation. Thus, heart rate tends to remain unchanged at rest, and exercise-induced increases are attenuated.[17] These agents may provide the vasodilating stimulus necessary to prevent coronary spasm or arteriolar constriction that occurs at rest and warrant trial in patients with these problems. Pindolol (Visken) is pending approval in this country for use in angina. Dosages range from 15 to 25 mg/day in three to four divided doses.

A new class of beta-adrenergic blocking agents also possesses alpha-blocking activity. Labetalol is the prototype agent of this class. In a recently published preliminary trial,[18] labetalol was reported effective in significantly reducing the frequency of effort and "spontaneous" angina episodes.

Platelet and Prostanoid-Active Agents

Recently, the role of prostaglandins in the pathogenesis of myocardial ischemia has been actively investigated.[9] In the presence of cyclo-oxygenase, arachidonic acid produces endoperoxides, which in turn are modified by specific synthetases to form either prostacyclin (PGI_2) or thromboxane (TXA_2). Formed within vascular walls, PGI_2 is a potent vasodilator and inhibits platelet aggregation. Thus, PGI_2 acts to increase regional myocardial blood flow. In contrast, TXA_2 synthesized by platelets is a potent vasoconstrictor and stimulates platelet aggregation. It has been suggested that, within a vascular bed, platelet aggregation, vasoconstriction, and vasodilatation can be altered by the relative balance between PGI_2 and TXA_2 production. With either reduced PGI_2 or increased TXA_2 production, the balance is shifted to favor vasoconstriction. Some investigators have proposed that such a mechanism may provoke coronary vasospasm, which could trigger acute myocardial ischemia.[20] Recently, marked elevation of thromboxane B_2, the major metabolite of TXA_2, was found during and after ischemia in patients with coronary spasm.

The observation that coronary spasm occurs frequently at sites of minimal atherosclerosis has led to the suggestion that vascular endothelium produces or releases deficient amounts of PGI_2 in atherosclerotic areas. Under conditions in which platelet adhesion and aggregation are increased, release of TXA_2 would result in vasoconstriction. Because of these findings, treatment with antiplatelet agents has been suggested, but early results have not been successful in preventing vasospastic angina.[22] Preliminary, acute studies found that aspirin, given in doses that reduced platelet TXA_2 production to negligible levels, did not prevent episodes of spontaneous angina in a small group of patients. Continuous intravenous infusion of PGI_2 in six patients with angina due to coronary spasm induced systemic vasodilation and reduced platelet aggregation but did not prevent ischemic episodes in five of the patients.[19] Nonetheless, various other methods to influence either platelet aggregation or prostanoids are possible. These methods include use of other nonsteroid anti-inflammatory agents, stable PGI_2 analogs, PGI_2-releasing agents, and specific inhibitors of TXA_2. It should also be mentioned that the first-generation calcium-channel antagonists, particularly verapamil and diltiazem, inhibit platelet aggregation. Studies using more specific platelet aggregation or TXA_2 inhibitors or PGI_2 activators are expected to shed new light on mechanisms of coronary constriction and may provide avenues for future treatment. At present, however, these agents are not recommended in the usual management of patients with angina.

Other Agents

There are several other agents that offer a possible beneficial pharmacologic approach for syndromes associated with restricted coronary blood flow and do not fit into a single general category outlined above. *Dipyridamole* is an example of such a drug. This agent inhibits platelet phosphodiesterase and could raise cyclic AMP levels.[23] When platelet cyclic AMP is increased, many platelet functions are altered. Studies with human platelets show that dipyridamole in combination with PGI_2, which stimulates adenylate cyclase, strongly inhibits platelet adherence to collagen and the subendocardium.[23] When used in combination with aspirin, inhibitory effects on thrombosis in small vessels in man appear potentiated. Recent studies also suggest an important effect of this combination on coronary saphenous vein bypass graft endothelium.[24] It is not clear whether this action on platelets and thrombosis relates to other effects, such as vasodilatation. Vasodilator effects result in an increase in total coronary blood flow and venous oxygen. In patients with angina due to coronary disease, we found that flow to both ischemic and nonischemic regions usually increases after dipyridamole. Regional flow increased within 1 minute after intravenous bolus infusion and persisted for approximately 15 minutes. In certain cases, however, ischemic region flow may also decrease without effect on coronary perfusion pressure, left ventricular pressure, or heart rate.[25] Results of clinical trials using intravenous or oral dipyridamole are conflicting. Uncontrolled trials often suggested potentially beneficial responses in certain patients with angina or acute myocardial infarction. A controlled trial in other patients with coronary disease failed to detect a beneficial response.[26] Usefulness of this agent in evaluation and management of patients with restricted coronary blood flow remains to be further defined.

Combination Approaches

Combinations of drugs have been used in patients with angina. The rationale for combination drug approaches is that because several different mechanisms are involved in transient myocardial ischemia, drug combinations that influence different mechanisms may be beneficial. There are some indications that combination drug therapy offers very beneficial responses or can lessen side effects. For example, use of *nitrates with beta-adrenergic blocking agents* represents a favorable combination.[27] Propranolol and nitrates exert certain opposite effects on $M\dot{V}O_2$, that is, nitrates induce reflex increases in cardiac contractility and rate, whereas propranolol blocks sympathetically mediated increases in heart rate and contractility, thus exerting favorable reduction of these oxygen-wasting parameters by a direct effect. Additionally, nitrates tend to decrease left ventricular ejection time and volume, whereas propranolol increases these determinants of $M\dot{V}O_2$. Though synergism in the pharmacologic sense is difficult to document in a clinical setting, overall results indicate that the combination of nitrates and propranolol produces a beneficial effect, delaying angina and improving exercise capacity. Objective documentation of these beneficial actions is provided by both reduction of pressure-rate product (for any given level of exertion) and improved ventricular function.[28]

Nitrates combined with calcium-channel antagonists represent another commonly used combination approach. However, since both agents are vasodilators, these agents may potentiate the hypotension and reflex tachycardia encountered when either agent is used alone. Because of this potentiation, dosage is usually reduced to avoid adverse reaction. Advantages of this combination are that sublingual nitrates have a much more rapid onset of action than the calcium-channel antagonists and can be used to relieve the acute ischemic episode. In addition, parenteral nitrates are readily available and when administered by this route, can be used in patients taking calcium-channel antagonists.

A final combination worthy of mention is that of a *calcium-channel antagonist with a beta-blocking agent.* The beta-blocking agent will attenuate the increase in heart rate encountered after administration of nifedipine. This drug combination has been shown to be clinically more beneficial than use of either agent alone. In patients with depressed left ventricular function, combination of a beta-adrenergic blocking agent with a calcium-channel antagonist that also depresses ventricular function, such as verapamil, could be potentially harmful. Likewise, in patients with AV conduction defects, combination of beta-adrenergic blocker and a calcium-channel blocker that alters AV conduction, like verapamil or diltiazem, could also be potentially deleterious.

SUMMARY AND CONCLUSIONS

Our current understanding of the pathophysiology of angina and myocardial ischemia includes both anatomic and dynamic mechanisms. The relative contribution made by hemo-

PREDOMINANT SYNDROME

Effort angina --	Beta blocker
	If intolerant or unsatisfactory response, add or substitute Ca++ - channel blocker.
Rest angina --	Ca++ - channel blocker
	If intolerant or unsatisfactory response, add or substitute another Ca++ - channel blocker.

Figure 2. Therapeutic strategy for patients with angina (in addition to nitrates).

dynamically important atherosclerotic obstruction and dynamic coronary artery obstruction, either by arterial spasm or arteriolar constriction, to the pathophysiology of ischemia in any given patient should be delineated. This information appears to be useful in identifying patients likely to achieve major benefit from vasodilators on the one hand or beta-adrenergic blocking agents on the other. A number of agents are now available within these two pharmacologic classes. There are some differences in action of these various agents that require thorough familiarity of effects of these drugs so that their action can be optimized.

Practically speaking, the large majority of patients with an angina syndrome will respond to nitrates. Nitrates are extremely safe and cheap; thus, their use for relief or prevention of the acute ischemic episode remains the initial treatment of choice. When symptoms are more than mild to moderate in severity, or unacceptably controlled in frequency using nitrates alone, other pharmacologic measures are needed (Fig. 2). In patients with a predominant symptom of *effort angina,* suggesting that a hemodynamically important atherosclerotic-type obstruction is responsible for the syndrome, beta-adrenergic blocking drugs can be very helpful. If effort angina remains unacceptably controlled or adverse effects occur, a calcium-channel antagonist may be added or substituted. These latter agents do not exacerbate bronchospasm or peripheral vascular disease, and they offer a distinct advantage over beta-adrenergic blocking agents in patients with angina who have such disorders. Where the predominant symptom is *rest angina,* or the patient has other evidence suggesting coronary spasm or arteriolar vasoconstriction, a calcium-channel antagonist may result in a very favorable response. This therapy should be extended not only to patients in whom coronary spasm occurs spontaneously but to those in whom it can be provoked by stimuli such as effort or cold. When spasm is superimposed upon hemodynamically important atherosclerotic obstruction, the favorable response does not seem to be as great as that seen when spasm exists alone. In these cases, coronary bypass surgery, plexectomy, and other nonpharmacologic approaches may have to be added to the pharmacologic regimen. Recommendations for such nonpharmacologic approaches, however, require a demonstration that spasm is occurring in and about the area of fixed atherosclerotic obstruction and not occurring in other vessels or over the entire course of the mid and distal coronary vessel.

We wish to emphasize that angina can be acceptably controlled in the vast majority of patients by using comprehensive drug management as outlined in this section. However, certain subsets of patients with angina will have improved life styles and even reduced mortality with bypass surgery. Thus, control of angina per se does not relieve the clinician of the obligation to pursue diagnostic measures aimed at defining the extent and severity of coronary artery disease.

REFERENCES

1. Pepine, CJ and Conti, CR: *Calcium blockers in coronary heart disease.* Mod Concepts Cardiovasc Dis 50:61, 72, 1981.
2. Feldman, RL, Whittle, JL, Pepine, CJ, et al: *Regional coronary angiographic observations during cold stimulation.* Am Heart J 102:822, 1981.
3. Epstein, SE and Talbot, TL: *Dynamic coronary tone in precipitation, exacerbation and relief of angina pectoris.* Am J Cardiol 48:797, 1981.
4. Abrams, J: *Nitroglycerin and long-acting nitrates.* N Engl J Med 302:1234, 1980.
5. Feldman, RL, Pepine, CJ, Curry, RC, et al: *Coronary artery response to graded doses of nitroglycerin.* Am J Cardiol 43:91, 1979.
6. Pepine, CJ, Feldman, RL, and Conti, CR: *Action of intracoronary nitroglycerin in refractory coronary artery spasm.* Circulation 65:411, 1982.
7. Mehta, J and Pepine, CJ: *Effect of sublingual nitroglycerin on regional coronary flow in patients with and without coronary disease.* Circulation 58:803, 1978.
8. Mason, DT, Zelis, R, and Amsterdam, EA: *Action of the nitrates on the peripheral circulation and myocardial oxygen consumption. Significance in relief of angina pectoris.* Chest 59:296, 1971.
9. Feldman, RL, Mad, D, Pepine, CJ, et al: *Analysis of coronary response to various doses of intravenous nitroglycerin.* Circulation 66:342, 1982.
10. Detry, JMR, Melin, J, Brasseur, L, et al: *Hemodynamic effects of molsidomine at rest and during submaximal and maximal exercise in patients with coronary artery disease limited to exertional angina pectoris.* Am J Cardiol 47:109, 1981.
11. Takeshita, A, Nakamura, M, Tajimi, T, et al: *Long-lasting effect of oral molsidomine on exercise performance.* Circulation 55:401, 1977.
12. Dwyer, EM Jr, Wiener, L, Cox, JW: *Effects of beta-adrenergic blockade (propranolol) on left ventricular hemodynamics and the electrocardiogram during exercise-induced angina pectoris.* Circulation 38:250, 1968.
13. Vatner, SF, Hintze, TH, and Macho, P: *Regulation of large coronary arteries by β-adrenergic mechanisms in the conscious dog.* Circ Res 51:56, 1982.
14. Macho, P, Hintze, TH, and Vatner, SF: *Regulation of large coronary arteries by increases in myocardial metabolic demands in conscious dogs.* Circ Res 49:594, 1981.
15. Schang, SJ and Pepine, CJ: *Effects of propranolol on coronary hemodynamic and metabolic responses to tachycardia stress in patients with and without coronary disease.* Cath Cardiovasc Diag 3:22, 1977.
16. Pepine, CJ and Conti, CR: *Acute and chronic heart disease—coronary artery spasm: An important pathophysiologic consideration.* In Rosen, KM (ed): *Current Cardiology.* Houghton Mifflin, Boston, 1980.
17. Frishman, WH, Kostis, J, Strom, J, et al: *Comparison of pindolol and propranolol in treatment of patients with angina pectoris.* In Frishman, WH (ed): *Clinical Pharmacology of the Beta-Adrenergic Blocking Drugs.* Appleton-Century-Crofts, New York, 1980.
18. Halparin, S, Frishman, W, Kirschner, M, et al: *Clinical pharmacology of the new beta adrenergic blocking drugs. Part II. Effects of oral labetalol in patients with both angina pectoris and hypertension. Preliminary experience.* Am Heart J 99:388, 1980.
19. Maseri, A, Chierchia, S, and L'Abbate, A: *Pathogenetic mechanism underlying the clinical events associated with atherosclerotic heart disease.* Circulation 62(Suppl V):3, 1980.
20. Lefler, A, Ogletree, M, Smith, J, et al: *Prostacycline: A potentially valuable agent for preserving myocardial tissue in myocardial ischemia.* Science 260:52, 1978.
21. Robertson, RM, Robertson, D, Roberts, LJ, et al: *Thromboxane A_2 in vasotonic angina pectoris: Evidence from direct measurements and inhibitor trials.* N Engl J Med 304:998, 1981.
22. Chierchia, S, de Caterina, R, Crea, F, et al: *Failure of thromboxane A_2 blockade to prevent attacks of vasospastic angina.* Circulation 66:702, 1982.
23. Packham, M and Mustard, JF: *Pharmacology of platelet-affecting drugs.* Circulation 62(Suppl V):26, 1980.
24. Chesebro, JH, Clements, IP, Fuster, V, et al: *A platelet-inhibitor-drug trial in coronary-artery bypass operations. Benefit of perioperative dipyridamole and aspirin therapy on early postoperative vein-graft patency.* N Engl J Med 307:73, 1982.
25. Feldman, RL, Nichols, WW, Pepine, CJ, et al: *Acute effect of intravenous dipyridamole on regional coronary hemodynamics and metabolism.* Circulation 64:333, 1981.

26. KINSELLA, D, TROUP, W, AND MCGREGOR, M: *Studies with a new coronary vasodilator drug, Persantin.* Am Heart J 63:146, 1962.

27. SCHANG, SJ AND PEPINE, CJ: *Coronary hemodynamic and metabolic effects of nitroglycerin in patients pretreated with propranolol.* Br Heart J 40:1221, 1978.

28. WEINER, L, DWYER, EM, AND COX, JW: *Hemodynamic effects of nitroglycerin, propranolol and their combination in coronary heart disease.* Circulation 32:623, 1969.

The Clinical Pharmacology of Antiarrhythmic Drugs

P.C. Adams, B.A., M.R.C.P., R.W.F. Campbell, F.R.C.P., and D.G. Julian, M.D., F.R.C.P.

Increased appreciation of the clinical importance of arrhythmias and mounting dissatisfaction with the efficacy and safety of currently available antiarrhythmic agents have led to a plethora of new drugs, many of which have yet to be fully evaluated. This chapter is concerned with the classification of both old and new drugs, and their pharmacokinetics, pharmacodynamics, and side effects.

CLASSIFICATION OF ANTIARRHYTHMIC DRUGS

Disorders of impulse generation and impulse conduction, together or separately, are responsible for the production of arrhythmias. Antiarrhythmic drugs alter both. They act in a number of different ways that have been variously classified by Hoffman and Bigger,[1] Touboul,[2] and Gettes.[3] However, the classification of antiarrhythmic actions suggested by Vaughan Williams[4] is the most popular and most clinically useful. This scheme classifies antiarrhythmic drug actions by their electrophysiologic effects on normal myocardial tissue in vitro. Four major classes of action, and possibly a fifth,[5] have been recognized by investigating the cellular electrophysiologic actions of antiarrhythmic drugs. Although the predominant possession of one of these classes of action explains the antiarrhythmic efficacy of currently available agents (Table 1), they have subsidiary actions on cellular electrophysiology and on autonomic tone that complicate prediction of their action on the intact circulation (Tables 2 and 3).

Class 1 Antiarrhythmic Action

Drugs with class 1 action depress the maximum rate of depolarization in atrial, His-Purkinje, and ventricular myocardial cells by reducing the magnitude of the inward sodium current during phase 0 of the action potential.[4] This action can be inferred from changes in action potential characteristics or, more directly, identified in voltage clamp experiments that can measure current flow accurately at different transmembrane potentials. This reduction in maximum rate of depolarization reduces conduction velocity and increases the size of a stimulus necessary to produce an action potential.

Drugs with class 1 action also alter the period for which cardiac tissue remains inexcitable following a depolarization. Following phase 0, sodium channels are inactivated to prevent further flux of sodium ions into the cell. Sufficient sodium channels have to recover from this inactivation before a further action potential can be produced. Two factors determine the rate of recovery. The first is the membrane potential. Recovery from inactivation does not occur

Table 1. The Vaughan Williams classification, applied to some antiarrhythmic drugs

	Class 1	*Class 2*	*Class 3*	*Class 4*	
Quinidine	+++		+		Group 1a
Procainamide	+++		+		
Disopyramide	+++		+		
Lidocaine	+++		−		Group 1b
Mexiletine	+++		−		
Diphenylhydantoin	+++		−		
Tocainide	+++		−		
Aprindine	+++		−		
Encainide	+++		0		Group 1c
Flecainide	+++		0		
Lorcainide	+++		0		
Amiodarone		±	+++		
Bretylium	±	+	+++		
Sotalol		+++	+++?		
Verapamil				+++	

Key:
+++ major antiarrhythmic property
+ subsidiary action
0 no effect
− opposite effect
± minor effect of uncertain significance

until the membrane potential has become more negative than −60 mV. Thus, during the plateau of the action potential, the sodium channels remain inactivated and the cell is inexcitable. Even if the membrane potential is abruptly changed to potentials more negative than −60 mV, however, there is a delay in the recovery from inactivation. This delay further extends the period during which the cell remains inexcitable. Drugs with class 1 action affect either the relationship between membrane potential and reactivation, or the time course of the recovery from inactivation.

Both the actions on depolarization and repolarization are antiarrhythmic. Changes in conduction velocity can abolish re-entrant arrhythmias that are dependent on critical conditions of conduction velocity for their maintenance. If the threshold for excitation is increased, abnormal impulses are less likely to propagate. An increase in the period during which cells remain inexcitable reduces the maximum frequency at which they can depolarize. Again, this alteration can change the critical properties of a re-entrant circuit.

Drugs with class 1 action have little effect on the resting potential of the cell, but diastolic (phase 4) depolarization, present in automatic cells, is reduced by concentrations of the drugs much lower than those needed to depress the maximum rate of depolarization. This action may abolish automatic rhythms.

Drugs With Class 1 Action

Three groups of drugs possess class 1 antiarrhythmic actions. Quinidine, procainamide, and disopyramide all lengthen action potential duration and effective refractory period. They do this in atrial, ventricular, and conducting system tissues. They are antiarrhythmic because they depress maximum rate of depolarization and also because they prolong refractoriness. This group of drugs is designated group 1a.

Lidocaine, tocainide, diphenylhydantoin, and mexiletine reduce action potential duration, by increasing outward potassium current. Despite prolonging the time dependence of the recovery from inactivation, the overall effective refractory period is shortened in ventricular

Table 2. Clinical electrophysiology

	Sinus Node		*AV Node*		*Refractoriness*				*Conduction Intervals*				
Drug	*Normal*	*Diseased*	*Normal*	*Diseased*	*Atria*	*AVN*	*HP*	*Vent*	*PR*	*QRS*	*QT*	*AH*	*HV*
Quinidine	+±	−	+	±	+	−	+	+	±	+	+	−	+
Procainamide	0	±	±	±	+	−	+	+	0	+	±	±	++
Disopyramide	±	±	±	±	±	±	+	+	±	+	+	±	+
with atropine	−	−	−	−	+	+	+	+	+	++	++	+	++
Lidocaine	0	−rare	0	−rare	0	0	−	−	0	0	0−	0− +rare	0 −rare
Mexiletine	0	−rare	0	−rare	0	0	±	±	0	0	0	0	0 −rare
Diphenylhydantoin	0	−rare	0	−rare	0	0	−	0−	0	0	0	0±	0
Tocainide	0−	−rare	0	−rare	0	0	0 −rare	0 −rare	0	0	0	0±	0
Aprindine	−	−	−	−	0	+	+	0	+	+	0	+	+
Encainide	0	?	0±	?	0	0	++	+	+	++	+	±	++
Flecainide	0	?	−	−	+	+	?	+	+	++	0+	+	+
Lorcainide	±	?	0	−	0	±	?	0	+	++	0+	0+	+
Amiodarone	−−	−	±	−−	++	+	+	++	+	0	++	+	0
Bretylium	Vary greatly due to autonomic effects												
Sotalol	−−	−−	−	−−	+	+	0?	++	0+	0	+	+	0
Verapamil	±	−	−	−−	0	+	0	0	0+	0	0	+	0

Key:
++ marked increase
\+ significant increase
± variable effect
0+ no or small change
0 no effect
− significant suppression
−− marked suppression
? unsure

Table 3. Autonomic effects of antiarrhythmic agents

	Sympathetic Effects	*Parasympathetic Effects*
Quinidine	Alpha blocking	Mild vagolytic
Procainamide	Ganglion blocking	
Disopyramide		Strongly vagolytic
Lidocaine		
Diphenylhydantoin	Sympathomimetic, by CNS effect	
Tocainide		
Mexiletine		
Encainide		Mild vagolytic
Flecainide		
Lorcainide		Mild vagolytic
Sotalol	Nonselective beta blockade	
Amiodarone	Noncompetitive sympatholytic	
Bretylium	Initial norepinephrine release; later depletion, thus sympatholysis	
Verapamil	Mild noncompetitive sympatholytic	

tissue.[6] This group of drugs is designated 1b. The antiarrhythmic actions of drugs in this group are enhanced by conditions that occur in association with or during arrhythmias. Class 1 action is enhanced at rapid rates of firing. Lidocaine markedly depresses the maximum rate of depolarization in ischemic tissue,[7] more so than in normal tissue. Its action on the effective refractory period is exaggerated by the high extracellular potassium concentrations that are a feature of both ischemic tissue and tissue that is firing rapidly.

A third group of drugs that depress maximum rate of depolarization has recently been undergoing clinical trials. This group includes lorcainide, flecainide, and encainide. These drugs have little or no effect on action potential duration in vitro,[8] and similarly little effect on measurements of refractory period in animals or humans.[9] They reduce conduction velocity in the specialized conduction system, increasing the H–V interval and producing fairly large increases in QRS duration during therapy.[10] Harrison has suggested this third group of drugs, characterized by a lack of effect on action potential duration and refractoriness, should be designated group 1c.[11]

Class 2 Antiarrhythmic Action

The second antiarrhythmic action in Vaughan Williams' classification is blockade of cardiac beta adrenoceptors by beta blockers, which reverses the arrhythmogenic effect of enhanced sympathetic stimulation. Catecholamines increase the slope of phase 4 depolarization in automatic tissue[12] and therefore increase sinus rate and enhance atrial, Purkinje, and ventricular automaticity, which are dependent on outward potassium currents. Reduction in sinus rate by beta blockade may be, in itself, antiarrhythmic. It may induce changes in refractoriness, secondary to rate-related changes in repolarization.

A further antiarrhythmic action of beta blockers may be to alter abnormal automaticity. Experimental evidence suggests that in some tissues abnormal automaticity, due to slow-channel calcium currents, may be produced by high potassium and catecholamine levels. These abnormal currents have been produced in a number of tissues, including Purkinje and mitral valve fibers.[13] They conduct with low velocity and are, therefore, suited to produce reentrant arrhythmias. Such slow responses may be responsible for some of the arrhythmias encountered in patients with ischemia. A drug action that blocks the effects of catecholamines in enhancing this abnormal automaticity would be antiarrhythmic. Slow currents are also responsible for triggered automaticity, which in some cases at least is enhanced by sympathetic stimulation.[14]

The antiarrhythmic properties of beta-adrenoceptor blockers are probably entirely due to a reversal of these effects of epinephrine. They can, therefore, be demonstrated in vitro only if epinephrine or another adrenergic agonist is added to the preparation. As beta blockers depend on reversal of the effects of epinephrine for their efficacy, they are most effective when an arrhythmia is associated with high levels of adrenergic drive.

Chronic treatment with beta blockers can also cause adaptive changes in repolarization in the myocardium.[15] After some weeks of treatment with beta blockers, action potential duration and Q–T interval increase slightly. This effect may confer an additional antiarrhythmic property on beta blockers.

Drugs With Class 2 Action

Many beta blockers are available, including propranolol, oxprenolol, metoprolol, atenolol, pindolol, acebutolol, and nadolol. They vary in their degree of selectivity in antagonizing $beta_1$ or $beta_2$ stimulation. They also possess varying degrees of agonist activity (intrinsic sympathomimetic activity). It is unlikely that these various properties are of significance in determining the drugs' antiarrhythmic efficacy. However, they may help the selection of an appropriate drug in a specific clinical context.

A small number of beta-blocking drugs, for example, propranolol and oxprenolol, also reduce the maximum rate of depolarization of the action potential (class 1 action) at very high drug concentrations. Although these concentrations are well above those reached in vivo in peripheral plasma, the local elevation of potassium concentration, hypoxia, and low pH associated with ischemia may all enhance the class 1 action of beta blockers sufficiently for this property to contribute to their antiarrhythmic action[16] despite low drug concentrations. However, there is no definite evidence that this phenomenon occurs in the clinical situation.

Class 3 Antiarrhythmic Action

Action potential duration determines the absolute refractory period of myocardial tissue because of the voltage dependence of the recovery from inactivation of sodium channels. Factors that increase action potential duration are antiarrhythmic, as the minimum interval between successive depolarizations is increased. The increase in action potential duration produced by antiarrhythmic drugs is termed class 3 action. Homogeneous prolongation of the action potential ensures a uniform change in refractoriness of the whole heart. Inhomogeneous prolongation of action potential duration leads to spatial variation in refractoriness, which can lead to arrhythmias, by favoring re-entry. Prolongation of maximum action potential duration increases the maximum interval between initial depolarization and final repolarization over the heart. Therefore, the Q–T interval is prolonged, whether the action potential prolongation is homogeneous or inhomogeneous. There is therefore no paradox in the association of arrhythmogenesis with long QT syndromes, and the association of class 3 antiarrhythmic action with Q–T prolongation of an apparently similar nature.[15]

Drugs With Class 3 Action

Amiodarone is a benzofuran derivative that has been used as an antianginal agent because of its vasodilator properties.[17] However, it was found also to have important antiarrhythmic properties. It prolongs action potential duration markedly, although to detect this effect in vitro, experiments have to be performed on tissue from animals chronically treated with amiodarone.[18] Prolongation of action potential duration is reflected during clinical use by a prolongation of the Q–T interval, mainly in the repolarization phase.

The drug has no significant effect on maximum rate of depolarization, but it does have a noncompetitive sympatholytic action.[18] This latter property is comparatively weak, and the clinical efficacy of amiodarone is remarkable,[19] certainly much greater than could be accounted for by its antisympathetic properties. The kinetics of its antiarrhythmic action are similar to the kinetics of the alterations in repolarization encountered during intravenous therapy. Some other influences that prolong action potential duration, for example, hypothyroidism, are associated with a low incidence of arrhythmia.

It is likely, then, that the antiarrhythmic properties of amiodarone are due to the increase in the action potential duration caused by the drug.

Other antiarrhythmic drugs possess this property to some extent. Bretylium prolongs the action potential duration strikingly in ventricular muscle but not in atrial muscle. It also has complex interactions with the sympathetic nervous system, with initial catecholamine release and later reduction in sympathetic activity, that complicate interpretation of its effects. However, it seems likely that the increase in action potential duration produced by bretylium is a significant factor in its antiarrhythmic efficacy, which may be high, even in resistant ventricular arrhythmias.[20] Sotalol is a beta blocker that prolongs action potential duration acutely to a much more marked extent than do other beta blockers. It is very likely that this property contributes to its antiarrhythmic efficacy, inasmuch as sotalol has recently been demonstrated to have marked effects on ventricular, accessory pathway, nodal, and atrial refractoriness.[21,22] This property is not shared by other beta blockers.

Class 4 Antiarrhythmic Action

The pacemaker cells of the sinoatrial node and conducting tissues within the atrioventricular node are dependent on action potentials that differ from those in atrial, Purkinje, and ventricular tissue by lacking an initial spike of sodium influx.[23] They are, thus, relatively insensitive to tetrodotoxin, which blocks sodium channels, and they are not rendered inactive by a less negative membrane potential. The action potentials depend on movement of ions through a channel with a low maximum rate of depolarization and a slow rate of inactivation. The current is conducted slowly, and the channels are therefore called slow channels. Slow-channel current is determined by the calcium-to-sodium ratio, but inasmuch as most of the charge is carried by the calcium ions, the currents have been termed calcium currents. As discussed previously, similar currents may be produced in conditions of high potassium and catecholamine concentrations. Drugs that block these currents are antiarrhythmic because they slow the sinus rate, depress AV nodal conduction, and abolish slow responses.

Drugs With Class 4 Action

Verapamil is a papaverine derivative that blocks the slow calcium current.[24] Its main clinical role as an antiarrhythmic agent is to depress AV nodal conduction. It is, therefore, effective in terminating nodal re-entrant tachycardias, and re-entrant arrhythmias involving the AV node and accessory pathway.[25] Thus, verapamil has become the drug of choice for the intravenous treatment of arrhythmias involving the AV node. It also slows the ventricular rate in atrial fibrillation.[26]

A number of other drugs, for example, diltiazem and nifedipine, interact with the role of calcium in the myocardium. These drugs have variable effects on electrophysiologic measurements.[27] Nifedipine has little action at the AV node, whereas diltiazem does depress AV nodal conduction, although not to the same extent as verapamil. Although they all interfere with the role of calcium in the myocardial cell, they act at somewhat different sites. Verapamil acts on the slow channel itself.[28] The exact site of action of nifedipine on the myocardium is not known, but it has been determined that felodipine, a derivative, relaxes smooth-muscle cells by interfering with the binding of calcium to calmodulin.[29] It is possible, by inference, that the action of nifedipine in the myocardium involves more than "calcium-channel blocking."

The Vaughan Williams Classification

A number of comments can be made about this classification system. It classifies drugs by their actions on normal myocardial tissue in vitro. Therefore, the effects on abnormal tissue are minimized, but as has been shown with lidocaine, they can be particularly important. It is quite difficult to reproduce in vitro the conditions found in ischemic tissue: reduced blood flow with metabolite accumulation, and local changes in potassium and hydrogen ion concentrations. It should be stressed, nonetheless, that the actions of antiarrhythmic drugs on normal tissue are important, as although in many cases the arrhythmia arises in abnormal tissue, it is clearly propagated through normal tissue.

The relationship between in vitro and in vivo electrophysiology is also altered by the autonomic effects of the drugs used (see Table 3). Disopyramide often shortens the effective refractory period of the AV node in vivo, despite its effects on the same tissue in isolated preparations. Studies performed in vivo on hearts denervated either temporarily by the use of atropine or in the rather unusual situation of the transplanted heart[30] suggest that the unexpected in vivo effect is due to a strong anticholinergic effect of the drug. The in vivo changes are the sum of the withdrawal of vagal tone and the direct effect of the drug on nodal tissue. Procainamide commonly causes hypotension when given intravenously, and this effect can stimulate baroreceptor reflexes that increase sympathetic stimulation to the heart. So the effects on cardiac tissue are the sum of the drug's direct and autonomic effects.

The Vaughan Williams classification as it currently stands fails to include all antiarrhythmic drugs. Digoxin is the most obvious example of a commonly used antiarrhythmic drug, the actions of which are not addressed. The classification covers only actions that are useful in the treatment of tachyarrhythmias; whereas the actions of those drugs used in bradyarrhythmias, for example, atropine and isoproterenol, are not mentioned. It would not be difficult to extend the classification and, indeed, Millar and Vaughan Williams have recently suggested[5] a fifth class of antiarrhythmic action, possessed by a new drug called alinidine, which is a derivative of clonidine. This drug depresses sinus rate, yet is neither sympatholytic nor vagomimetic. It has no effect on the relationship between extracellular calcium concentration and sinus node frequency, nor does it depress sodium current in atrial fibers. Thus, it has none of the antiarrhythmic actions associated with the other four classes. It has been suggested that the slowed sinus rate is due to a restriction of chloride current, and this may constitute a fifth class of antiarrhythmic action.

These considerations must not allow the classification to be extended indefinitely so that it becomes unwieldy.

PHARMACOKINETIC CONSIDERATIONS

After selection of a drug with an appropriate qualitative effect on cardiac electrophysiology, quantitative considerations become important. To achieve the desired therapeutic effect, adequate drug concentration must be present at the receptor. This concentration is difficult to measure, but for antiarrhythmic drugs in many cases it correlates well with plasma concentration, and the latter is usually accepted as the active concentration, especially when free drug levels are measured. For many drugs, estimates of plasma concentration are widely available. It is the most commonly available quantitative information and forms the basis of the study of a drug's pharmacokinetics. However, in both the clinical and the investigational context, the plasma level has to be interpreted critically.

Table 4. Elimination and the importance of metabolites

Drug	Half-life	Site of Elimination	Metabolites	Activity of Metabolite		
				Antiarrhythmic	*Side Effects*	*In Assay System*
Quinidine	6–8 hr	90% hepatic 10% renal	Mono- and dihydroxyquinidine	Minimal		Some measure a proportion of metabolite
Procainamide	3–4 hr	40–60% hepatic 40–60% renal	N-acetyl procainamide	Active	Less severe than parent; ? no LE	Separable
Disopyramide	7–10 hr	20% hepatic 80% renal	Mono-N-dealkylated disopyramide	50% activity of parent	More anticholinergic	Variable, can be separated
Lidocaine	1–2 hr	70% first pass, hepatic	Numerous	MEGX in animals	More CNS than parent	
Diphenylhydantoin	24 hr	95% hepatic 5% renal	Parahydroxyphenylhydantoin	Probably not	?	No
Tocainide	13 hr	40% renal 25% hepatic ? rest	N-carboxytocainide glucuronide Lactoxyxylidide	No No	No No	No No
Mexiletine	8–12 hr 12–16 hr (pts)	85% hepatic 15% renal	Para-hydroxymexiletine Hydroxymethyl mexiletine	Not known	Not known	GLC separates

Aprindine	50 hr	95% hepatic 5% renal	Desethylaprindine	Active in animals, small amount in man	Probably not	Not relevant
Encainide	1–2 hr (parent)	95% hepatic	O-demethyl-encainide 3-methoxy-O-demethyl-encainide	Very likely	Unknown, but likely	No(HPLC) No(RIA)
Flecainide	14 hr 20 hr (pts.)	75% hepatic 25% renal	?			
Lorcainide	5–10 hr	Variable hepatic	Norlorcainide	Yes	Probably	Can be separated
Amiodarone	50 days	?	Desethylamiodarone	?	Possibly	No(HPLC)
Sotalol	12 hr	60–75% renal	Excreted unchanged	—	—	—
Bretylium	4–16 hr	70–80% renal	Excreted unchanged	—	—	—
Verapamil	2–10 hr acutely, longer chronic	95% hepatic 5% renal unchanged	Norverapamil	Possibly	?	No

HPLC = high performance liquid chromatography; RIA = radioimmunoassay; MEGX = monoethylglycine xylidide

Antiarrhythmic Activity and Plasma Levels

Variable Activity of Metabolites

Almost all antiarrhythmic drugs are metabolized to compounds with varying toxicity, varying antiarrhythmic efficacy, and varying activity in drug assays (Table 4). All these factors affect the relationship between plasma level and patient response. Drug assays generally have two components, a separation phase and a detection phase. The former usually depends on chemical properties of the drug, although it may depend on differential solubility. The detection phase often depends on physical properties of the molecule, for example, the ability of desaturated parts of the molecule to absorb specific wavelengths of ultraviolet light (when using UV spectrophotometry).

Drug metabolites may well separate with the parent compound and then be detected along with it; for example, hydroxyquinidine separates with quinidine in the older extraction method of Brodie,[31] giving a value for plasma concentration that exceeds the true level. If the ratio of metabolite to active compound is always constant, this would not be a problem, but there is considerable variation in this relationship among individuals and in different disease states. In the assay of Sokolow and Edgar,[32] the extraction removes some of the inactive metabolites of quinidine but only a proportion of the active parent compound. In this case, the total drug concentration may, indeed, reflect activity in plasma as the metabolites substitute for the parent compound lost in the extraction procedure, being detected as parent compound in the method. In renal failure, however, hydroxyquinidine accumulates, and the ratio of hydroxyquinidine to quinidine concentrations rises. The measurement of total quinidine produced by this accumulation produces a falsely high estimate of plasma antiarrhythmic activity.

As well as assay measurement of inactive metabolites, the failure of an assay to determine the quantity of active metabolites may be important. N-acetylprocainamide (NAPA) is a major metabolite of procainamide with marked antiarrhythmic activity.[33] The modified spectrophotometric assay technique[34] does not quantify this compound and therefore underestimates the amount of antiarrhythmic substance in the plasma. If the relationship between the concentrations of NAPA and the parent compound were always constant, this would not be a problem. About 50 percent of procainamide ingested is normally excreted unchanged in the urine. In renal failure, the procainamide is retained and metabolized to NAPA, with a consequent rise in NAPA-to-procainamide ratio. If the assay used measures only the amount of procainamide, both the total antiarrhythmic activity and the concentration of substances able to cause toxicity would be much higher than suggested by the procainamide level. It is preferable to follow procainamide levels in renal failure with an assay technique that quantifies the two compounds separately.[35]

The mono-N-dealkylated metabolite of disopyramide, which has almost 50 percent the antiarrhythmic efficacy of the parent compound and is more strongly anticholinergic, tends to accumulate in renal failure. Fluorometric assays do not generally detect the metabolite. Therefore, in renal failure particularly, a quoted disopyramide concentration using such techniques will underestimate both the tendency of the patient to suffer from side effects and also the level of active drug present.

More specific assays, for example, gas-liquid chromatography and high-performance liquid chromatography, depend upon the retention time on a column to characterize a molecular species. As various compounds elute, they are detected, for example, by UV photometry or fluorometry. The position of the peak is determined by the chemical structure of the drug, and the size of the peak by quantity. Such assays can usually separate different metabolites and, therefore, the true situation may be resolved. It is clear that it is important to understand the contribution of metabolites, both to the result of the assay used and to the drug's antiarrhythmic effects and production of side effects, in order for the value received from the laboratory to be interpreted appropriately.

Drug Binding

Drug activity depends on free drug concentration, but assays usually measure total drug concentration. Many antiarrhythmic drugs are bound to plasma proteins to varying extents. In most cases, the relationship between free and protein-bound drug concentrations is constant, and total drug concentration is an adequate index of plasma activity. However, the situation is more complex with some drugs, for example, disopyramide, which shows saturable protein binding. At low total drug concentrations, protein binding is high for the parent compound, but at high total concentrations it is reduced to 5 percent.[36] So a small increase in total drug concentration can cause a relatively large increase in free drug concentration. The clinical relevance of the findings in this particular example is debated, inasmuch as over the clinical dose range, yielding plasma levels of 2 to 5 μg/ml, the changes in binding are relatively small.

Determinants of Plasma Level

With intravenous therapy, drug delivery to the circulation is 100 percent. However, when a drug is given orally (the other major route for the delivery of antiarrhythmic drugs), a more complex process occurs, at various stages of which drug may be lost. Variable drug loss may occur during the movement of drug from gut to circulation. There are differences both among drugs and among individuals in the ratio of drug delivered to the circulation when the oral and intravenous routes are compared. If this ratio is expressed as a percentage, it is known as bioavailability. It is usually determined by comparing the plasma concentration against time curves following single intravenous and oral doses. The rate of drug delivery to the circulation may also be important for compounds with a narrow therapeutic index, that is, those with small difference between toxic and therapeutic blood levels.

Absorption

Most antiarrhythmic drugs are relatively well absorbed, dissolving rapidly in the gut and undergoing little loss by degradation, for instance, by gastric acid. The half-time for absorption is generally relatively short—20 to 30 minutes in normal persons—and high peak concentrations can, therefore, be produced.

First-Pass Metabolism

Once a drug has dissolved in the gut, it is absorbed through the gut wall. Some drugs, for instance, isoproterenol, are metabolized in the gut wall. However, the majority are absorbed into the splanchnic circulation and pass to the liver where, if hepatic clearance is high, a substantial proportion of the drug absorbed may be metabolized. This phenomenon is called first-pass metabolism, and it reduces the drug's bioavailability.

A number of antiarrhythmic drugs with high hepatic clearance undergo fairly extensive first-pass metabolism. A useful antiarrhythmic effect of orally administered lidocaine is almost completely precluded by hepatic first-pass metabolism, although gastrointestinal irritation is also a major problem. The metabolites produced in this first pass are toxic to the central nervous system but have low antiarrhythmic activity.[37] Propranolol is extensively metabolized during its first pass, although a proportion of the metabolites produced block beta receptors. Verapamil undergoes extensive first-pass metabolism; although almost completely absorbed, it is only 10 to 20 percent bioavailable. The major metabolite norverapamil, however, is active.[38] Variation in first-pass metabolism is a major cause of differences among individuals in pharmacokinetic responses to antiarrhythmic drugs.

Table 5. Parenteral therapy

Drug	*Loading Dose*	*Maintenance Dose*	*Volume of Distribution*	*Comments*
Quinidine	6–10 mg/kg I.V. over 22–45 min	Not used	2–4 L/kg	Risk of VF with I.V. quinidine
Procainamide	100 mg over 1 min, I.V. every 5 min until control 50 mg/min until control 5 mg/kg bolus, 25 mg/min infusion for 15 min, then 2.5 mg/kg bolus	Infusion 2–7 mg/min	2–3 L/kg	Hypotension common
Disopyramide	1.5–2 mg/kg (total less than 150 mg). May repeat × 1 in hour. Less in AMI.			
Lidocaine	50 mg bolus, repeat after 2 min	4 mg/min for 30 min, 3 mg/min for 30 min, 2 mg/min maintenance	1–2 L/kg	
Diphenylhydantoin	3.5–5 mg/kg, less than 50 mg/min 100 mg q 5 min until control, total less than 1000 mg	Usually repeat × 1, and use oral therapy	0.5–1 L/kg	Peripheral vein infusion causes phlebitis
Tocainide	500–750 mg I.V. injection or as infusion over 15–30 min	1.2–1.5 gm daily by infusion	1 L/kg	No real advantage over lidocaine if infusion necessary
Mexiletine	150–250 mg @ 25 mg/min, then 250 mg @ 4 mg/min for 1 hr, 250 mg @ 2 mg/min for 2 hr	0.5–1 mg/kg	5 L/kg	

Aprindine	200 mg @ 2 mg/min, 30-min gap 100 mg @ 2 mg/min, 6-hr gap 100 mg @ 2 mg/min	Injection of 50–75 mg q 6 hr, @ 2 mg/min	2–4 L/kg	
Encainide	50–100 mg over 15–20 min 0.6–0.9 mg/kg over 15 min	Not usually given I.V.	Variable	Wide variation in dose needed
Flecainide	1.5 mg/kg over 30 min, 1 mg/kg/hr over 4 hr	0.2 mg/kg/hr	8–9 L/kg	
Lorcainide	2 mg/kg over 5 min	Not usually given I.V.	7–15 L/kg	Hepatic clearance is saturable
Amiodarone	5–10 mg/kg over 5–10 min	(1500 mg less loading) over remainder of 24 hrs	80+ L/kg	Central line needed for infusion to avoid phlebitis
Sotalol	100 mg over 5–10 min or 1.5 mg/kg over 5 min	10 mg/hr	1–2 L/kg	
Bretylium	500 mg over 5 min bolus 500 mg in 50 ml dextrose over 10 min 2 × 250 mg intramuscular	1–2 mg/min infusion Repeat q 6–8 hr		May be 20 min to 1 hr before effect seen, peaks after several hr.
Verapamil	0.1–0.15 mg/kg over 5 min	0.005 mg/kg/min	2–4 L/kg	Great care with beta blockers May give 0.0001mg/kg/min, but probably best avoided unless no other therapy available.

Distribution and Elimination

Drug distribution throughout the body is usually rapid compared with elimination, but both clearly determine plasma concentration–time relationships. If the body behaves as a single homogeneous unit, or compartment, initial plasma concentration after intravenous administration is simply determined by drug dosage and total volume to which the drug distributes. If elimination is slow compared with distribution, this model of the body's behavior as a single unit may give a reasonably accurate guide to drug levels. This is called a one-compartment model. This simple model of drug distribution suggests the concept of volume of distribution. The latter is an imaginary volume given by the drug dose administered divided by the plasma concentration. Although in most cases it does not represent a real volume, volume of distribution is a useful concept. The volume of distribution of many antiarrhythmic drugs is large—of the order of 2 to 5 L/kg. This means the drugs have a lower concentration in plasma than expected on the one-compartment model, owing to tissue and protein binding. So a quotation of volume of distribution for a drug gives some information as to its tissue binding (Table 5).

According to a one-compartment model, the concentration-versus-time curve is exponential, inasmuch as the rate of elimination for most drugs is dependent on their concentration. Therefore, the plot of logarithm of concentration versus time is linear. In both these models, the rate of drug elimination is conveniently estimated from the slope of the terminal phase of the log concentration-time curve. Half-life is a simple measure of the rate of elimination and is the time taken for the drug concentration to drop by 50 percent.

Although the one-compartment model is adequate in some circumstances, a two-compartment model is increasingly used to describe drug behavior.[39] According to this model, drug is administered into a central compartment in which equilibration is rapid. This represents plasma and interstitial fluid in well-perfused tissue. A second compartment is in equilibrium with the central compartment, but movement between the two is relatively slow. The second compartment reflects both tissue binding and drug distribution to poorly perfused tissues. For antiarrhythmic drugs with their apparent high volume of distribution, this second peripheral compartment is large. The two-compartment model accurately describes the plasma concentration–time curve of many drugs, including antiarrhythmic drugs, following intravenous injection. The curve of plasma concentration versus time is made up of two components. There is an initial rapid fall in plasma concentration, the alpha phase, reflecting distribution from the central to the peripheral compartment. The second slope represents the rate of elimination from the central compartment, modified by movement of drug from the peripheral back to the central compartment. This is the beta phase or elimination phase.

In the two-compartment model, there are therefore both alpha and beta half-lives, the alpha half-life being the half-life of distribution and the beta half-life that of elimination. Thus, the beta half-life is estimated from the terminal part of the slope. Although a strict quantitative treatment is needed to describe accurately plasma concentration–time relationships, the use of the simple concepts of volume of distribution and of distribution and elimination half-lives is often adequate to design appropriate dosing techniques.[40]

Table 4 gives information about the elimination of the various drugs under discussion.

Principles of Dosage

Intravenous Therapy

The intravenous route is used for the acute treatment of arrhythmias and in situations where absorption is suspect as, for example, in acute myocardial infarction. With some drugs, such as lidocaine, intravenous administration is the only route in general use. Inasmuch as most antiarrhythmic drugs are both distributed and eliminated rapidly, a single intravenous bolus injection produces therapeutic levels only for a short time. Larger single doses that would give a longer duration of action can be given but risk toxicity at peak concentrations because the therapeutic ratio is rather small.

An alternative is a constant infusion of drug. Using this mode of delivery, the time taken to reach an equilibrium level designed to be within the therapeutic range varies directly with drug elimination half-life and inversely with the volume of distribution. Lidocaine has a short half-life, and 5 to 6 hours are necessary before a plasma concentration that is 90 percent of the steady state is achieved. Mexiletine has a much longer half-life, 14 hours, and it may take as long as 2 days for a level of 90 percent of the steady state to be achieved. There is, therefore, a long period at the beginning of therapy during which subtherapeutic levels are produced. Clearly, the latter situation is undesirable in the treatment of acute arrhythmias. The combination of bolus and infusion produces a satisfactory compromise. Recommended dosages for various drugs, along with volumes of distribution, are given in Table 5.

Oral Therapy

Chronic therapy for arrhythmias is usually given orally. The pharmacokinetic principles described for intravenous therapy apply to oral treatment. However, the situation is complicated by the introduction of the gut as a further compartment of drug distribution. Thus, a three-compartment model may be used to describe oral drug dosage more accurately, gut compartment equilibrating with the central compartment, which again equilibrates with the peripheral compartment. The important kinetic variable in this model is the rate at which drug transfers from the gut to the central compartment, and a useful descriptor of this rate of transfer is the time taken to reach half the peak plasma levels. The latter is called the half-time of absorption and is fairly short for most antiarrhythmic drugs. The peak concentrations occur 30 minutes to 1½ hours after drug ingestion.

Half-life of elimination again determines the time to steady state, and again loading doses may have to be given, for example, with mexiletine and disopyramide (see Table 5). If absorption is slowed (half-life of absorption increases), the difference between peak and trough levels during chronic therapy, which is important for the use of drugs with a narrow therapeutic ratio, is minimized. This effect can be achieved by the use of slow-release preparations that extend the absorption time and reduce fluctuations in serum levels. A further advantage is an increase in dosage intervals. Slow-release preparations are unfortunately less reliably absorbed and can be affected by gastrointestinal upsets, for example, to a greater extent than standard preparations. Nevertheless, the slow-release preparations of quinidine, procainamide, mexiletine, and disopyramide may be advantageous in some situations.

Table 6 gives oral regimens and other information about oral therapy.

Individual Differences in Drug Response

Individuals differ in their response to standard drug doses. Because antiarrhythmic drugs have such a narrow therapeutic ratio, this can mean the difference between subtherapeutic dosing and catastrophic toxicity. These differences may be pharmacokinetic, determined by differing plasma levels with the same dosage, or pharmacodynamic, depending upon a different response to the same plasma level. Both types of difference between individual response occur with antiarrhythmic drugs.

Variations in Bioavailability

Drug absorption differs little from individual to individual but may be affected by disease states. The absorption of many drugs, for example, procainamide, disopyramide, mexiletine, aprindine, and propranolol, is unpredictable and erratic in patients with acute myocardial

Table 6. Oral therapy

Drug	*Daily Oral Dose*	*Dose Interval*	*Bioavailability*	*Slow-Release Form*	*Comments on Slow-Release Form*
Quinidine	125–200 mg test dose 1.2–2.4 gm	6 hr	60–70%	Quinidine Durules 200 mg quinidine base	B.i.d. dosage
Procainamide	3–6 gm	3–4 hr	75–90%	Procainamide Durules 500 mg	Every 6–8 hr dosage
Disopyramide	300–800 mg	6–8 hr	Almost 100%	Available in Europe 250 mg	B.i.d. dosage
Lidocaine	Not used orally				
Mexiletine	600–750 mg loading dose 400–600 mg single dose	8 hr	Almost 100%	Slow-release form available	Reduces side effects
Diphenylhydantoin	200–300 mg, occ more Loading: 15 mg/kg day 1 7.5 mg/kg day 2	24 hr	Slow, erratic absorption	—	—
Tocainide	1.2–2.4 gm	8–12 hr	Almost 100%	—	—
Aprindine	50–200 mg	12–24 hr	100%	—	—
Encainide	75–300 mg	6–12 hr	18–66%	—	Parent has short half-life, active metabolites prolong action
Flecainide	200–600 mg	12 hr	95%	—	
Lorcainide	200–400 mg	8–12 hr	Low at onset of therapy, rises to almost 100%		
Amiodarone	Usually 100–200 mg (larger dose for VA) Loading: 600 mg o.d. 1 wk 400 mg o.d. 1 wk May give up to 1400 mg daily for rapid onset of effect	Up to alternate day	40%	—	
Sotalol	160–640 mg	12–24 hr	Almost 100%		
Bretylium	Oral use unusual		Less than 50%		
Verapamil	120–360 mg, up to 720 mg used	8 hr	10–20%	Verapamil retard 240 mg	Elimination slows with chronic therapy, so short half-life not a disadvantage

infarction.[41] Although this variable absorption may reflect changes in splanchnic blood flow, the use of narcotics and consequent retarded gastric emptying also contribute. This altered absorption has been shown to lead to subtherapeutic levels for mexiletine, for example,[42] and to failure of therapy.

Drug absorption is unpredictable in malabsorption states. For example, practolol is poorly absorbed in patients with celiac disease, but propranolol absorption is increased. Bioavailability is also affected by changes in hepatic first-pass metabolism consequent upon alterations in hepatic blood flow. Inasmuch as the latter also affects drug elimination, it will be discussed below.

Variation in Distribution

The circulatory changes associated with acute myocardial infarction or congestive failure, secondary to low cardiac output, include peripheral vasoconstriction with preservation of blood flow to central organs, for example, myocardium and brain. The apparent volume of distribution of drugs is reduced by these changes, leading to higher-than-expected levels in the central compartment. For lidocaine, quinidine, procainamide, disopyramide, and mexiletine, this increase in plasma levels has been noted in patients with acute myocardial infarction.

Hepatic blood flow is an important determinant of rate of elimination for drugs with a high hepatic extraction, the best examples being lidocaine and propranolol. Changes in liver blood flow correlate well with whole-body lidocaine clearance. Liver blood flow is decreased in congestive failure and also in hypotension, as elegantly shown in recent experiments using patients with autonomic neuropathy.[44] Even in acute myocardial infarction without overt hypotension or congestive failure, the elimination half-life of lidocaine is increased. For example, Prescott[41] found this half-life to be an average 1.4 hours in normal subjects, and 4.3 hours in patients with myocardial infarction with no heart failure. However, when congestive failure was present, the elimination half-life was prolonged to 10.4 hours. If cardiogenic shock occurs, lidocaine elimination may almost cease. Not only disease states but also other drugs may cause a reduction in liver blood flow. Propranolol and cimetidine both decrease liver blood flow and have been shown to lead to accumulation of lidocaine in patients treated with either of the drugs.[45,46]

Variation in Rates of Elimination

The elimination of water-soluble drugs by renal excretion is sensitive to changes in renal function. Drug elimination usually correlates well with creatinine clearance. Sotalol is a water-soluble drug, 60 to 75 percent of which is excreted unchanged by renal mechanisms. Sotalol elimination varies with renal function, and with a creatinine clearance of greater than 39 ml/min, the mean elimination half-life is 8 hours; but if creatinine clearance falls to between 8 and 38 ml/min, the elimination half-life is extended to a mean of 24 hours.[47] Sites of elimination and drug half-lives of elimination are given in Table 6.

Many drugs are made more water-soluble by hepatic metabolism, usually involving two steps.[48] In the first step, functionally reactive groups are added to the drug molecule (oxidation, reduction, and hydrolysis). During the second step, the active group is conjugated to make the molecule into a more water-soluble moiety (glucuronidation, acetylation, and sulfation). Rates of hepatic metabolism vary significantly among individuals, even those with normal hepatic function and blood flow. Variability in oxidation of diphenylhydantoin produces widely varying plasma concentrations following the same dose. For example, the oral administration of 300 mg diphenylhydantoin daily can produce plasma levels varying from 4 to 40 μg/ml.[49] Encainide is another drug with which pharmacokinetics vary dramatically among individuals. Bioavailability ranges from 7 to 82 percent. Plasma concentration at which arrhythmias returned following single intravenous or oral doses were very different in one study, varying from 39 ± 54 ng/ml with intravenous therapy and 14 ± 16 ng/ml with oral therapy.[50] The assay used in the latter study was almost specific for encainide, suggesting that metabolites produced by oral dosing contributed to antiarrhythmic efficacy when the oral route was used. Most subjects form at least two metabolites in significant quantities, that is, O-demethyl-encainide (ODE) and 3-methoxy-O-demethyl-encainide (MODE). It is several hours before these metabolites are detectable following intravenous administration, but following oral administration they are present after a short time. The suggestion that these metabolites are active and produced during oral administration is supported by the kinetic features of this study. Although encainide has a short half-life (1.3 ± 0.9 hr), ODE and MODE have long half-lives, and MODE concentrations hardly changed over 24 hours following encainide withdrawal. Arrhythmia suppression persists for a median of 14 hours following drug withdrawal despite the short half-life of the parent compound. Taken together, these findings suggest that the metabolites are active, although the findings could be explained by prolonged myocardial binding of the parent drug. Roden and coworkers[51] reported one patient who formed no detectable ODE and MODE at normal encainide doses. Antiarrhythmic efficacy in this patient was low. These observations emphasize the possible variations that can occur among members of an apparently homogeneous group of subjects.

Acetylation is also variable, and for some drugs at least under clear genetic control. The acetylation rates of isoniazid and hydralazine are clearly bimodally distributed in the population, with an antimode containing very few individuals. Procainamide metabolism to NAPA is by acetylation, but there is controversy as to whether procainamide rates are bimodally distributed throughout the population.[52] Nevertheless, acetylation rates for procainamide do vary between individuals, considerably affecting the NAPA-to-procainamide ratio, which can vary from less than 1 to 1 in slow acetylators to 6 to 1 in fast acetylators.

The importance of liver disease per se in altering drug elimination has been debated.[53] Many patients with liver disease have been exposed to a variety of drugs that are enzyme inducers, and changes in distribution secondary to liver disease may also occur so that tissue penetration is more rapid. There is little doubt that enhanced portacaval shunting increases the delivery of oral propranolol to the systemic circulation with liver disease. Hypoalbuminemia reduces the available binding protein for some drugs and, therefore, the volume of distribution.

Lidocaine dosage should be halved in patients with liver disease. Procainamide and quinidine are unaffected. Diphenylhydantoin metabolism may be impaired in liver disease.

Variation Due to Age

Differences among individuals owing to aging also affect drug response. Although usually kinetic, pharmacodynamic effects have been described, for example, the enhanced efficacy of digoxin in inhibiting red cell sodium-potassium ATPase in elderly subjects.[54] Variation in pharmacokinetics with age is better recognized. Ochs and associates[55] have demonstrated reduced quinidine clearance in the elderly compared with young subjects. Renal clearance of quinidine was 35 percent lower in the elderly subjects. This correlated with creatinine clearance. On the other hand, lidocaine kinetics are unchanged in the elderly.[56]

Secular Changes in Drug Metabolism

Most pharmacokinetic studies are performed using acute dosing. They describe drug behavior over short periods of time, often following single doses. Information obtained from these studies is valuable as a guide to therapy for the urgent use of antiarrhythmic drugs. However, many patients need chronic treatment, and pharmacokinetic properties may change during such therapy.

During lidocaine infusion, lidocaine levels often rise if infusion continues for more than 24 hours.[45] Elimination is two to three times more prolonged at the end than at the beginning of the infusion. This may be due to product inhibition, that is, inhibition of the hepatic metabolism of lidocaine by the accumulation of metabolites, particularly of monoethylglycine xylidide.[57] Similar increases in elimination half-life occur during chronic verapamil therapy. After a single dose, the mean elimination half life is 6.4 hours in patients with atrial fibrillation, and 10.3 hours for the active metabolite, norverapamil. After 10 to 12 weeks of therapy with from 40 mg to 120 mg every 6 hours, the values rise to 12 hours and 16.5 hours, respectively.[58] This change has been attributed to a decrease in hepatic blood flow during chronic therapy, and indeed two of the patients in this latter study developed congestive failure. However, this phenomenon is unlikely to be the entire explanation, as similar findings were obtained after seven doses in a group of patients with supraventricular tachycardia, who did not have myocardial impairment.[59]

These findings are of clinical significance. Care must be taken during prolonged lidocaine infusion. The changes in verapamil pharmacokinetics are probably an advantage, as the dose interval can be increased, but care must be taken to avoid accumulation.

ADVERSE REACTIONS TO ANTIARRHYTHMIC DRUGS

Rawlins and Thompson have recently suggested that adverse drug reactions are of two major types.[60] One group of adverse effects (augmented or Type A) is determined by a normal pharmacologic action of the drug, usually to excess. The second group of adverse effects (bizarre or Type B) is due to a novel and totally abnormal response to the drug and is independent of its pharmacologic action. It seems to be an expression of the presence of the drug as a foreign molecule in the body. Some Type A reactions are due to the normal pharmacologic properties of the drugs, acting on the normal target organ. Such reactions would include beta blocker–induced cardiac failure or bradycardia. In this case the adverse effect is merely an exaggeration of the normal, desirable therapeutic effect of the molecule. However, a further normal pharmacologic action of nonselective beta blockers is the production of peripheral vasoconstriction by the release of unopposed alpha effects. This effect is clearly due to the drug's standard pharmacologic action, although it is undesirable. However, it does not fall into the same category as the former Type A reaction, as it is not acting on the intended target organ. We propose that Type A adverse reactions can, therefore, be subdivided into target organ and non–target organ effects (Table 7).

A Type B reaction caused by a beta blocker is the oculomucocutaneous syndrome,[61] an idiosyncratic reaction to practolol that led to its withdrawal from oral use. This adverse effect

Table 7. Classification of adverse drug reactions

	Type A		
	Target Organ	*Non–Target Organ*	*Type B*
Incidence	High	High	Usually low
Relation to normal pharmacology	Strong	Fairly strong	Weak or absent
Mortality	Low	Lower	May be higher
Occurrence	Predictable	Fairly predictable	Unpredictable
Drug withdrawal	May be necessary, and effective	Effective, often unnecessary	May be ineffective, sometimes unnecessary

Table 8. Adverse effects

	Type A				Type B	
	Cardiovascular					
Drug	*Electrophysiologic*	*Hemodynamic*	*Neurologic*	*Gastrointestinal*	*Hematologic*	*Miscellaneous*
Quinidine	Inc QRS, inc QT Arrythmia aggravation "Quinidine syncope" Inc rate in A flutter Occ AV block Dec sinus function occ.	Small negative inotropic effect Peripheral vasodilatation	Cinchonism, tinnitus, hearing loss, visual problems, headache, photophobia	Nausea, vomiting Diarrhea	Hemolysis (G6PD) Thrombocytopenia Agranulocytosis	Pain on I.M. injection
Procainamide	Inc QRS Inc QT occ. may be associated with arrhythmia aggravation AV block	Small negative inotropic effect Hypotension with I.V. use	Insomia	Anorexia, nausea, vomiting Occ diarrhea	ANF positive in 60–70% after 1 yr 20–30% lupus after 1 yr Agranulocytosis	Granulomatous hepatitis
Disopyramide	Inc QT, occ inc QRS Arrhythmia aggravation Variable dec sinus function Inc V rate in A flutter	Produces CHF Hypotension I.V.	Minor	Minor		Anticholinergic: blurred vision, prostatism
Lidocaine	Occ dec automaticity and conduction in ischemia	Minor	Drowsiness, confusion, coma, respiratory depression, seizures	Not given orally as produces severe GI upset		
Diphenylhydantoin	Ditto	Minor	Nystagmus, ataxia, drowsiness, resp arrest	Gum hyperplasia (40–80%), 10% if good oral care and levels well controlled	Pseudolymphoma Risk of true lymphoma inc 2–4 fold	Rash Sterile abscess after IM use, phlebitis with infusions
Tocainide	Minor Occasional aggravation of arrhythmias	Minor	Tremor Similar to lidocaine	Nausea and vomiting		Rash ± fever Immune-complex nephritis Interstitial pneumonitis
Mexiletine	Some sinus or conduction impairment Probable aggravation of arrhythmias	Minor, but occ CHF and hypotension I.V.	Dizziness, seizures, tremor, vomiting partly CNS	Nausea and vomiting	Rarely thrombocytopenia	Rash, possibly photosensitive

Aprindine	Impairs AH and HV conduction Arrhythmia aggravation	Mild negative inotropic, mild hypotension	Tremor, ataxia, dizziness, visual difficulty	Nausea, diarrhea	Agranulocytosis, 0.1–1% may be reversible	Hepatitis, early, often reversible
Encainide	Impairs HV conduction, 20–25% arrhythmia aggravation, problems with resuscitation	Dec preload with hypotension	Tremor, visual blurring, dizziness	Nausea		
Flecainide	Inc PR, inc QRS Inc QT with VT c10% arrhythmia aggravation	Minor	Blurred vision, dizziness, metallic taste			
Lorcainide	Inc QRS, impairs HV and causes distal block if disease in conducting system	Inc systemic resistance, negative inotrope	Marked sleep disturbance (up to 40%) Blurred vision, dizziness with injection			
Amiodarone	Inc QT Arrhythmia aggravation unusual AV block with high doses, Sinus rate depressed	Vasodilatation with I.V., can give hypotension Well tolerated orally, even if poor LV function	Headache, sleep disturbance Peripheral neuropathy, proximal muscle weakness	Constipation		Goiter, hypothyroidism, hyperthyroidism Photosensitive dermatitis and blue pigmentation Corneal deposits, pneumonopathy
Sotalol	Dec SN function Dev AVN cond. Inc QT, with arrhythmia provocation at high doses	LV impairment Hypotension				Asthma, cold extremities, proximal myopathy
Bretylium	No conduction delay Possible arrhythmia aggravation, uncommon	Initially, unimportant hypertension Hypotension in 50–75% patients Not negative inotrope	Nausea and vomiting after I.V. injection			Parotid pain and swelling common with chronic therapy
Verapamil	Dec sinus automaticity Produces AV block	Peripheral vasodilatation, transient hypotension I.V. Negative inotrope	Headache	Constipation		Flushing

is not encountered with other beta blockers, emphasizing that it is not due to beta-receptor blockade.

Target Organ Type A Effects

Certain Type A adverse effects tend to be common to antiarrhythmic drugs of a given class, and these are shown in Table 8, along with the wide variety of other adverse effects encountered with antiarrhythmic drugs.

Conduction Disorders

It is not surprising that most antiarrhythmic agents cause conduction disorders, as many of their actions on cardiac conducting tissue are depressant.

Depression of conduction velocity and excitability are the fundamental actions of the class 1 agents. The anticholinergic effect of disopyramide and quinidine may protect, to some extent, against the production of AV block, but it does occur despite this effect. Lidocaine and other drugs with class 1b actions tend to be relatively safe from the point of view of conduction defects, but inasmuch as they clearly do depress conduction in ischemic tissues, problems may occur.

Infra-His block is encountered with quinidine, procainamide, and disopyramide and more often with encainide, lorcainide, and flecainide. This difference reflects the greater efficacy of the latter group of drugs on H–V and intraventricular conduction. For example, Bär and coworkers[62] described two patients with pre-existing right bundle branch block, left axis deviation, and an H–V interval of 130 msec who developed in one case complete infra-His block, and in the other 2:1 infra-His block. In the same study, two individuals with previous normal H–V times developed right bundle branch block. These findings contrast with those in two patients with AV nodal and intra-His block prior to treatment with lorcainide, in whom there was no deterioration in conduction at this level after drug administration. We have not observed any cases of conduction disturbance due to encainide, except one instance of transient AV block during catheter removal. The Stanford experience with encainide is similar.[50]

The depressant effects of beta blockers on AV nodal conduction and sinus rate are well recognized.

Amiodarone has, in our experience, produced a few cases of transient AV conduction defects when used in high doses at the onset of treatment for ventricular tachycardia. This effect seems relatively unusual at standard doses, although the drug produces a predictable reduction in sinus rate in most patients.

The main electrophysiologic effects of verapamil are on the sinus and AV nodes, and so it is not surprising that the drug can produce bradyarrhythmias. Although class 4 effects suppress sinus node rate in isolated tissue, this suppression is less pronounced in vivo. In sinus rhythm, there is often little effect on rate after verapamil administration. The latter is likely to be due to the reflex sympathetic activity associated with the peripheral vasodilating effects of the drug. The major problem with the use of verapamil occurs with concurrent beta-blocker therapy.

Arrhythmia Aggravation

Conduction disturbances have been recognized for many years as a common problem with the use of antiarrhythmic agents. It is only relatively recently, however, that the problem of arrhythmia aggravation has been recognized to be as important as it seems to be with a wide variety of antiarrhythmic drugs.

Quinidine syncope, due to ventricular arrhythmias occurring during chronic quinidine therapy, has been recognized for some years.[63] Although more common in the setting of a high quinidine level, with QRS and Q–T prolongation, it may occur in the individual with apparently normal plasma levels. Patients with Q–T prolongation may be at particular risk. Torsade de pointes is the arrhythmia often produced. The latter is a form of ventricular tachycardia with continuous axis shift during the arrhythmia. It originates from a late ventricular ectopic depolarization and occurs in the setting of a prolonged Q–T interval. Fortunately, this arrhythmia is often self-terminating, but it may degenerate into ventricular fibrillation.

Quinidine may also provoke monomorphic ventricular tachycardia in the setting of a normal Q–T interval, or an increase in the number of PVCs and of repetitive forms without progression to sustained ventricular tachycardia.[64] A dose-response relationship occurs (suggesting a Type A reaction), with a progressive increase in ectopic activity noted following a single oral dose (600 mg) in 75 percent of 20 patients who developed arrhythmia aggravation. In five cases, however, as the quinidine concentration increased and reached a maximum, ventricular ectopic activity was suppressed 1 to 2 hours after the dose. After 2 to 4 hours, despite quinidine concentrations still being in the "therapeutic range," rebound aggravation of ectopic activity occurred.

There have been relatively few reports of arrhythmia aggravation caused by procainamide, but in one study procainamide was arrhythmogenic in up to 9 percent of subjects to whom the drug was administered.[64] It has also caused Q–T prolongation and torsade de pointes.[65] Disopyramide produces arrhythmias fairly commonly, particularly at high blood levels. Lo and colleagues[66] described a patient with Q–T prolongation and high disopyramide levels who developed ventricular tachycardia. In their case, the arrhythmia responded promptly to lidocaine and DC shock. High levels of disopyramide were produced by excessive prescription of disopyramide in the context of congestive heart failure and mildly impaired renal function. Tzivoni and coworkers[67] also described four patients with a long Q–T and a ventricular tachycardia of torsade de pointes morphology. Meltzer and associates[68] report a further case associated with high disopyramide levels. The anticholinergic properties of these drugs may contribute to their arrhythmogenic potential. When they are used to treat atrial tachyarrhythmias, both disopyramide and quinidine can produce marked acceleration of the ventricular rate by simultaneously slowing atrial rate and enhancing AV nodal conduction via their vagolytic action.[69] There is strong evidence for a protective effect of vagal tone in the acute phase of acute myocardial infarction, especially in the presence of enhanced sympathetic tone. Bailey and coworkers[70] have shown that in the presence of isoproterenol and acetylcholine, both disopyramide and quinidine shorten action potential duration in Purkinje fibers by blocking the effects of acetylcholine, which were to prolong the action potential. Shortening of action potential duration could be arrhythmogenic in this situation, inasmuch as it increases the likelihood for re-entrant arrhythmias to re-invade the His-Purkinje system. Anticholinergic actions can then be arrhythmogenic.

These properties are not the entire explanation of antiarrhythmic drug-induced arrhythmogenesis. This is shown by the arrhythmogenic potential of drugs with class 1c activity, especially with encainide. In a study of intravenous encainide in our department, 21 patients were given encainide in doses of 0.9 to 1.8 mg/kg, 15 out of 21 receiving 1 mg/kg, as an infusion over 10 minutes. In three patients, encainide had no effect on the arrhythmia. In 12 patients, encainide either abolished or slowed ventricular tachycardia or abolished echo beats occurring during electrophysiology study. In six patients, however, the rate of ventricular tachycardia increased, nonsustained ventricular tachycardia changed to sustained ventricular tachycardia, or ventricular tachycardia or echo beats became apparent after encainide was given. These changes suggest that arrhythmia aggravation had occurred. We were unable to define pharmacokinetic or electrophysiologic properties that would predict which patients would respond with arrhythmia aggravation.

Other workers[71] have reported a similar problem with encainide. Winkle and associates[71] also quote two cases of deterioration with lorcainide. The problem of arrhythmia aggravation by group 1c agents has been reviewed by Camm,[72] who also mentions that out of 40 cases treated with flecainide, three sustained marked arrhythmia deterioration. The various reports are difficult to handle together inasmuch as they use different criteria for arrhythmia exacerbation, but most suggest a 10 percent incidence of severe arrhythmia aggravation.

Although the new drugs may produce Q–T prolongation and torsade de pointes,[73] they usually produce monomorphic ventricular tachycardia, which may be self-terminating but may be sustained and resistant to treatment, including DC cardioversion.

Inasmuch as group 1c agents have little effect on ventricular, His-Purkinje, or atrial refractoriness, it is likely that the pronounced slowing of His-Purkinje conduction produced by the drugs is the property that renders them liable to produce arrhythmias. It is not clear at present whether these drugs are more prone to cause arrhythmia aggravation than other antiarrhythmic agents.

Although Q–T prolongation on the surface ECG is associated with an increased incidence of arrhythmias,[15] class 3 drug action is not necessarily arrhythmogenic, as the increases in refractoriness produced may be homogeneous. Amiodarone has been reported to produce ventricular fibrillation, and it has also been found to have increased the ventricular rate in a case of atrial fibrillation associated with the Wolff-Parkinson-White syndrome.[74] It has also been suggested to produce incessant ventricular tachycardia, and to enhance the production of native ventricular tachycardia in recent reports,[75] and has been associated with torsade de pointes.

The situation with bretylium is more complex inasmuch as the properties of this drug include sympathomimesis, which is known to be arrhythmogenic. Anderson and colleagues[76] described two cases in which bretylium seemed to exacerbate arrhythmias. In the first, rechallenge reproduced the arrhythmia, although subsequent control with propranolol suggests a sympathetic component. Allen and associates[77] described bretylium-induced enhancement of Harris second-stage arrhythmias in a dog infarct model.

High plasma levels of sotalol produce concentration-dependent Q–T prolongation that has been associated with ventricular arrhythmias. Elonen and coworkers[78] described two cases of sotalol intoxication. In the first, ventricular fibrillation occurred on two occasions, once terminating spontaneously, but on the second occasion terminating "with pacing." In a second case, typical torsade de pointes was initiated by a late ventricular ectopic beat. This arrhythmia was associated with Q–T prolongation, which reverted to normal as sotalol concentration fell.

Verapamil has not been reported to aggravate common tachyarrhythmias, but its use in atrial fibrillation complicating the Wolff-Parkinson-White syndrome may on occasion increase ventricular rate by shortening the anterograde effective refractory period of the accessory pathway. Two patients have been reported in whom cardioversion was necessary.[79] This problem can be avoided if verapamil is not used in atrial fibrillation where the ventricular complexes are predominantly pre-excited.

Hemodynamic Effects

The net hemodynamic effects of an antiarrhythmic agent may be due to alterations of heart rate, the contractile state of the myocardium, and the state of the peripheral circulation. Adverse effects are more pronounced in patients with poor cardiac function, and inasmuch as many patients needing antiarrhythmic treatment fall into this category, it is important that hemodynamic effects are assessed in this group of subjects as well as in normal subjects during drug testing. Most antiarrhythmic drugs have the capacity to depress myocardial function to some extent at least, but the relationship between antiarrhythmic action and myocardial depression varies with the electrophysiologic actions of the drug.

Class 1 Drugs

Drugs with class 1a action depress myocardial function, but there is variation in the clinical picture produced, depending on the actions on the peripheral circulation (see Table 8). At high doses, quinidine decreases myocardial contractility, but the main hemodynamic problem clinically with this drug is the production of hypotension, probably due to blockade of alpha receptors in peripheral arterioles. The effects of procainamide are similar, the peripheral actions being due either to a ganglion-blocking property or to a direct effect on smooth muscle. As a consequence, procainamide commonly produces hypotension, in up to two thirds of patients in some series.[80] Disopyramide seems to have potent negative inotropic effects when compared with other agents.[81] Direct depression of the myocardial contractile state causes congestive heart failure even in patients with no prior history of cardiac decompensation. When given intravenously, left ventricular contractility (measured as dp/dt) is impaired, although there is a tendency for peripheral resistance to increase as well, producing an increase in afterload that will also be deleterious.[82] The reason for the apparent severity of the myocardial depression produced by disopyramide is unclear. It has been suggested that the class 1 action of these drugs[83] is the basis of the negative inotropic effects. However, the d and l isomers of disopyramide have different effects on some electrophysiologic properties at least (QTc), whereas they have the same effect on echocardiographic measurements of myocardial contractility.[84]

Drugs with class 1b properties are less negatively inotropic. Lidocaine is probably the least depressant of all the drugs possessing class 1 action, but even this drug may depress left ventricular function that is already severely compromised. Life-threatening cardiovascular complications were reported in only 5 of 750 patients with various cardiovascular diseases by the Boston Collaborative Drug Surveillance Program,[85] four of which involved hypotension or conduction disturbance. When given orally, mexiletine rarely produces heart failure, even in high-risk patients following myocardial infarction,[86] but it can certainly depress left ventricular function following parenteral administration in the presence of pre-existing cardiac disease.[87] Tocainide[88] is similarly relatively safe, even in patients with acute myocardial infarction. Recent evidence[89] suggests that encainide decreases preload and therefore reduces cardiac output and blood pressure but has little effect on the contractile state of the myocardium.

The marked variation in hemodynamic effects between the different drugs suggests that class 1 activity per se is not the only explanation for myocardial depression by class 1 agents.

Class 2 Drugs

The beta-blocking effects of class 2 agents are well recognized to cause heart failure. In a study of the use of propranolol by the Boston Collaborative Drug Surveillance Program,[90] 4.2 percent of 800 inpatients treated with propranolol developed heart failure or severe hypotension. Dangerous reactions could develop with small dosages; 70 percent occurred in patients given less than 40 mg of propranolol per day, although this small dosage probably reflects their physicians' concern for their cardiovascular status and defines a high-risk population, rather than suggesting that the effect is not dose-related. Severe effects tend to be encountered within the first 24 hours, but may develop insidiously.

Parenteral beta-blocker therapy for arrhythmias may produce hypotension, particularly following cardiac surgery. Clearly, the balance between the advantage gained by arrhythmia control has to be set against the risks of myocardial depression. In this context, the greater efficacy of verapamil against supraventricular tachycardia deserves comment. In one study, 19 of 20 arrhythmias reverted to sinus rhythm with the calcium-channel blocking agent, whereas only 8 of 20 reverted to sinus rhythm following practolol administration.[91]

Class 3 Drugs

The hemodynamic effects of sotalol are mainly due to beta blockade. There is considerable controversy about the hemodynamic effects of amiodarone when given intravenously. However, there is no doubt that the latter drug is one of the least cardiodepressant antiarrhythmic drugs in chronic oral use.

In a dog infarct model,[92] amiodarone in the large dose of 10 mg/kg given as a bolus over 3 minutes (dissolved in distilled water) caused a reduction in heart rate, maximum aortic pressure, left ventricular peak pressure, and left ventricular dp/dt. There was no significant change in left ventricular end-diastolic pressure, although it did increase slightly, below the level of statistical significance, suggesting that there was possibly even a beneficial effect of amiodarone on afterload that could, in some circumstances, produce hypotension. Côté and coworkers[93] confirmed these findings when amiodarone was given to men with coronary artery disease. Other workers have suggested that some of the effect is due to the detergent that is added to help dissolve the very insoluble drug.[94] This suggestion is unlikely for two reasons: the detergent, Tween 80, has only a short duration of action on the peripheral circulation, and the findings of DeBoer and associates[92] suggest the drug itself can produce hypotension.

Heart failure is an unusual problem with oral amiodarone therapy and, indeed, it may be difficult to determine any improvement following amiodarone withdrawal because of the drug's extremely long duration of action following withdrawal.

The effects of bretylium are more dependent on its interactions with the sympathetic nervous system than on its class 3 effect. Initial dosage produces a rise in blood pressure. Postural hypotension occurs in up to 50 percent of patients with chronic therapy. It seems unlikely that the class 3 action of these drugs is inherently negatively inotropic.

Class 4 Agents

Myocardial contraction is dependent on the release of sarcolemmal calcium proportional to the influx of calcium through the slow channels. The major antiarrhythmic activity of verapamil is to block these channels,[27] and it is likely, therefore, that verapamil could be negatively inotropic. Indeed, in isolated preparations, verapamil reduces myocardial contractility. Its effects on the peripheral circulation are, however, of relevance. It causes peripheral arteriolar vasodilatation, presumably by a reduction of available intracellular calcium in the smooth muscle cells of the arterioles. However, the net cardiovascular effects are the result of an interaction between heart rate, peripheral and coronary vasodilatation, and myocardial performance. The combination of these effects on the intact circulation usually produces hypotension, with negative inotropic effects at large doses (greater than 0.2 mg/kg). Smaller doses tend to produce only very small changes in dp/dt. Cardiac output may rise following verapamil administration, but left ventricular end-diastolic pressure may also rise.[95] Clinical studies suggest that hemodynamic effects are generally relatively slight, but problems can occur, particularly in patients with cardiomegaly given large doses of verapamil intravenously.[96]

The hemodynamic effects of antiarrhythmic drugs are very variable and are profoundly determined mainly by the pre-existing state of the myocardium. Overall, class 1b and class 3 drugs are the safest, although quinidine and procainamide do not often precipitate congestive failure during chronic oral use.

Non–Target Organ Type A Adverse Effects

Autonomic Effects

The autonomic effects of the various antiarrhythmic agents mentioned may cause adverse effects; for example, the anticholinergic effects of disopyramide can produce urinary retention, glaucoma, and constipation. Table 3 summarizes the autonomic effects of a range of antiarrhythmic agents.

Central Nervous System Effects

Central nervous system side effects are typical non–target organ Type A problems that are possibly the commonest side effects of class 1 antiarrhythmic drugs. The mechanism of their production is probably in some way related to antiarrhythmic mechanisms.

The neurologic side effects of lidocaine are well recognized. At low drug levels, dizziness, nausea, and irritability occur, progressing to confusion and even respiratory depression, seizures, and coma in unusual cases with very high blood levels. These effects on the central nervous system occurred in 7 to 39 percent of patients treated with lidocaine in trials for the prophylaxis of primary ventricular fibrillation following acute myocardial infarction.[97] Careful attention to dosage adjustment during prolonged infusion, with older patients, and in the presence of decreased hepatic blood flow will reduce the likelihood of these effects. In a trial of mexiletine for prophylaxis of sudden death in a group of high-risk patients following acute myocardial infarction,[86] neurologic side effects were encountered in a large number of patients treated with 200 to 250 mg of mexiletine three times daily. For instance, insomnia and tremor were noted in one fourth to one third of all patients on mexiletine but in only 10 percent receiving placebo. Similar neurologic side effects have been encountered with tocainide. Tremor is a common problem during aprindine therapy. Our experience with flecainide suggests a relatively low incidence of CNS disturbance, although a metallic taste is an occasional problem. Quinidine does not seem to produce such marked effects, which may relate to its lower lipid solubility in comparison to these other drugs. However, quinidine does produce occasional cases of cinchonism, a toxic reaction including neurologic manifestations ranging from tinnitus and hearing loss to confusion and psychosis. Encainide produces dizziness at high blood levels, which may be moderate to severe in up to 25 percent of patients. These neurologic side effects can be serious for unstable patients, for example, those with acute myocardial infarction, inasmuch as they have secondary undesirable effects on the cardiovascular status of the patient, by increasing restlessness and sympathetic drive. They therefore increase myocardial oxygen consumption and the tendency to arrhythmias. During chronic therapy, neurologic adverse effects also produce morbidity and can be a hindrance to compliance.

Gastrointestinal Problems

Gastrointestinal adverse effects, including nausea, vomiting, and dyspepsia, are quite common with antiarrhythmic drug therapy. Much of the nausea encountered is, in fact, secondary to central nervous system stimulation; for example, it occurs promptly following intravenous injection of mexiletine. In fact, most drugs are able to produce nausea and vomiting in susceptible individuals. Class 1 agents again tend to be particularly bothersome; for example, gastrointestinal upset with quinidine and procainamide may lead to drug intolerance in up to 40 percent of individuals. Diarrhea is occasionally troublesome with quinidine and procainamide but not particularly with the other drugs possessing class 1 activity. Indeed, constipation may be encountered with disopyramide. Verapamil and amiodarone also produce this problem. Beta blockers may cause either constipation or excessive looseness of stool.

Type B Adverse Reactions

Immunologic Problems

Antiarrhythmic drugs produce a number of bizarre (Type B) adverse reactions, some of which have an immunologic basis.

Long-term therapy with oral procainamide is limited by the development of a positive antinuclear factor in 60 to 70 percent of patients after a year's treatment, 20 to 30 percent of whom develop a frank lupus syndrome, with arthralgia, fever, pleurisy, and pericarditis. Although more common with higher doses, this adverse reaction may occur at low plasma levels. There is controversy as to whether acetylator status determines the risk that a positive antinuclear factor or lupus will develop. Originally, it was believed that slow acetylators were relatively protected against the development of lupus,[98] but doubt has been cast on this contention.[99] Indeed, Giardina and coworkers[52] could find no clear evidence that the rate of procainamide acetylation was distributed in a bimodal fashion. The differences between these studies may be due to the different ways of determining acetylator status. Immunologic problems have also been seen with tocainide, which has been reported to produce rash, hepatitis, polyarthritis with a positive antinuclear factor, an interstitial pneumonitis, and immune complex glomerulonephritis.[100] The rash has been reproduced by rechallenge. These reactions have been of low frequency and reversible.

Hematologic Problems

Depression of the formed elements of the blood by drugs, although an uncommon side effect of any one particular drug, is reported occasionally with most. Antiarrhythmic drugs are no exception, and the use of some is particularly commonly associated with blood dyscrasias.

The effects of quinidine have been thoroughly investigated.[101] Both autoimmune hemolytic anemia and thrombocytopenia are due to destruction of formed elements in the peripheral circulation. The drug, or a metabolite, complexes with a component of the membrane of the cells and a hapten-mediated immunologic reaction occurs, causing cytolysis. This may be a very specific reaction. For example, the antibodies produced by quinine and quinidine in the purpura produced by these agents are not cross-reactive, despite the very similar structure of the offending agents. Blood dyscrasias can also be produced by direct marrow toxicity. Although this toxicity may be immunologically mediated in many cases, it can also be due to an effect on stem cell metabolism. Aprindine lowers the white count to less than $1500 \times 10^9/L$ in almost 3 percent of patients, with frank agranulocytosis in 0.1 to 1 percent of patients. This syndrome is usually reversible, but fatalities caused by infection have occurred.[102]

Hepatic Problems

Nine to 10 percent of all adverse effects reported to the British Committee on Safety of Medicines from 1964 to 1971 were of hepatic disorders. The role of the liver in detoxification makes it likely that hepatic drug reactions will occur. Aprindine has been reported to cause reversible hepatitis in a number of patients. In one case, rechallenge was associated with a further deterioration in liver function.[103] This effect usually occurs within 3 weeks of starting therapy. Procainamide and quinidine can also produce granulomatous hepatitis.

Miscellaneous Effects of Amiodarone

Antiarrhythmic agents produce a number of other miscellaneous effects, some of which may be difficult to classify. Amiodarone is probably associated with the greatest variety. As it is one of the most powerful of the new antiarrhythmic drugs, its side effects are important and must be put in a proper perspective. It would be quite wrong to deprive patients of the marked clinical efficacy of this drug because of the risk of side effects that may occur at a low incidence or be themselves treatable.

The most commonly detectable unwanted effect of amiodarone therapy is the deposition of brown pigment in the lower part of the cornea.[104] This corneal change is visible only with slit-lamp examination, and only in rare cases affects vision. Although slit-lamp examination at intervals has been recommended in the past, we have discontinued this practice and recommend ophthalmologic assessment only if the patient complains of visual difficulties. No retinal toxicity has been encountered despite the similarity of the corneal deposit to cornea verticulata caused by chloroquine therapy, which may cause severe retinal changes.

The most common problems of which patients complain are cutaneous. A self-limiting maculopapular erythematous rash occurs in some 9 percent of patients in the first 6 weeks of treatment. Although not usually a problem, the rash may be very itchy. Photosensitivity is more troublesome, causing erythema and marked pruritus in parts of the body exposed to sun. Some degree of photosensitivity occurs in 75 percent of patients after 2 years' treatment,[105] and protective measures are required in almost 30 percent. Even in our practice in a relatively unsunny area of Britain, photosensitivity seems to be very common. There seems to be geographic variation in the incidence of this reaction, inasmuch as it is relatively unusual in South Africa, despite the high incidence of other photosensitivity disorders. In those patients more mildly affected by amiodarone-induced photosensitivity, the tanning produced may be acceptable. A peculiar type of slate gray pigmentation may also occur, which is less acceptable. This pigmentation is probably preceded by sunburn in most cases and takes more than a year to develop. It is confined to light-exposed areas, usually the nose and upper face, sparing the skin folds, but the backs of the hands may be involved. Histologic examination in our cases has revealed brown pigment granules in macrophages in the dermis, which are not present in unpigmented skin from the same patient. These granules have some of the staining properties of lipofuscin. However, we have found that concentrations of the drug and its major metabolite, desethylamiodarone, are much higher in pigmented than in unpigmented skin, suggesting that at least some of the discoloration reflects local drug and metabolite accumulation.[106] Because many patients taking amiodarone are relatively resistant to treatment with other agents, it is often necessary to continue the amiodarone despite this inconvenient but apparently not dangerous side effect. Avoiding light exposure is helpful, but the use of standard sunscreens is not particularly valuable because they do not cut out the appropriate wavelengths. More help may be gained by the use of broad-spectrum sunscreens. It is our clinical experience that these screens reduce the photosensitivity, but it is not yet known if the pigmentation is reliably reduced.

There are now reports of a number of cases in which the association of pneumonitis or pulmonary fibrosis with amiodarone therapy has been made.[107,108] In some patients, this association has occurred within 6 weeks of starting therapy. The reaction in these cases has responded to steroids, but in others where the reaction has occurred later, no response is found. We have seen one patient in the former group. High drug doses have been used in some cases, but this has not been a uniform finding. Other antiarrhythmic drugs, for example, tocainide, may cause an interstitial pneumonitis, and may have played a part in two of the reported cases. However, it seems likely that amiodarone can indeed induce pulmonary damage.

Clinical hypothyroidism and hyperthyroidism have been reported in up to a few percent of cases receiving treatment with amiodarone. Goiter may occur, although thyroid function remains normal. It is likely that both hypothyroid and hyperthyroid states are precipitated by the iodine content of the molecule, which also affects the PBI estimation and blocks thyroid uptake of radioiodine.

Diagnosis of the extent of disturbance of thyroid metabolism is difficult, because even in clinically euthyroid patients there are predictable changes in thyroid function tests due to the amiodarone itself.[109] They are not reproduced by dosing with an appropriate amount of free iodine. Most patients show an increase in total serum concentration of thyroxine (T_4), with an increase in reverse triiodothyronine (rT_3). These alterations may be due to a peripheral action of amiodarone, inhibiting T_4 to T_3 conversion, with diversion of T_4 to rT_3. In keeping with this, free T_3 is depressed. Thyroid-stimulating hormone levels may rise a little, even with no clinical or other laboratory evidence of hypothyroidism. This effect may reflect a reduced pituitary receptor delivery of T_3, by the same mechanism as above. There seems to be no consistent change in the results of the TRH test.

The ability of the drug to predictably increase rT_3 levels seems to correlate with both antiarrhythmic efficacy and with side effects. Measurements of rT_3 concentration may be a useful way to monitor therapy with amiodarone.[110]

DRUG INTERACTIONS

When drugs are given concurrently, the quantitative and qualitative effects on the patient may differ, both from the effects expected from the separate actions of the drugs and from a simple sum of their effects. Interactions may occur via a number of mechanisms, and often more than one mechanism is acting at the same time. The result may benefit the patient, or, more commonly, be to his or her detriment.

Similar Drug Effects

Drugs with similar effects given together produce an exaggeration of the expected effects. This occurs relatively commonly with antiarrhythmic drugs. The interaction between verapamil and beta blockers is one of the more dramatic examples. When given to patients receiving chronic beta-blocker therapy, intravenous verapamil can produce marked sinus slowing and complete AV block.[111] Fatalities have occurred. This complication is due to a combined effect of the drugs on both sinus node automaticity and AV nodal conduction. Combined oral therapy may be useful in some patients with angina pectoris, with no particular problems from cardiac failure or bradycardia.[112] However, sporadic cases of severe myocardial depression needing treatment with inotropic agents have been described,[113] suggesting that caution is necessary. The anticholinergic side effects of disopyramide would be expected to be additive with anticholinergic effects of other drugs, for example, tricyclics or antihistamines. Although this interaction has not been reported, it seems very likely that such an effect could be encountered and lead to problems.

Opposing Drug Effects

A reduction in drug effect can occasionally occur when drugs with opposing effects are given. There is a beneficial interaction between the effects of digitalis and disopyramide or quinidine on the AV node. Both quinidine and disopyramide can lead to acceleration of the ventricular rate during atrial tachyarrhythmias, an effect that is prevented by prior treatment with digoxin, which slows AV nodal conduction.

Pharmacokinetic Interactions

The aforementioned interactions are pharmacodynamic in nature. A number of pharmacokinetic interactions also occur. Drug absorption can be affected by the concomitant administration of a second drug. For example, narcotics reduce the absorption of various oral antiarrhythmics in patients after acute myocardial infarction, adding to the effects of decreased cardiac output. Metoclopramide also increases quinidine absorption during chronic therapy.[114] The concomitant administration of antacids with various drugs has been shown to retard their absorption, and care should always be taken when this is a possibility.

Changes induced by drug distribution by a second drug may change drug levels, with unexpected toxicity. If quinidine is given to patients established on digoxin therapy, a rise in digoxin level of some twofold to threefold is commonly seen.[115] This rise in serum digoxin level is not due to assay interference and is associated with an increase in digoxin effects, so that digoxin toxicity can be produced. A number of suggestions have been made as to the cause of this interaction,[116] but certainly a major factor is a reduction in the volume of distribution of digoxin, possibly caused by competition for binding sites in tissue. There are certainly secondary changes in rate of elimination of digoxin, and it is likely that there are direct effects on renal clearance of digoxin by inhibition of tubular secretion. Amiodarone causes a similar degree of elevation of the serum digoxin concentration,[117] and again displacement from tissue binding has been suggested as the mechanism.

A common mechanism of drug interaction is the change in metabolism produced by the administration of a second drug. Such interactions are relatively unusual with antiarrhythmic drugs. However, both amiodarone and disopyramide increase the effect of warfarin. Amiodarone probably halves warfarin requirements in most patients.[118] Quinidine increases the action of warfarin in some patients, but not all. Procainamide seems to be safe in this situation. A common cause of interaction is enzyme induction. Rifampicin is a potent inducer of hepatic enzymes and can increase the metabolism of quinidine so that arrhythmia control is lost.

The renal excretion of a number of antiarrhythmic drugs and their metabolites is affected by urinary pH. A rise in urinary pH due to antacids or to acetazolamide therapy can reduce the excretion of quinidine, thereby producing quinidine toxicity. The extent of changes in urinary pH determine whether the interaction is significant or not. Interaction at active sites of tubular secretion also changes drug elimination, and it may be that the renal clearance of digoxin is reduced by quinidine by competition for a tubular secretory site.

Drugs acting on the sympathetic system may interact at various sites around the adrenergic neurone. For example, bretylium enhances the response to infused sympathetic agents.

ASSESSMENT OF ANTIARRHYTHMIC DRUG EFFICACY

During drug use, patient response has to be monitored to ensure adequate doses of the correct drug are being given. For some drugs, this assessment is straightforward, but with others, there is a greater problem in assessing the adequacy of therapy. This difficulty often applies to antiarrhythmic drugs. The efficacy of antiarrhythmic drugs can be monitored in a number of ways depending on the individual patient, the arrhythmia being treated, and, indeed, the drug being used. When a patient is suffering from frequent attacks of symptomatic palpitations, it is easy to assess control by the relief of symptoms. However, this is so in relatively few cases where antiarrhythmic drugs are used. Symptoms may be difficult to interpret for both patient and physician. When the arrhythmia is an infrequent and unpredictable event, a symptom-free interval is not necessarily indicative of therapeutic success. One major goal of antiarrhythmic therapy is the suppression of asymptomatic arrhythmias that may be the harbingers of sudden death. Although the evidence that suppression of these arrhythmias is actually beneficial is rather controversial, a considerable amount of effort is expended in their control. There are therefore two areas where special techniques have to be used to assess the efficacy of antiarrhythmics. The first is where arrhythmias are severely symptomatic or life-threatening but occur only infrequently; the second is when they are common but asymptomatic and their suppression is thought to be associated with the prevention of more serious arrhythmias.

Holter Monitoring

Continuous ECG recording by portable monitoring has now become a standard part of cardiologic practice. Reliable analysis of the recordings made has been facilitated by the development of automatic arrhythmia analyzing computers in systems where quality control is maintained. It is relatively easy using such techniques to produce results for counts of premature ventricular complexes (PVCs) occurring per hour in association with background heart rate. The simplest form of analysis of drug efficacy depends on comparison of recordings made while the patient is not being treated with those made during a period when the patient is receiving adequate drug doses. The frequency of arrhythmia, the duration of taping, and the amount of spontaneous variability demonstrated in control tapes all determine the degree of PVC reduction that is accepted as showing a real drug effect, as opposed to an effect of spontaneous variability that may have occurred naturally. Although a number of statistical techniques have been used to assess whether a treatment tape actually shows a drug effect when it is compared with a placebo tape, for most purposes a reduction of 85 percent of the control PVC rate is a reasonable guide that the drug regimen being used is efficacious.[119] It is important to ensure that the drug has been given for a long enough time for steady-state levels to have been achieved, and, therefore, it would appear sensible for drug levels to be obtained at the same time when this is possible.

Holter monitoring can also be useful in assessing the response of supraventricular arrhythmias that are associated with sinus node disease. Many of the drugs that can be used to suppress these supraventricular arrhythmias can also cause excessive sinus slowing. Evidence that undue slowing can occur at presymptomatic levels can be obtained using Holter monitoring. Information as to ventricular rate control in atrial fibrillation can be obtained using this technique.

Exercise Testing

Where an arrhythmia is infrequent, it may be possible to provoke it by an intervention, and once it has been established that this intervention can reliably provoke the arrhythmia, the effects of an antiarrhythmic drug can be assessed. Exercise testing can be used in this context to assess the efficacy of agents that are intended to suppress exercise-induced arrhythmias. The applicability of this technique as part of a program for assessing the control of sudden death has been investigated by Lown's group with apparent success.[120] Exercise can induce arrhythmias by a number of mechanisms including enhanced sympathetic drive, increase in heart rate per se, and also by the production of ischemia. Exercise testing is most useful when the arrhythmia under discussion is clearly exercise-provoked, for example, 1:1 atrial flutter induced by exercise, or right ventricular outflow tract ventricular tachycardia,[121] but it may also be of value for an ischemic population in general.

Invasive Electrophysiologic Testing

For many paroxysmal arrhythmias, exercise testing and Holter monitoring are inadequate to assess the efficacy of a drug schedule. For patients who have been resuscitated from sudden death, or those who have ventricular tachycardia or rapid supraventricular arrhythmias with hemodynamic compromise, the controlled production of an arrhythmia in the catheterization laboratory during an invasive electrophysiology study allows the administration of a number of different drugs and the assessment of their efficacy. It also provides further information as to the mechanism of the arrhythmia in question, which may be of both academic and practical value. There is a considerable body of evidence[122] suggesting that control of ventricular tachycardia or supraventricular arrhythmias by a drug regimen in the electrophysiology laboratory is also associated with clinical control. For example, Mason and Winkle[123] found that 68 percent of the group of patients successfully treated in the catheterization laboratory maintained control after 18 months, whereas only 11 percent of those in whom the regimen eventually chosen was found to be ineffective in the catheterization laboratory remained controlled after 18 months followup. Similarly, Bauernfeind and associates[124] found that if drug therapy prevented the induction of paroxysmal atrial fibrillation by atrial pacing, then the drug would be efficacious in clinical use.

A number of objections have been raised to this technique, which is invasive, expensive, and time consuming. It is invaluable in the assessment of antiarrhythmic agents experimentally, but there is some question about its value in routine clinical use.[125] The procedure must be complete, the arrhythmia produced must represent the clinical problem, and the design of the study must take into account the possibility that drug therapy can aggravate the arrhythmia. One particularly valuable use of this technique is the determination of the safety of digoxin in patients with accessory pathways.

Drug Levels

It is important that the results of all these techniques are related to the drug dose used and, where possible, to the drug's plasma levels.

Miscellaneous Ways of Assessing Therapeutic Efficacy

The antiarrhythmic effects of some drugs are correlated with predictable changes on the surface ECG. Class 1c agents generally produce QRS prolongation that serves as a "bioassay" for the drug's antiarrhythmic efficacy. Similarly, the failure of amiodarone to induce Q–T prolongation on the surface ECG suggests that its antiarrhythmic effect has not had time to develop fully. It is possible that in the future other more subtle surface electrocardiographic measurements may be made after drug therapy, and therapeutic efficacy then assessed. Examples might include measurements of conduction intervals or possibly of late ventricular depolarization, which are now possible using signal averaging techniques applied to surface ECGs.

For amiodarone, one nonelectrophysiologic method has been suggested. Nademanee and coworkers[110] have found that the increase in reverse T_3 levels found during amiodarone therapy correlates well with the drug's antiarrhythmic efficacy. This way of assessing efficacy is, of course, not applicable to other drugs.

ANTIARRHYTHMIC DRUGS AND PREGNANCY

Adverse drug reactions may not be restricted to the patient. When a pregnant woman is treated for an arrhythmia, the drug used may cross the placenta and affect the fetus. If therapy continues to delivery, the neonate is also affected.

Controversy has surrounded the use of beta blockers during pregnancy, and in particular their effect on the neonate. Both bradycardia and hypoglycemia have been reported in neonates born to mothers treated with beta blockers.[126] However, it is difficult to be certain that these reactions, which are fairly common in infants born to mothers with hypertension, are definitely due to the drug in question. Another important consideration is that even in reports in which propranolol has been associated with neonatal bradycardia and hypoglycemia, the babies have been well at hospital discharge.[127]

Other antiarrhythmic agents cross the placenta and have been used to the fetus' advantage. Procainamide, propranolol, and digoxin have all been used to control fetal tachycardias causing congestive failure in utero.[128]

Although antiarrhythmic drugs are not used very often in women exposed to the likelihood of pregnancy, it is important to bear in mind possible teratogenic effects or cardiac effects on the fetus. Diphenylhydantoin probably causes an increased incidence of fetal malformation, especially oral clefts. It also predisposes to neonatal hemorrhage, by interfering with the metabolism of vitamin K. Local anesthetics, when given for paracervical or epidural block, may produce neonatal hypotension and bradycardia; so lidocaine, used as an antiarrhythmic, would be expected to have the same effects.

ACKNOWLEDGMENTS

Sincere thanks are due to Mrs. Joan Gray for invaluable secretarial assistance.

REFERENCES

1. HOFFMAN, BF AND BIGGER, JT JR: *Antiarrhythmic drugs.* In DIPALMA, JR (ED): *Drill's Pharmacology in Medicine,* ed 4. McGraw-Hill, New York, 1971, p 824.
2. TOUBOUL, P: *An electrophysiological classification of antiarrhythmic drugs.* In *Antiarrhythmic and Antianginal Drugs with Cumulative Effects.* Sanofi Pharma International, Paris, 1981, p 27.
3. GETTES, LS: *On the classification of antiarrhythmic drugs.* Mod Concepts Cardiovasc Dis 48:13, 1979.
4. VAUGHAN WILLIAMS, EM: *Anti-arrhythmic Action and the Puzzle of Perhexiline,* ed 1. Academic Press, London, 1980.
5. MILLAR, JS and VAUGHAN WILLIAMS, EM: *Anion antagonism; a fifth class of antiarrhythmic action?* Lancet 1:1291, 1981.
6. YAMAGUCHI, I, SINGH, BN, AND MANDEL, WJ: *Electrophysiological actions of mexiletine on isolated rabbit atria and canine ventricular muscle and Purkinje fibres.* Cardiovasc Res 13:288, 1979.
7. LAZARRA, R, HOPE, RR, EL-SHERIF, N, ET AL: *Effects of lidocaine on hypoxic and ischemic cardiac cells.* Am J Cardiol 41:872, 1978.
8. GIBSON, JK, SOMANI, P, AND BASSETT, AL: *Electrophysiological effects of encainide (MJ 9067) on canine Purkinje fibres.* Eur J Pharmacol 52:161, 1978.
9. NICHOLSON, MR, CAMPBELL, RWF, AND JULIAN, DG: *Ventricular tachycardia—management with encainide.* Circulation 64:37, 1981.
10. JACKMAN, WM, ZIPES, DP, NACCARELLI, GV, ET AL: *Electrophysiology of oral encainide.* Am J Cardiol 49:1270, 1982.
11. HARRISON, DC, WINKLE, RA, SAMI, M, ET AL: *Encainide: a new and potent antiarrhythmic agent.* In HARRISON, DC (ED): *Cardiac Arrhythmias:A Decade of Progress.* GK Hall, Boston, 1981, p 315.
12. NOBLE, D: *The Initiation of the Heart Beat,* ed 2. Clarendon Press, Oxford, 1979, p 109.
13. ARONSON, RS AND CRANEFIELD, PF: *The electrical activity of canine cardiac Purkinje fibres in sodium free, calcium rich solutions.* J Gen Physiol 61:786, 1973.
14. WIT, AL AND CRANEFIELD, PF: *Triggered and automatic activity in the canine coronary sinus.* Circ Res 41:435, 1977.
15. VAUGHAN WILLIAMS, EM: *QT and action potential duration.* Br Heart J 47:513, 1982.
16. VAUGHAN WILLIAMS, EM: *Some factors that influence the activity of antiarrhythmic drugs.* Br Heart J 40(Suppl):52, 1978.
17. VASTESAEGER, M, GILLOT, P, AND RASSON, G: *Etude clinique d'une nouvelle médication anti-angoreuse.* Acta Cardiol 22:483, 1967.
18. SINGH, BN AND VAUGHAN WILLIAMS, EM: *The effect of amiodarone, a new antianginal drug, on cardiac muscle.* Br J Pharmacol 39:657, 1970.
19. NADEMANEE, K, HENDRICKSON, JA, CANNOM, DS, ET AL: *Control of refractory life-threatening ventricular tachyarrhythmias by amiodarone.* Am Heart J 101:759, 1981.
20. KOCH-WESER, J: *Drug therapy: Bretylium.* N Engl J Med 300:473, 1979.
21. NATHAN, AW, HELLESTRAND, KJ, BEXTON, RS, ET AL: *Electrophysiological effects of sotalol—just another beta-blocker?* Br Heart J 47:515, 1982.
22. BENNETT, DH: *Acute prolongation of myocardial refractoriness by sotalol.* Br Heart J 47:521, 1982.
23. BIGGER, JT JR AND HOFFMAN, BF: *Antiarrhythmic drugs.* In GILMAN, AG, GOODMAN, LS, AND GILMAN, A (EDS): *The Pharmacological Basis of Therapeutics,* ed 6. Macmillan, New York, 1980, p 763.
24. KOHLHARDT, M, BAUER, M, KRAUSE, B, ET AL: *Selective inhibition of the transmembrane calcium conductance of mammalian myocardial fibres.* Pfluegers Arch 338:115, 1973.
25. KRIKLER, DM AND SPURRELL, RAJ: *Verapamil in the treatment of paroxysmal supraventricular tachycardia.* Postgrad Med J 50:447, 1974.
26. SCHAMROTH, L: *Immediate effects of intravenous verapamil on atrial fibrillation.* Cardiovasc Res 5:419, 1971.
27. SINGH, BN: *Pharmacological basis for the therapeutic applications of slow-channel blocking drugs.* Angiology 33:492, 1982.
28. GLOSSMAN, H, FERRY, DR, LUBBECKE, F, ET AL: *Calcium channels: Direct identification with radioligand binding studies.* Trends in Pharmacological Sciences 3:431, 1982.
29. BOSTROM, SL, LJUNG, B, MAORDH, S, ET AL: *Interaction of the anti-hypertensive drug felodipine with calmodulin.* Nature 292:777, 1981.
30. BEXTON, RS, HELLESTRAND, KJ, CORY-PEARCE, R, ET AL: *The direct electrophysiologic effects of disopyramide phosphate in the transplanted human heart.* Circulation 67:38, 1983.

31. BRODIE, BB, BAER, JE, AND CRAIG, LC: *Metabolic products of the cinchona alkaloids in human urine.* J Biol Chem 188:567, 1951.

32. SOKOLOW, M AND EDGAR, AL: *Blood quinidine concentrations as a guide in the treatment of cardiac arrhythmias.* Circulation 1:576, 1950.

33. DRAYER, DC, REIDENBERG, MM, AND SEVY, RW: *N-acetylprocainamide. An active metabolite of procainamide.* Proc Soc Exp Bio Med 146:358, 1974.

34. SITAR, DS, GRAHAM, DN, RANGNO, RE, ET AL: *Modified colorimetric method for procainamide in plasma.* Clin Chem 22:379, 1976.

35. GIBSON, TP: *The use of antiarrhythmic drugs in renal failure.* Ration Drug Ther 13:1, 1979.

36. HINDERLING, PH, BRES, J, AND GARRETT, ER: *Protein binding and erythrocyte partitioning of disopyramide and its monodealkylated metabolite.* J Pharm Sci 63:1684, 1974.

37. BURNEY, RG, DIFAZIO, CA, PEACH, MJ, ET AL: *Anti-arrhythmic effects of lidocaine metabolites.* Am Heart J 88:765, 1974.

38. SINGH, BN, COLLETT, JT, AND CHEW, CYC: *New perspectives in the pharmacologic therapy of cardiac arrhythmias.* Prog Cardiovasc Dis 22:243, 1980.

39. WINKLE, RA, GLANTZ, SA, AND HARRISON, DC: *Pharmacologic therapy of ventricular arrhythmias.* Am J Cardiol 36:629, 1975.

40. BIGGER, JT JR: *Management of arrhythmias.* In BRAUNWALD, E (ED): *Heart Disease. A Textbook of Cardiovascular Medicine.* WB Saunders Co, Philadelphia, 1980, p 691.

41. PRESCOTT, LF: *Pharmacokinetic abnormalities in myocardial infarction.* In SANDØE, E, JULIAN, DG, AND BELL, JW (ED): *Management of Ventricular Tachycardia—Role of Mexiletine.* Excerpta Medica, New York, 1978, p 465.

42. POTTAGE, A, CAMPBELL, RWF, ACHUFF, SC, ET AL: *The absorption of oral mexiletine in coronary care patients.* Eur J Clin Pharmacol 13:393, 1978.

43. ZITO, RA AND REID, PR: *Lidocaine kinetics predicted by indocyanine green clearance.* N Engl J Med 298:1160, 1978.

44. FEELY, J, WADE, D, MCALLISTER, CB, ET AL: *Effect of hypotension on liver blood flow and lidocaine disposition.* N Engl J Med 307:866, 1982.

45. OCHS, HR, CARSTENS, G, AND GREENBLATT, DJ: *Reduction in lidocaine clearance during continuous infusion and by coadministration of propranolol.* N Engl J Med 303:373, 1980.

46. FEELY, J, WILKINSON, GR, MCALLISTER, CB, ET AL: *Increased toxicity and reduced clearance of lidocaine by cimetidine.* Ann Intern Med 96:592, 1982.

47. BLAIR, AD, BURGESS, ED, MAXWELL, BM, ET AL: *Sotalol kinetics in renal insufficiency.* Clin Pharmacol Ther 29:457, 1981.

48. WILLIAMS, RJ: *Comparative patterns of drug metabolism.* Fed Proc 26:1029, 1967.

49. LOESER, EW: *Studies on the metabolism of diphenylhydantoin (Dilantin).* Neurology (Minneap) 11:424, 1961.

50. WINKLE, RA, MASON, JW, KATES, RE, ET AL: *Encainide.* In COLTART, J AND JEWITT, DE (EDS): *Recent Developments in Cardiovascular Drugs.* Churchill Livingstone, New York, 1982, p 102.

51. RODEN, DM, REELE, SB, HIGGINS, SB, ET AL: *Total suppression of ventricular arrhythmias by encainide: Pharmacokinetic and electrocardiographic characteristics.* N Engl J Med 302:877, 1980.

52. GIARDINA, EGV, STEIN, RM, AND BIGGER, JT JR: *The relationship between the metabolism of procainamide and sulfamethazine.* Circulation 55:388, 1977.

53. CURRY, SH: *Drug Disposition and Pharmacokinetics, With a Consideration of Pharmacological and Clinical Relationships,* ed 2. Blackwell Scientific, Boston, 1977, p 121.

54. KELLY, JG AND MCDEVITT, DG: *Erythrocyte cation transport and age: Effects of digoxin and frusemide.* Br J Clin Pharmacol 15:129P, 1983.

55. OCHS, HR, GREENBLATT, DJ, WOO, E, ET AL: *Reduced quinidine clearance in elderly persons.* Am J Cardiol 42:481, 1978.

56. TRIGGS, EJ: *Pharmacokinetics of lignocaine and chlormethiazole in the elderly; With some preliminary observations on other drugs.* In CROOKS, J AND STEVENSON, IH (EDS): *Drugs and the Elderly: Perspectives in Geriatric Clinical Pharmacology.* Macmillan, New York, 1979.

57. LENNARD, MS, BAX, NDS, TUCKER, GT, ET AL: *Product-inhibition of hepatic lignocaine metabolism.* Clin Sci Mol Med 55:5P, 1978.

58. SCHWARTZ, JB, KEEFE, DL, KIRSTEN, E, ET AL: *Prolongation of verapamil elimination kinetics during chronic oral administration.* Am Heart J 104:198,1982.

59. SHAND, DG, HAMMILL, SC, AANONSEN, L, ET AL: *Reduced verapamil clearance during long-term oral administration.* Clin Pharmacol Ther 30:701, 1981.

60. RAWLINS, MD AND THOMPSON, JW: *Pathogenesis of adverse drug reactions.* In DAVIES, DM (ED): *Textbook of Adverse Drug Reactions,* ed 2. Oxford University Press, Oxford, 1981, p 11.

61. WRIGHT, P: *Untoward effects associated with practolol administration: Oculomucocutaneous syndrome.* Br Med J 1:595, 1975.

62. BÄR, FW, FARRÉ, J, ROSS, D, ET AL: *Electrophysiological effects of lorcainide, a new antiarrhythmic drug. Observations in patients with and without pre-excitation.* Br Heart J 45:292, 1981.

63. SELZER, A AND WRAY, HW: *Quinidine syncope. Paroxysmal ventricular fibrillation occurring during treatment of chronic atrial arrhythmias.* Circulation 30:17, 1964.

64. VELEBIT, V, PODRID, P, LOWN, B, ET AL: *Aggravation and provocation of ventricular arrhythmias by antiarrhythmic drugs.* Circulation 65:886, 1982.

65. STRASBERG, B, SCLAROVSKY, S, ERDBERG, A, ET AL: *Procainamide-induced polymorphous ventricular tachycardia.* Am J Cardiol 47:1309, 1981.

66. LO, KS, GANTZ, KB, STETSON, PL, ET AL: *Disopyramide-induced ventricular tachycardia.* Arch Intern Med 140:413, 1980.

67. TZIVONI, D, KEVEN, A, STERN, S, ET AL: *Disopyramide-induced torsade de pointes.* Arch Intern Med 141:946, 1981.

68. MELTZER, RS, ROBERT, EW, MCMORROW, M, ET AL: *Atypical ventricular tachycardia as a manifestation of disopyramide toxicity.* Am J Cardiol 42:1049, 1978.

69. ROBERTSON, CE AND MILLER, HC: *Extreme tachycardia complicating the use of disopyramide in atrial flutter.* Br Heart J 44:602, 1980.

70. BAILEY, JC, MIRRO, MJ, AND ZIPES, DP: *The possible arrhythmogenic potential of the anticholinergic properties of quinidine and disopyramide.* In SANDØE, E, JULIAN, DG, AND BELL, JW (EDS): *Management of Ventricular Tachycardia—Role of Mexiletine.* Excerpta Medica, New York, 1978, p 293.

71. WINKLE, RA, MASON, JW, GRIFFIN, JC, ET AL: *Malignant ventricular tachyarrhythmias associated with the use of encainide.* Am Heart J 102:857, 1981.

72. CAMM, AJ: *Proarrhythmic effects of Class IC agents.* Current Medical Literature—Cardiovascular Medicine RSM 1:117, 1982.

73. LUI, HK, LEE, G, DIETRICH, P, ET AL: *Flecainide-induced QT prolongation and ventricular tachycardia.* Am Heart J 103:567, 1982.

74. SHEINMAN, BD AND EVANS, T: *Acceleration of ventricular rate by amiodarone in atrial fibrillation associated with the Wolff-Parkinson-White syndrome.* Br Med J 285:999, 1982.

75. MCGOVERN, B, GARAN, H, KELLY, E, ET AL: *Life-threatening reactions during amiodarone therapy.* Circulation 66(Suppl II):224, 1982.

76. ANDERSON, JL, POPAT, DK, AND PITT, B: *Paradoxical ventricular tachycardia and fibrillation after intravenous bretylium therapy.* Arch Intern Med 141:801, 1981.

77. ALLEN, JD, ZAIDI, SA, SHANKS, RG, ET AL: *The effects of bretylium on experimental cardiac dysrhythmias.* Am J Cardiol 29:641, 1972.

78. ELONEN, E, NEUVONEN, PJ, TARSANNEN, L, ET AL: *Sotalol intoxication with prolonged QT interval and severe tachyarrhythmias.* Br Med J 1:1184, 1979.

79. GULAMHUSEIN, S, KO, P, CARRUTHERS, SG, ET AL: *Acceleration of the ventricular response during atrial fibrillation in the Wolff-Parkinson-White syndrome after verapamil.* Circulation 65:348, 1982.

80. KOCH-WESER, J AND KLEIN, SW: *Procainamide dosage schedules, plasma concentrations and clinical effects.* JAMA 215:1454, 1971.

81. PODRID, PJ, SCHOENEBERGER, A, AND LOWN, B: *Congestive heart failure caused by oral disopyramide.* N Engl J Med 302:614, 1980.

82. NAQUI, N, THOMPSON, DS, MORGAN, WE, ET AL: *Haemodynamic effects of disopyramide in patients after open heart surgery.* Br Heart J 42:587, 1979.

83. NAYLER, WG: *The cellular basis for anti-arrhythmic therapy.* In KRIKLER, DM AND GOODWIN, JF (EDS): *Cardiac Arrhythmias: The Modern Electrophysiological Approach.* WB Saunders, Philadelphia, 1975, p 212.

84. POLLICK, C, GIACOMINI, KM, BLASHKE, TF, ET AL: *The cardiac effects of d-and l-disopyramide in normal subjects: A noninvasive study.* Circulation 66:447, 1982.

85. PFEIFER, HJ, GREENBLATT, DJ, AND KOCH WESER, J: *Clinical use and toxicity of intravenous lidocaine. A report from the Boston Collaborative Drug Surveillance Program.* Am Heart J 92:168, 1976.

86. CHAMBERLAIN, DA, JEWITT, DE, JULIAN, DG, ET AL: *Oral mexiletine in high-risk patients after myocardial infarction.* Lancet 2:1324, 1980.

87. BERNARD, R, DE HEMPTINNE, J, GILLET, JM, ET AL: *Mexiletine in acute myocardial infarction—tolerance and haemodynamic effects.* In SANDØE, E, JULIAN, DG, AND BELL, JW (EDS): *Management of Ventricular Tachycardia—Role of Mexiletine.* Excerpta Medica, New York, 1978, p. 324.

88. NYQUIST, O, FORSSELL, G, NORDLANDER, R, ET AL: *Hemodynamic and antiarrhythmic effects of tocainide in patients with acute myocardial infarction.* Am Heart J 100:1000, 1980.

89. TUCKER, CR, WINKLE, RA, PETERS, FA, ET AL: *Acute hemodynamic effects of intravenous encainide in patients with heart disease.* Am Heart J 104:209, 1982.

90. GREENBLATT, DJ AND KOCH WESER, J: *Adverse reactions to propranolol in hospitalized medical patients: A report from the Boston Collaborative Drug Surveillance Program.* Am Heart J 86:478, 1973.

91. HARTEL, G AND HARTIKAINEN, M: *Comparison of verapamil and practolol in paroxysmal supraventricular tachycardia.* Eur J Cardiol 4:87, 1976.

92. DEBOER, LWV, NOSTA, JJ, KLONER, RA, ET AL: *Studies of amiodarone during experimental myocardial infarction: Beneficial effects on hemodynamics and infarct size.* Circulation 65:508, 1982.

93. CÔTÉ, P, BOURASSA, MG, DELAYE, J, ET AL: *Effects of amiodarone on cardiac and coronary hemodynamics and on myocardial metabolism in patients with coronary artery disease.* Circulation 59:1165, 1979.

94. LOTTO, A, SATOLLI, R, AND BALDINI, MR: *Hemodynamic effects of amiodarone.* Circulation 60:666, 1979.

95. SINGH, BN AND ROCHE, AHG: *Effects of intravenous verapamil on haemodynamics in patients with heart disease.* Am Heart J 94:593, 1977.

96. WICHITZ, S, HAIAT, R, TARRADE, T, ET AL: *Accidents cardio-vasculaires au cours des traitements par le verapamil. A propos de 6 observations.* Nouv Presse Med 4:337, 1975.

97. DESILVA, RA, HENNEKENS, CH, LOWN, B, ET AL: *Lignocaine prophylaxis in acute myocardial infarction: An evaluation of randomised trials.* Lancet 2:855, 1981.

98. DAVIES, DM, BEEDIE, MA, AND RAWLINS, MD: *Antinuclear antibodies during procainamide treatment and drug acetylation.* Br Med J 3:682, 1975.

99. WOOSLEY, RL, DRAYER, DE, REIDENBERG, MM, ET AL: *Effect of acetylator phenotype on the rate at which procainamide induces antinuclear antibodies and the lupus syndrome.* N Engl J Med 298:1157, 1978.

100. WINKLE, RA, MASON, JW, AND HARRISON, DC: *Tocainide for drug-resistant ventricular arrhythmias: Efficacy, side-effects and lidocaine responsiveness for predicting tocainide success.* Am Heart J 100:1031, 1980.

101. WORRLLEDGE, SM: *Immune drug-induced haemolytic anaemias.* Semin Hematol 10:327, 1973.

102. STOEL, I AND HAGEMEIJER, F: *Aprindine: A review.* Eur Heart J 1:147, 1980.

103. HERLONG, HF, REID, PR, BORTNOTT JK, ET AL: *Aprindine hepatitis.* Ann Intern Med 89:359, 1978.

104. D'AMICO, DJ, KENYON, KR, AND RUSKIN, JN: *Amiodarone keratopathy: Drug induced lipid storage disease.* Arch Ophthalmol 99:257, 1981.

105. CHALMERS, RJG, MUSTON, HL, SRINIVAS, V, ET AL: *High incidence of amiodarone-induced photosensitivity in North-West England.* Br Med J 285:341, 1982.

106. ADAMS, PC, NICHOLSON, MR, STOREY, CGA, ET AL: *Amiodarone tissue distribution—relation to adverse effects.* Br Heart J 49:297, 1983.

107. SOBOL, SM AND RAKITA, L: *Pneumonitis and pulmonary fibrosis associated with amiodarone treatment: A possible complication of a new antiarrhythmic drug.* Circulation 65:819, 1982.

108. ROTMENSCH, HH, LIRON, M, TUPILSKI, M, ET AL: *Possible association of pneumonitis with amiodarone therapy.* Am Heart J 100:412, 1980.

109. BURGER, A, DINICHERT, D, NICOD, P, ET AL: *Effect of amiodarone on serum triodothyronine, reverse triodothyronine, thyroxine and thyrotropin. A drug influencing peripheral metabolism of thyroid hormones.* J Clin Invest 58:255, 1976.

110. NADEMANEE, K, SINGH, BN, HENDRICKSON, JA, ET AL: *Pharmacokinetic significance of serum reverse T_3 levels during amiodarone treatment: A potential method for monitoring chronic drug therapy.* Circulation 66:202, 1982.

111. BOOTHBY, CB, GARRARD, CS, AND PICKERING, D: *Verapamil in cardiac arrhythmias.* Br Med J 2:349, 1972.

112. SUBRAMANIAN, B, BOWLES, MJ, DAVIES, AB, ET AL: *Combined therapy with verapamil and propranolol in chronic stable angina.* Am J Cardiol 49:125, 1982.

113. WAYNE, VS, HARPER, RW, LAUFER, E, ET AL: *Adverse interaction between beta-adrenergic blocking drugs and verapamil—report of three cases.* Aust NZ J Med 12:285, 1982.

114. GUCKENBIEHL, W, GILFRICH, HJ, AND JUST, H: *Einfluss von Laxantien und Metaclopramid auf die Chinidin-Plasmakonzentration während Langzeittherapie bei Patienten mit Herzrhythmusstorungen.* Med Welt 27:1273, 1976.

115. BIGGER, JT JR: *The quinidine-digoxin interaction—what do we know about it?* N Engl J Med 301:779, 1979.

116. BUSSEY, HI: *The influence of quinidine and other agents on digitalis glycosides.* Am Heart J 104:289, 1982.

117. Moysey, JO, Jaggarao, NSV, Grundy, EN, et al: *Amiodarone increases plasma digoxin concentrations.* Br Med J 282:272, 1981.

118. Rees, A, Dalal, JJ, Reid, PG, et al: *Dangers of amiodarone and anticoagulant treatment.* Br Med J 282:1756, 1982.

119. Morganroth, J, Michelson, EL, Horowitz, LN, et al: *Limitations of routine long-term electrocardiographic monitoring to assess ventricular ectopic frequency.* Circulation 58:408, 1978.

120. Lown, B: *Management of patients at high risk of sudden death.* Am Heart J 103:689, 1982.

121. Palileo, EV, Ashley, WW, Swiryn, S, et al: *Exercise provocable right ventricular outflow tract tachycardia.* Am Heart J 104:185, 1982.

122. Horowitz, LN, Spielman, SR, Greenspan, AM, et al: *Role of programmed stimulation in assessing vulnerability to ventricular arrhythmias.* Am Heart J 103:604, 1982.

123. Mason, JW and Winkle, RA: *Accuracy of the ventricular tachycardia induction study for predicting the long-term efficacy and inefficacy of antiarrythmic drugs.* N Engl J Med 303:1073, 1980.

124. Bauernfeind, RA, Swiryn, SP, Strasberg, B, et al: *Electrophysiologic drug testing in prophylaxis of sporadic paroxysmal atrial fibrillation: Technique, application and efficacy in severely symptomatic preexcitation patients.* Am Heart J 103:941, 1981.

125. Surawicz, B: *Intracardiac extrastimulation studies: How to? where? by whom?* Circulation 65:428, 1982.

126. Dumez, Y, Tchobroutsky, C, Hornych, H, et al: *Neonatal effects of maternal administration of acebutolol.* Br Med J 283:1077, 1981.

127. Rubin, PC: *Current concepts: Beta-blockers in pregnancy.* N Engl J Med 305:1323, 1981.

128. Dumesic, DA, Silverman, NH, Tobias, S, et al: *Transplacental cardioversion of fetal supraventricular tachycardia with procainamide.* N Engl J Med 307:1128, 1982.

Management of Serious Cardiac Arrhythmias With Drugs

Debra S. Echt, M.D., and Jay W. Mason, M.D.

Improved in-hospital and out-of-hospital recognition, monitoring, and treatment of lethal cardiac arrhythmias have resulted in increased interest in management of patients susceptible to recurrent, life-threatening arrhythmias.[1] Despite recent advances in the understanding of cardiac electrophysiology and use of clinical cardiac stimulation techniques, antiarrhythmic drug therapy remains empirical because the mechanisms governing ventricular tachyarrhythmias are largely unknown.[2] Treatment choices have expanded to include investigational antiarrhythmic agents, pacemaker and defibrillator implantation, and surgical ablative therapy. In the face of managing an unknown entity with any of a wide variety of therapies, it is difficult to treat rationally. The purpose of this chapter is to discuss the contemporary management of lethal arrhythmias with drugs, emphasizing practical applications in the rapidly evolving area of electrophysiology.

Consideration of the following aspects can guide management: (1) Specific characterization of the arrhythmia. The nature of the arrhythmia may be apparent from an ECG monitoring strip or 12-lead electrocardiogram, but an invasive electrophysiologic test may be required for accurate diagnosis. For example, an ECG with wide-complex tachycardia and disassociated atrial activity is virtually diagnostic of ventricular tachycardia, whereas QRS duration greater than 140 msec, left axis deviation, and ventricular rate less than 170 beats per min during tachycardia are only suggestive of a ventricular origin.[3] (2) The presence of underlying heart disease. Infrequent ventricular premature contractions occur in normal subjects. Although these subjects are at increased risk of sudden death, the risk is small, and they do not require therapy. Sustained ventricular tachycardia, on the other hand, is an unusual occurrence in patients with otherwise normal hearts but, when present, should be treated. The urgency of initiating treatment is determined in each case. (3) Correlation of symptoms with the occurrence of arrhythmia. Do the patient's symptoms require therapy, and can they be used as an indicator of therapeutic success? (4) The setting in which the arrhythmia occurs. Treatable conditions such as hypoxia, electrolyte imbalance, or acidosis should be sought. Because all antiarrhythmic agents can cause arrhythmias even at therapeutic doses and blood levels,[4] drug-induced arrhythmia is a diagnostic consideration in any patient receiving these drugs. (5) The likelihood of arrhythmia chronicity. Tachyarrhythmias occurring during the acute phase of myocardial infarction often do not recur. However, tachyarrhythmias occurring more than 7 days after myocardial infarction usually recur chronically.

Which Arrhythmia to Treat

Patients with documented, recurrent, sustained ventricular tachycardia or ventricular fibrillation, without evidence of acute myocardial infarction or other inciting events, require chronic therapy. Patients with complex ectopy or unsustained ventricular tachycardia require therapy if they are symptomatic, or if their cardiac condition is associated with a significantly increased incidence of lethal cardiac arrhythmias, for example, advanced cardiomyopathy, coronary artery disease, or valvular heart disease. The occurrence of lethal ventricular arrhythmias is closely associated with conditions causing poor left ventricular function.[5] Numerous studies have demonstrated the relationship between left ventricular dysfunction after myocardial infarction, ventricular premature contractions, and sudden cardiac death.[6] Because 80 percent of patients experiencing sudden cardiac death have underlying coronary artery disease, this group is of greatest clinical concern. In patients surviving an episode of sudden cardiac death and subsequently undergoing electrophysiologic study for ventricular tachyarrhythmia induction, the arrhythmia initiated in the majority of patients is ventricular tachycardia.[7]

The treatment of atrial arrhythmias in the Wolff-Parkinson-White syndrome will be considered in a later section.

Alternative Therapies

In addition to antiarrhythmic drugs, antitachycardia pacemakers and map-guided surgical ablation techniques are effective therapies, either alone or in combination with drug therapy, but will not be discussed in this chapter. Coronary revascularization in patients with severe coronary artery disease and ventricular arrhythmias has also been attempted to prevent lethal ventricular arrhythmias. Although studies comparing coronary artery bypass surgery with medical therapy have shown a lower incidence of sudden death in surgical patients, the trials were either not randomized or not prospective, or the patients were not matched for important clinical variables.[8,9] The potential mechanism(s) responsible for the prevention of sudden death by revascularization is unknown. In patients with recurrent, sustained ventricular tachycardia, coronary artery bypass grafting alone rarely prevents arrhythmia recurrence.[10] Likewise, blind aneurysmectomy for the prevention of malignant ventricular arrhythmia is inadequate therapy.[11]

The remainder of this chapter is devoted to the choice and use of antiarrhythmic drugs for treatment of ventricular tachyarrhythmias in a variety of settings and of atrial tachyarrhythmias in the Wolff-Parkinson-White syndrome. Methods of assessing the efficacy of therapy will be considered individually.

DRUGS FOR VENTRICULAR TACHYARRHYTHMIAS

Electrophysiologic mechanisms potentially responsible for the genesis and perpetuation of ventricular tachycardia are discussed in detail in other publications and are beyond the scope of this discussion.[12,13] At this time, our knowledge of underlying mechanisms is not sufficient to accurately predict which antiarrhythmic drug will be successful without some form of trial.[2] Even though we cannot match an antiarrhythmic drug to an individual based on its electrophysiologic actions, knowledge of the electrophysiologic actions of specific drugs is nevertheless useful in managing these patients. Electrocardiographic and electrophysiologic variables are as important as blood levels in determining therapeutic and toxic effects. For example, agents with similar electrophysiologic effects may cause toxicity if given together in "therapeutic" doses. If a patient has failed to respond to antiarrhythmic agents of one type, it may be advantageous to use one of a different type. The antiarrhythmic drug classification most often used is based on certain effects on the action potential of normal tissue.[14,15]

Although this classification ignores important features of drug action, it is widely acknowledged. Class 1 drugs decrease the rate of rise of phase 0 of the action potential. Class 1 may be subdivided: 1a drugs prolong action potential duration, 1b agents shorten the action potential, and 1c drugs do not affect action potential duration. Class 2 drugs are competitive inhibitors of beta-adrenergic receptor sites. Class 3 drugs prolong the action potential with no effect on phase 0. Class 4 drugs selectively block the calcium channel. Table 1 lists standard and investigational agents according to this classification and summarizes their effects on the cardiac action potential and surface electrocardiogram, and their clinical electrophysiology.[15–17]

The therapy for lethal ventricular arrhythmias is separated into acute treatment and chronic preventive therapy. Table 2 provides a guide for administration of standard and investigational antiarrhythmic drugs. For the acute treatment of ventricular tachycardia, intravenous lidocaine is the drug of choice, followed by procainamide and bretylium.[18] Procainamide has proven to be highly effective in the acute treatment of ventricular tachycardia.[19] Intravenous bretylium is effective in the treatment of drug-resistant ventricular tachycardia and ventricular fibrillation, particularly in acute myocardial infarction;[18] however, a common adverse effect is orthostatic hypotension, which may be ameliorated by concomitant protriptyline or ephedrine administration.[20,21] Quinidine is not generally used owing to fear of adverse negative inotropic effects. However, quinidine can be safely administrated intravenously, even in patients with congestive heart failure, if precautions are taken:[22] We recommend an intravenous loading dose of 5 to 10 mg/kg administered at 0.25 to 0.5 mg/kg/min with concomitant saline administration to maintain an adequate arterial pressure. Phenytoin and propranolol are less effective acute agents.

Of the investigational agents listed for the acute treatment of ventricular arrhythmia, amiodarone, flecainide, encainide, lorcainide, aprindine, disopyramide (parenteral), and verapamil have been proven effective in acute testing.[16,20,23–30]

Oral quinidine, procainamide, disopyramide, propranolol, and phenytoin are standard agents with proven efficacy for chronic suppression of ventricular ectopy. Procainimide and quinidine have been shown to decrease ectopy in approximately 62 percent of patients.[31] Long-term therapy with procainamide is limited by the development of serious side effects.[19] An uncommon but potentially lethal adverse effect of quinidine is *torsade de pointes* ventricular arrhythmias. The latter may be an idiosyncratic reaction or a result of toxic serum quinidine levels.[32] However, all antiarrhythmic agents that prolong the Q–T interval can cause *torsade de pointes* arrhythmias. Oral disopyramide has proven effective in control of ventricular ectopy including ventricular tachycardia,[24,25] but its use is limited by negative inotropic and anticholinergic side effects. Although phenytoin demonstrates acute efficacy, long-term suppression of ventricular tachycardia is less likely.[33]

Propranolol is currently the only beta-adrenergic blocking drug approved in the United States for treatment of arrhythmia. However, several beta blockers, including alprenolol, practolol, timolol, and most recently propranolol, have been shown to prevent mortality in patients after myocardial infarction.[21] The reason for this protection is unknown, but the improved survival correlates with both fewer sudden deaths and a reduction in subsequent myocardial infarctions. Cardioprotection may be due to ventricular antiarrhythmic effects, which have been demonstrated for propranolol and acebutolol.[34]

The availability of investigational antiarrhythmic agents has increased the potential for successful therapy. All drugs listed in Table 2 have demonstrated chronic efficacy in the treatment of sustained ventricular tachyarrhythmias. The efficacy of individual drugs varies among studies, probably owing to differing patient populations and drug assessment protocols. No single agent has emerged as unequivocally superior. However, the various investigational antiarrhythmic drugs have some unique properties. Amiodarone has an extremely long half-life, perhaps 30 days, allowing long dosing intervals and better patient compliance. On the other hand, the oral loading period preceding attainment of steady state is several weeks, during which time patients are not fully protected against lethal tachyarrhythmias and often

Table 1. Electrophysiologic effects

	Intracellular			
Drug	Class	Action Potential Effects	ECG Effects	Clinical Electrophysiologic Effects
Quinidine	1a	↓Rate phase 0, prolong action potential	↑QT	↑AH, ↑HV, ↑A-ERP, ↑V-ERP, ↓AVN-ERP, ↑HPS-ERP, ↓WCL
Procainamide	1a	" " " "	↑QRS, ↑QT	↑HV, ↑A-ERP, ↑V-ERP, ↓AVN-ERP, ↑HPS-ERP, ↓WCL
Dysopyramide	1a	" " " "	↑SR, ↑QRS, ↑QT	↑HV, ↑A-ERP, ↑V-ERP, →↓AVN-ERP, ↑HPS-ERP
*Imipramine	1a	Not available	↑PR, ↑QRS, ↑QT	Human data not available
*Pirmenol				
Lidocaine	1b	↓Rate phase 0, shorten action potential		→↓AVN-ERP, →↓HPS-ERP, →↓WCL
Phenytoin	1b	" " " "	↓SR	→↓AVN-ERP, ↓HPS-ERP
*Aprindine	1b	" " " "	↓SR, ↑PR, ↑QRS	↑AH, ↑HV, ↑A-ERP, ↑AVN-ERP, ↑HPS-ERP, ↑WCL
*Ethmozin	1b	" " " "	None	
*Mexiletine	1b	" " " "	None	→↑AH, →↑AV, →↑AVN-ERP, →↑HPS-ERP
*Tocainide	1b	" " " "	None	→↑AH, →↓A-ERP, →↓V-ERP, →↓AVN-ERP, →↓ HPS-ERP
*Encainide	1c	↓Rate phase 0	↑QRS	↑HV

*Flecainide	1c	" " , prolong action potential(?)	$\overline{\uparrow \text{QRS}}$	↑HV, ↑V-ERP (incomplete data)
*Lorcainide	1c	" "	$\overline{\uparrow \text{QRS}}$	↑HV (↑AH, ↑A-ERP, ↑V-ERP with chronic oral)
*Propofenone	1c	" "	$\overline{\uparrow \text{QRS}}$ $\overline{\uparrow \text{PR}}$	↑HV, ↑AH
*Propranolol	2	↓Rate phase 4, shorten action potential at high concentration	↓SR	↑AH, ↑AVN-ERP, ↑WCL
*Amiodarone	1+3	↓Rate phase 4, ↓rate phase 0, prolong action potential	↓SR, $\overline{\uparrow \text{QRS},}$ $\overline{\uparrow \text{QT}}$	↑AH, ↑A-ERP, ↑V-ERP, ↑AVN-ERP, ↑HPS-ERP, ↑WCL
Bretylium	3	↑Rate phase 4, " " "	$\overline{\uparrow \text{QRS}}$	
*N-acetylprocainamide	3	Prolong action potential	$\overline{\uparrow \text{QT}}$	↑A-ERP, ↑V-ERP
*Verapamil	4	↓Rate phase 4 ↑Duration phases 1,2	↓SR(chronic)↑PR	↑AH, ↑AVN-ERP, ↑WCL

*Investigational agents, i.e., investigational use only for ventricular arrhythmias.

↑ increase; ↓ decrease; → no change.

AH: Interval from atrial to His spike measured from the His bundle electrogram.

HV: Interval from the His spike measured from the His bundle electrogram to the onset of the QRS complex from the superficial ECG leads.

A-ERP: Longest interval between atrial drive and atrial premature extrastimulus in which the extrastimulus fails to capture the atrium.

V-ERP: Longest interval between ventricular drive and ventricular premature extrastimulus beats in which the extrastimulus fails to capture the ventricle.

AVN-ERP: Longest interval between atrial drive and atrial premature extrastimulus beats in which the extrastimulus fails to elicit a His spike.

HPS-ERP: Longest interval between the His spikes of the atrial drive and atrial premature extrastimulus beats in which the extrastimulus fails to depolarize the ventricle.

WCL: Longest atrial cycle length with 1:1 ventricular capture resulting from rapid atrial pacing.

Table 2. Therapeutic guidelines

Drugs	*Usual Dose and Administration*	*Blood Levels*	*Limiting Adverse Effects*
A. Standard Drugs			
Bretylium	1200–1400 mg,qd,po* 5 mg/kg load and 5–10 mg/kg q 6–8 h I.V.	0.5–1.0 μg/min	Orthostatic hypotension
Disopyramide	100–200 mg q 6–8 hr po 2 mg/kg I.V.	2–8 μg/ml	Negative inotropic effects
Lidocaine	100 mg and 50 mg 5 min later I.V. load, then 2 mg/min I.V.	1.4–6.0 μg/ml	Neurologic
Phenytoin	200–500 mg/day po 1 gm at 20 mg/min I.V.	10–20 μg/ml	Neurologic
Procainamide	250–1000 mg q 4 h po 13 mg/kg at 50 mg/min I.V.	4–12 μg/ml	Hypotension (I.V.); lupus-like syndrome
Propranolol	20–160 mg q 6 h po 0.15 mg/kg at 1 mg/min I.V.	—	Negative inotropic effects; bradycardia
Quinidine	300–600 mg q 6 h po 5–10 mg/kg over 20 minutes I.V.	2.0–5.0 μg/ml	Gastrointestinal
B. Investigational Drugs			
Amiodarone	200–800 mg qd po 5 mg/kg over 1 to 15 min I.V.	0.15–4.5 mg/ml	Pulmonary infiltrates; neurologic
Aprindine	50–100 mg q 6 h po 200 mg and 100 mg 30 min later at 2 mg/min to load	1–3 μg/ml	Neurologic; hepatotoxicity; agranulocytosis
Encainide	25–60 mg q 6–8 h po 1 mg/kg over 15–30 min I.V.	0.6–400 μg/ml	Neurologic
Ethmozin	75–400 mg q 8 h po	0.25–1.3 μg/ml	Neurologic
Flecainide	200–400 mg q 12 po 1–2 mg/kg I.V.	0.8–1.6 μg/ml	Neurologic
Imipramine	50–100 mg q 12 h po	0.15–0.25 μg/ml	Neurologic
Lorcainide	100–200 q 12 h or 100 q 8 h po 2–6 mg/kg over 15–45 min I.V.	0.1–0.4 μg/ml	Sleep disturbance
Mexiletine	150–400 mg q 8 h po	0.50–3.0 μg/ml	Neurologic
N-Acetyl procainamide	0.5–2.5 gm q 6–8 h po	9.4–19.5 μg/ml	Gastrointestinal
Propofenone	150–300 mg q 8 h po 1.0–2.0 mg/kg I.V. over 10 min	—	Neurologic
Tocainide	400–800 mg q 8 h po 750 mg over 15 min I.V.	3.5–10 μg/ml	Neurologic
Verapamil	80–120 mg q 6–8 h po 0.25 mg/kg over 15 min I.V.	0.5–3.0 μg/ml	AV block; hypotension (I.V.)

*No longer available po.

remain hospitalized. In addition, if amiodarone is discontinued because of toxicity or inefficacy, tissue stores take many days to clear.[34] Encainide produces marked prolongation of the QRS complex on ECG recordings. Encainide is well tolerated and reasonably effective in short- and long-term followup.[2,19] Oral encainide therapy results in at least two metabolites with electrophysiologic activity, each differing somewhat from that of the parent compound.[35] Lorcainide has been shown to be effective in the treatment of recurrent ventricular tachycardia[26] and has at least one known active metabolite, norlorcainide. Lorcainide may cause a sleep disturbance characterized by nightmares and reduced sleep time. The latter may be prevented by flurazepam administration. Tocainide has been shown to be most often effective in patients responsive to lidocaine.[36] Lidocaine responsiveness may also predict a favorable response to mexiletine. Experience with flecainide has been encouraging because it produces a prolonged antiarrhythmic response and low incidence of toxicity, and has proven to be a highly effective drug.[37] In a report of the chronic use of flecainide for ventricular ectopy and unsustained ventricular tachycardia, an increase in arrhythmia frequency was observed early in therapy in 4 of 11 patients. However, patients were subsequently effectively treated for a mean followup of 12 months.[38]

There are several cardiac conditions in which specific agents have been shown to have greater efficacy. *Torsade de pointes*, a pleomorphic ventricular tachycardia that is usually unsustained and characterized by 180-degree changes in the QRS complex vector (Fig. 1), is most often associated with Q–T interval prolongation and class 1a drug toxicity. In the latter setting, the appropriate treatment is withdrawal of all antiarrhythmic drugs and institution of overdrive pacing.[39–41] Arrhythmias occurring in association with Q–T interval prolongation respond best to propranolol or phenytoin.[42] Phenytoin and propranolol are also effective in the therapy for ventricular arrhythmias associated with digitalis toxicity. Propranolol is the drug of choice for exercise-induced arrhythmias.[43] Several authors also recommend propranolol for

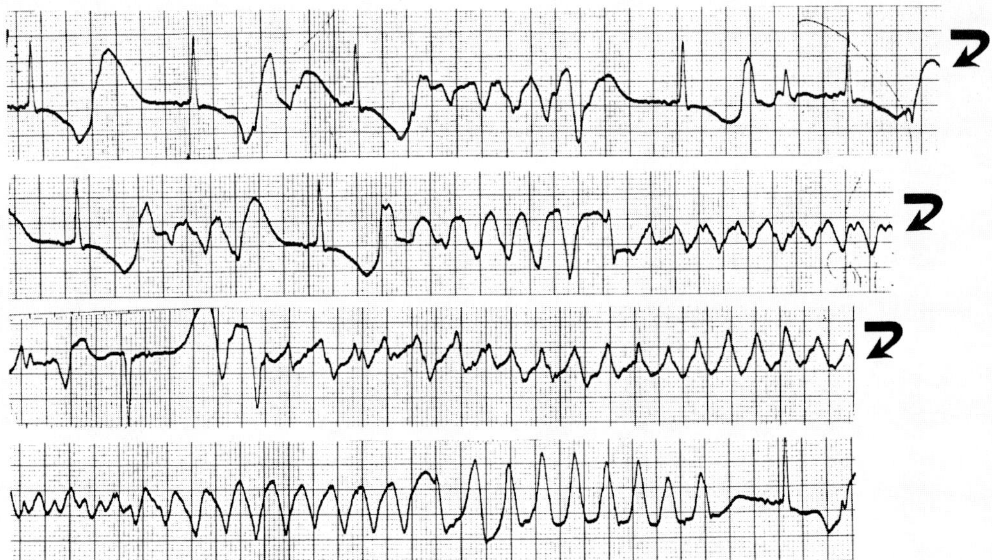

Figure 1. Continous ECG rhythm strip of *torsade de pointes* ventricular arrhythmias in a patient with a long Q–T interval. In the top panel, the sinus beats have markedly prolonged Q–T interval with giant, bizarre T waves. Runs of ventricular tachycardia are initiated when premature ventricular beats occur on the T waves of antecedent sinus beats. Note that the ventricular tachycardia is self-terminating and demonstrates 180-degree changes in QRS vector. (From Swerdlow, CD and Mason, JW: *Emergency treatment of ventricular tachycardia.* In Scheinman, MM (ed): *Cardiac Emergency.* Lange, Los Altos, Calif, with permission.).

the ventricular arrhythmias encountered with mitral valve prolapse.[44] The specific drug treatment of serious ventricular arrhythmias in acute myocardial infarction is discussed in another chapter.

DRUGS FOR ATRIAL FLUTTER-FIBRILLATION IN THE WOLFF-PARKINSON-WHITE SYNDROME

Wolff-Parkinson-White syndrome is a condition in which one or more accessory pathways allow pre-excitation of ventricular myocardium. There are two distinct supraventricular arrhythmias that commonly occur in the Wolff-Parkinson-White (WPW) syndrome: atrial fibrillation (or flutter) and reciprocating tachycardia. The reciprocating tachycardia usually uses the AV node for antegrade conduction and the accessory pathway for retrograde conduction. Because the tachycardia rate is limited by conduction velocity over a spatially large re-entry circuit, this arrhythmia is generally not lethal. Conversely, antegrade conduction in atrial fibrillation (or flutter) can be conducted at high frequency over an accessory pathway with a short refractory period, because decremental conduction is usually absent (Fig. 2). In the latter situation, the rapid ventricular response may be intolerable or may be complicated by degeneration to ventricular fibrillation.

Direct-current cardioversion is the appropriate immediate therapy for rapid atrial fibrillation in patients with WPW syndrome and a very rapid ventricular response rate. The effect of antiarrhythmic agents on the refractory period of the accessory pathway is variable.[45] Lidocaine or procainamide may increase antegrade accessory pathway refractoriness, but even lidocaine may be deleterious.[46] Propranolol and digoxin, common acute treatment choices in atrial fibrillation, are generally ineffective in WPW syndrome. Digoxin administration is dangerous because it may decrease refractoriness of bypass fibers.

One criterion used to direct chronic therapy in patients with the WPW syndrome who are prone to atrial fibrillation is the determination of the R–R interval during atrial fibrillation. Gallagher and coworkers[45] analyzed data from 163 patients with WPW syndrome, 18 of whom presented with ventricular fibrillation, presumably complicating atrial fibrillation. In

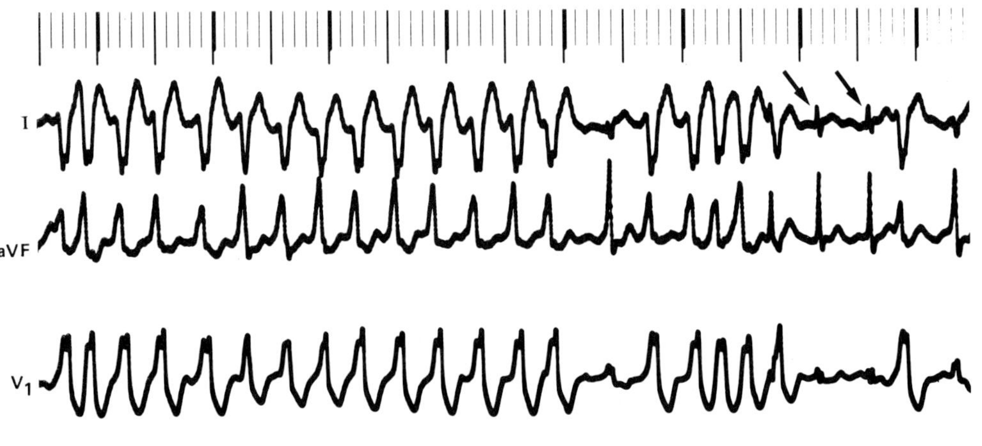

Figure 2. Atrial fibrillation in a patient with Wolff-Parkinson-White syndrome. Recordings are from surface ECG leads I, aVF, and V_1. The tachycardia is irregularly irregular with marked beat-to-beat variation of QRS complexes. The beats designated by arrows are morphologically identical to normally conducted sinus beats. (From Swerdlow, CD and Mason, JW: *Emergency treatment of ventricular tachycardia.* In Scheinman, MM (ed): *Cardiac Emergency.* Lange, Los Altos, Calif, with permission.)

this group of 18, the shortest R–R interval during atrial fibrillation was less than 205 msec. Identification of patients with rapid ventricular conduction during atrial fibrillation is presumed to distinguish those at high risk for lethal arrhythmias. However, it is not certain whether the episodes of ventricular fibrillation were precipitated by atrial fibrillation. Thus, we do not know how often the presence of short R–R intervals during atrial fibrillation is a false-positive indication for therapy. Despite the uncertainty, we recommend induction of atrial fibrillation during electrophysiology study in patients with WPW syndrome who have experienced syncope or ventricular fibrillation. Antiarrhythmic drug response should include measurement of the shortest R–R interval during atrial fibrillation and of the antegrade refractory period of the accessory pathway.

Be wary that the brief period of observation of atrial fibrillation in the electrophysiology laboratory may not give an accurate representation of the clinical arrhythmia inasmuch as the electrophysiologic properties of accessory pathways vary under autonomic and other influences. Wellens and associates evaluated the effect of isoproterenol on the antegrade refractory period of the accessory pathway.[47] In six of seven patients tested, the refractory period shortened during infusion of isoproterenol. The effect was greatest in patients with longer control values. The authors suggest that any factor causing enhancement of beta-adrenergic stimulation may lead to more rapid atrial fibrillation rates. Surgical therapy for accessory pathway ablation should be considered in patients with atrial fibrillation conducting rapidly over the accessory bypass. For the chronic control of atrial fibrillation, drug therapy should be aimed at suppression of ectopic beats as well as increasing refractoriness of the accessory pathway.

Amiodarone is the agent that is most consistently effective in treating atrial fibrillation in the WPW syndrome by suppressing ectopic beats and increasing the refractory period of the accessory pathway.[48] Quinidine, disopyramide, procainamide, aprindine, encainide, and other agents[15,16,45,49,50] often slow the ventricular response or shorten the duration of the episodes, but these same agents may occasionally accelerate the ventricular response.[46,49–51] Verapamil may produce differing effects on refractoriness of the AV node and the accessory pathway, thereby resulting in an unpredictable net effect. For instance, in a study of eight patients with WPW syndrome, induction of atrial fibrillation was used to evaluate the response to verapamil.[51] The shortest R–R interval increased in three patients, decreased in four others, and was unchanged in one. Patients primarily conducting via the accessory pathway during atrial fibrillation were more likely to demonstrate acceleration of the ventricular response in this study.

To summarize, cardioversion is the treatment of choice for the acute management of rapid atrial fibrillation in patients with WPW syndrome. The long-term therapy for atrial or ventricular fibrillation and the evaluation of syncope require electrophysiologic testing for guidance. Drug selection is determined by effects on the shortest pre-excited R–R interval during atrial fibrillation and the refractory period of the accessory pathway. Surgical ablation of the accessory pathway is a consideration in patients with rapid ventricular response over the accessory pathway.

ASSESSMENT OF DRUG THERAPY

Role of Electrophysiologic Studies

Electrophysiologic studies with programmed stimulation provide for correct identification of wide-complex tachycardias as either ventricular or supraventricular in origin; induction of suspected but undocumented ventricular tachyarrhythmias; evaluation of the prophylactic efficacy of antiarrhythmic drugs; and performance of activation sequence mapping for future surgical ablative therapy. Electrophysiologic studies are indicated for antiarrhythmic drug selection in those patients in whom arrhythmias are life-threatening or refractory to conven-

Table 3. Ventricular tachyarrhythmia induced with programmed stimulation

Clinical Arrhythmia	*No. Patients*	*Induced Arrhythmia (%)* Sustained VT	*Unsustained VT*	*VF*	*None*
Sustained VT	241	76	8	6	7
Unsustained VT	42	19	36	7	40
VF	28	14	18	36	29
Survivor of sudden death	104	58	12	15	15

VT = ventricular tachycardia; VF = ventricular fibrillation.

From Mason, JW, Swerdlow, CD, Winkle, RA, et al: *Ventricular tachyarrhythmia induction for drug selection: Experience with 311 patients. NIH Symposium on Antiarrhythmic Drug Therapy.* Raven Press, New York (in press), with permission.

tional therapy, or if trial-and-error therapy is not efficient because of infrequent arrhythmia occurrence.

Evaluation of potential therapies with electrophysiologic testing requires that the arrhythmias be inducible. Patients most likely to benefit from electrophysiologic testing are those with recurrent, sustained ventricular tachycardia. Results of a series of 311 patients with life-threatening ventricular tachyarrhythmias undergoing ventricular tachyarrhythmia induction study at our institution are summarized in Table 3.[52] Patients with clinical sustained ventricular tachycardia demonstrated a 90 percent incidence of inducible arrhythmias. In patients with documented, recurrent ventricular tachycardia, the clinical arrhythmia has been shown to be reproducibly inducible by programmed stimulation in 80 to 95 percent of cases in other series.[53–55] The lowest incidence of inducibility (60 percent) in our 311 patients was found in those in whom the clinical arrhythmia was unsustained ventricular tachycardia. Other authors have found a similar low inducibility rate in patients with unsustained ventricular tachycardia.[56]

In patients surviving sudden cardiac death, only 50 to 80 percent have inducible arrhythmias at electrophysiologic study.[7,57,58] A large series evaluated 52 patients resuscitated from cardiac arrest and in whom ECG documentation of ventricular tachyarrhythmia was available.[7] Using programmed stimulation technique, ventricular tachycardia or fibrillation was induced in only 63 percent of patients. Of the 30 cases found to be in ventricular fibrillation at the time of arrest, only 13 (43 percent) had either ventricular tachycardia or fibrillation induced with programmed stimulation. A significant proportion of patients surviving sudden cardiac death, particularly those with clinical ventricular fibrillation, did not have inducible sustained ventricular arrhythmias with programmed stimulation. Therefore, therapy directed by programmed stimulation was not possible in a significant portion of the sudden cardiac death survivors with documented arrhythmias. In a series of 104 patients studied following an episode of sudden cardiac death at our institution, 85 percent of patients had an arrhythmia induced at electrophysiologic study. The majority (58 percent) of the induced arrhythmias were ventricular tachycardias.[52]

Electrophysiologic studies have been used to uncover ventricular tachycardia in patients with unexplained syncope and with negative ambulatory monitoring studies and neurologic evaluations. In a series of 25 patients with unexplained syncope undergoing electrophysiologic testing,[59] the cause was found in 17, nine of whom had inducible ventricular tachycardia. Drug therapy selected by programmed stimulation resulted in successful treatment in seven of those nine patients for a mean followup of 18 months. It appears that in a significant minority of patients, ventricular tachyarrhythmias rather than bradyarrhythmias are responsible for syncopal episodes. Electrophysiologic studies may be of both diagnostic and therapeutic benefit in these patients.

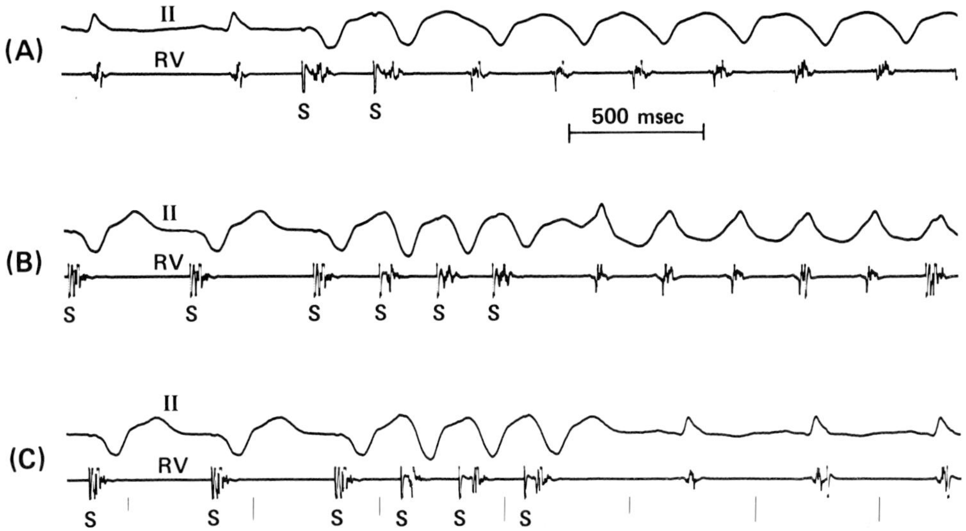

Figure 3. Arrhythmia induction before and after drug administration in a patient with recurrent, sustained ventricular tachycardia. Surface ECG lead 2 (top tracing in each panel) and right ventricular apical electrogram (bottom tracing in each panel) are shown. *A*, In the control state, two extrastimuli (S) delivered during sinus rhythm initiate ventricular tachycardia. *B*, During lidocaine administration, three extrastimuli delivered during ventricular paced rhythm initiate ventricular tachycardia. *C*, After intravenous quinidine, ventricular tachycardia was not inducible with three extrastimuli delivered during ventricular pacing.

Drug Assessment Using Programmed Stimulation

General Principles

In patients with documented spontaneous ventricular arrhythmias in whom arrhythmias are reproducibly inducible during electrophysiologic testing, arrhythmia reinduction with acute drug administration is an accepted method to evaluate drug therapy.[52–55,60]

To ensure reproducibility, we routinely induce three episodes of the suspected clinical ventricular arrhythmia prior to drug administration. Several of the antiarrhythmic agents, for instance, lidocaine, quinidine, propranolol, verapamil, phenytoin, and procainamide, can be given intravenously and evaluated during the initial electrophysiology procedure. However, only lidocaine has a sufficiently short half-life to allow subsequent testing of single agents (Fig. 3). Results of intravenous drug testing may differ from those of chronic oral therapy. Plasma concentrations attained, degrees of tissue saturation, and formation of active metabolites may alter electrophysiologic parameters. Therefore, oral therapy should also be evaluated by a repeat induction study. Oral antiarrhythmic drug testing with programmed stimulation should be performed under steady-state conditions, preferably during the latter part of a dosing interval. Ideally, the plasma drug concentration from a sample drawn at the conclusion of the induction study should be similar to levels attained chronically.

Long-term Effectiveness

Drug therapy guided by programmed stimulation has been shown to predict long-term drug effectiveness.[52,60,61] In a study of 51 patients, we compared long-term treatment with drugs predicted to be effective to treatment with drugs predicted to be ineffective.[60] After a followup period of 6 months, 80 percent of patients treated with positively predicted drugs were free from recurrence of arrhythmias compared with 33 percent without recurrence in the group treated with negatively predicted drugs. We have now analyzed the incidence of late ventricular tachyarrhythmia recurrence in 170 patients.[52] After 2 years of drug therapy, 78 percent of patients treated with drugs predicted to be effective were without arrhythmia recurrence, compared with 59 percent treated with drugs predicted to be ineffective.

Patient Selection

Therapy directed by programmed stimulation is desirable, but facilities and personnel to perform electrophysiologic evaluation are not presently available in many hospitals. Inasmuch as many antiarrhythmic agents studied are investigational and the techniques require trained electrophysiologists, it seems appropriate that the centers performing such procedures be limited.[5] How, then, can a cardiologist or internist without electrophysiology facilities manage these patients? Must the patients all be referred to a center and undergo lengthy, stressful procedures, or can management be successful by other means?

We have attempted to evaluate the question of whether clinical factors can be helpful in deciding which patients are most likely to benefit from programmed stimulation for drug selection.[62] Stepwise logistic regression was applied to 22 clinical variables to construct a predictor function. Variables determined to be predictive of finding an effective drug were absence of structural heart disease, female sex, absence of left ventricular aneurysm, and a lower number of empiric drug trial failures prior to electrophysiologic testing. The validity of the regression function was successfully tested using a method to correct for bias, and by applying the equation prospectively to 25 patients undergoing electrophysiologic testing for drug selection. The logistic regression function can determine the probability of a successful electrophysiologic-pharmacologic study in any given patient. In the equation, variables are weighted to maximally separate the probability of responding or not responding to low-, intermediate-, and high-probability groups. As an example, a woman with a single 90 percent coronary artery stenosis and three episodes of arrhythmia has a probability score of 0.73. In other words, this patient has a high probability of having an effective drug determined by programmed stimulation testing.

Programmed Stimulation Techniques

There is considerable variation and controversy regarding programmed stimulation protocols. The induction technique used influences the results of drug testing. Increasing the number of extrastimuli introduced increases the percentage of patients in whom arrhythmias are inducible but could also lead to induction of nonclinical arrhythmias, such as ventricular fibrillation in a patient with a history of recurrent ventricular tachycardia. Similarly, a very aggressive testing protocol could lead to reinduction of the tachyarrhythmia in the presence of a potentially clinically effective antiarrhythmic agent. In our analysis of 234 patients undergoing electrophysiologic drug testing, the limitations of an aggressive protocol were demonstrated. A total of 541 drug trials were performed using 15 different drugs alone and in combination[52] (Table 4). The incidence of acute antiarrhythmic drug efficacy for each drug tested was low. The range of acute efficacy rates for individual drugs was 8 to 33 percent, with at least one effective drug identified in 49 percent of patients. We believe that this low rate is partly due to the practice of evaluating drug efficacy using three premature ventricular extrastimuli in instances in which only one or two extrastimuli were required to induce the ventricular arrhythmia before drug administration, as demonstrated in Figure 4. The addition of a third extrastimulus to the ventricular tachycardia induction protocol was instituted in our laboratory after a published analysis of patients undergoing drug testing.[61] In that series, an effective agent was identified in 71 percent of patients in whom a maximum of two extrastimuli were used. Results of drug testing in the aforementioned 234 patients were retrospec-

Table 4. Efficacy of antiarrhythmic drugs with programmed stimulation

Drug Tested	*No. Patients*	*Percentage Effective Tests*
Lidocaine	136	13
Quinidine	97	22
Procainamide	66	20
Propranolol	20	25
Disopyramide	12	33
Phenytoin	7	14
All other drugs	203	9
Investigational drugs (incl. amiodarone)	155	9
Amiodarone	37	8

From Mason, JW, Swerdlow, CD, Winkle, RA, et al: *Ventricular tachyarrhythmia induction for drug selection: Experience with 311 patients. NIH Symposium on Antiarrhythmic Drug Therapy.* Raven Press, New York (in press), with permission.

tively analyzed to compare the effect of adding the third ventricular extrastimulus.[63] An acutely effective drug was found in 32 percent of patients when using a third ventricular extrastimulus. If only two extrastimuli had been used, an effective drug would have been identified in 68 percent of patients. Other investigators have reported similar findings of 67 to 70 percent acute drug efficacy using a maximum of two extrastimuli[53,64] and 51 percent

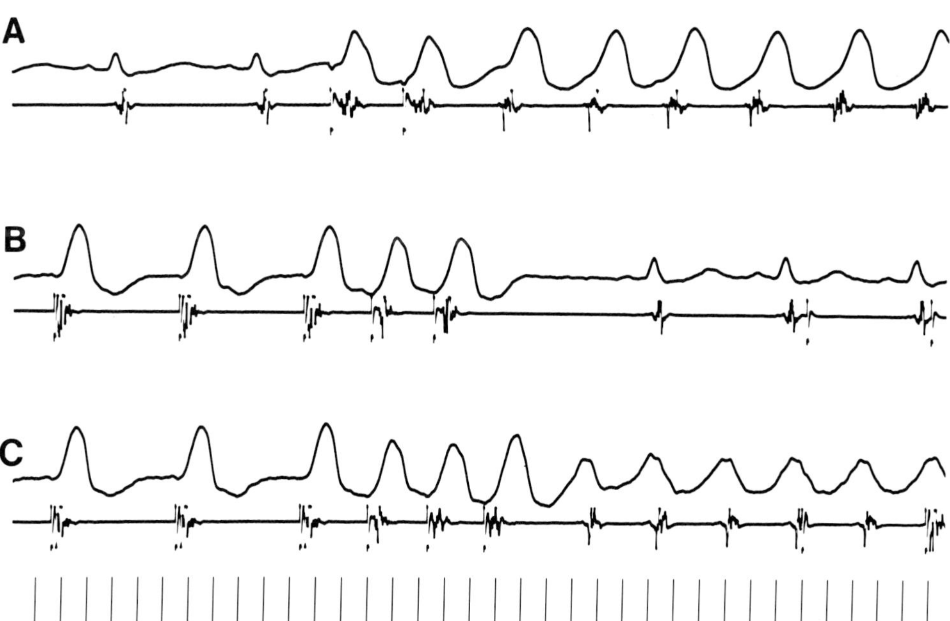

Figure 4. Arrhythmia induction before and after drug administration in a patient with recurrent ventricular tachycardia (VT). Surface ECG lead 1 (top tracing in each panel) and right ventricular apical electrogram (bottom tracing in each panel) are shown. *A*, Prior to drug administration, two extrastimuli (V_2V_3) delivered during sinus rhythm initiate sustained VT. *B*, After administration of a lidocaine loading dose and infusion, two extrastimuli delivered in ventricular drive rhythm ($V_1V_2V_3$) fail to initiate VT. *C*, Three extrastimuli delivered in ventricular drive rhythm ($V_1V_2V_3V_4$) initiate VT in the presence of lidocaine. (From Swerdlow, CD, Blum, J, Winkle, RA, et al: *Decreased incidence of antiarrhythmic drug efficacy at electrophysiologic study associated with use of a third extrastimulus.* Am Heart J 104:1004, 1982, with permission.)

using a third extrastimulus when necessary.[65] Therefore, the addition of the third extrastimulus may exclude some drugs with which the patient would potentially be effectively treated.

In addition to the differences in the specific induction methods utilized, there is variability in the criteria used to assess drug efficacy with electrophysiologic testing.[56,66] For instance, in our laboratory, a drug was deemed effective against sustained ventricular tachycardia only if fewer than six ventricular beats were induced with programmed stimulation. These were excessively strict criteria. In a recent analysis of Swerdlow and associates,[67] inducibility of 10 or fewer beats was associated with a low 2-year incidence of sudden death compared with patients with greater than 10 beats induced. There was no difference in outcome if no beats to 10 beats remained inducible.

Amiodarone Testing

One special case to be noted is the use of programmed stimulation in the testing of oral amiodarone. There is evidence that inducibility of ventricular tachyarrhythmias in the presence of amiodarone does not predict clinical inefficacy. In one study of nine patients, ventricular tachycardia was inducible in seven patients both before and after a range of 7 to 20 weeks of amiodarone therapy.[68] No patient had evidence of arrhythmia recurrence at 1-year followup. In another series, 18 to 19 patients still had inducible tachyarrhythmias after amiodarone therapy.[69] Thirteen of 19 patients were without evidence of recurrent ventricular tachycardia at a mean followup of 17 months. Most studies in patients taking amiodarone were conducted after only 2 to 4 weeks of therapy. Failure to attain steady state may have caused the low efficacy rates with electrophysiologic testing. The utility of programmed stimulation for evaluating drug response of amiodarone is unclear at this time. Similar uncertainty exists regarding other investigational agents.

Drug Combinations

There is disagreement over the utility of drug combinations in the therapy of ventricular tachycardia. Analysis with programmed stimulation testing by Ross and coworkers[70] of 110 antiarrhythmic drug combination trials revealed that the combination of lidocaine or propranolol with a class 1a agent was not likely to be acutely effective if both agents failed in single testing. Although we no longer routinely test drug combinations in our laboratory based on this analysis, other drug combinations were not analyzed. Other authors have recommended the use of drug combinations, but have cautioned that reports of efficacy are based on small numbers of patients,[71] and that a second agent may antagonize a useful electrophysiologic action of the first.[72]

ROLE OF AMBULATORY ECG MONITORING

Indications

ECG monitoring can be used successfully in selected patients as the primary method of drug assessment. It is most effective in patients with frequent episodes of ventricular tachycardia (one or more per day). Ambulatory ECG monitoring should be the primary method of drug efficacy assessment in patients with frequent episodes of unsustained ventricular tachycardia, in patients with spontaneous ectopy in whom electrophysiologic studies are contraindicated or of very low yield, and in those patients without inducible tachyarrhythmias at electrophysiologic study. The greatest utility of ambulatory monitoring is in the evaluation of new investigational drugs as potentially effective agents.[73]

Management

Therapy directed by ambulatory monitoring includes acquiring baseline studies for a minimum of 24 hours. We recommend longer periods of monitoring in patients with low numbers of ectopic beats, because ectopy in this group demonstrates greater variability. Several studies have demonstrated the need for more than 24 hours of ECG monitoring or the requirement of at least 80 percent suppression of ectopy, rather than 50 percent or 80 percent, in order to decrease the likelihood of spontaneous variation.[74] Although there is a direct correlation between the occurrence of salvos, complex ectopy, and the total number of premature ventricular beats, ventricular salvos and complex forms are less frequent and demonstrate greater spontaneous variability than total ventricular ectopic beats. Therefore, caution must be used in evaluating the ability of a drug to reduce the number of episodes of nonsustained ventricular tachycardia by ambulatory monitoring. Care must be taken to obtain recordings at appropriate times. When drug dosage is changed, recordings are best made during steady-state conditions, after a minimum of five drug half-lives.

Alternative ECG Monitoring

For patients with less frequent ventricular arrhythmias that do not lead to circulatory collapse, other forms of ECG recording devices are useful.[73] Symptomatic events can be documented with a battery-operated recording device activated by the patient and later transmitted via telephone. Longer-lasting events can be transmitted while they occur via telephone to an answering service for immediate evaluation. Other intermittent recorders can be worn for several days with recordings taken at preselected intervals or only during tachycardia or bradycardia.

ROLE OF EXERCISE TESTING

In patients with coronary artery disease, mitral valve prolapse, or idiopathic hypertrophic cardiomyopathy, electrophysiologic studies and ambulatory ECG monitoring are more sensitive and, therefore, superior means of diagnosing and managing ventricular arrhythmias than exercise testing.[76] Studies in patients with coronary artery disease have shown that ambulatory monitoring is about twice as sensitive as treadmill testing in the detection of ventricular arrhythmias, and even more sensitive in identification of complex ventricular ectopy.[77] In addition, the occurrence of complex ectopy with exercise testing is not as reproducible as ambulatory ECG monitoring.[78] However, in a small subgroup of patients, clinical arrhythmias are induced by exercise or stress. In this population, exercise testing may be more useful than ambulatory monitoring. We recommend obtaining an exercise test (treadmill or bicycle) in any patient in whom there is an association of arrhythmia with emotion or physical activity or in whom documented, sustained ventricular tachyarrhythmias are not inducible by programmed stimulation techniques. Some authors believe that catecholamines (circulatory and neurogenic) are contributing factors in all patients with ventricular arrhythmias, and advocate inclusion of exercise testing for therapeutic management.[79]

LONG-TERM IMPLICATIONS

A substantial number of patients are effectively treated with drug therapy alone. In the remainder, antitachycardia pacemakers, defibrillator devices, or surgical myocardial ablation guided by mapping techniques are often successful, either alone or in combination with drugs. The ultimate question is whether any intervention improves long-term patient survival. We have evaluated the determinants of survival in patients with sustained ventricular tachycardia

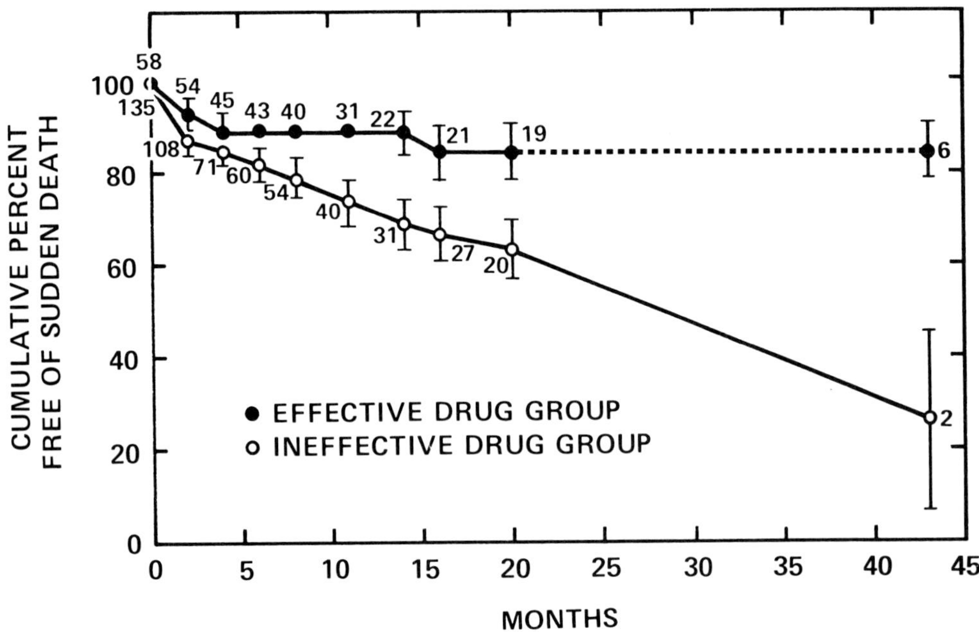

Figure 5. Life-table analysis of sudden death in patients with ventricular tachycardia treated with antiarrhythmic drugs. Closed-circle curve represents sudden death–free survival in 58 patients treated with drugs predicted to be effective with electrophysiologic testing. Open-circle curve represents sudden death–free survival in 135 patients for whom no effective antiarrhythmic drug could be identified at electrophysiologic testing. Cumulative percentages with standard errors are shown. The incidence of sudden death was significantly lower ($p<.04$) in the effective drug group after 8 months of follow-up. Numbers at each circle represent the numbers of patients remaining in each group at various follow-up intervals. (From Swerdlow, CD and Mason, JW: *Emergency treatment of ventricular tachycardia.* In Scheinman, MM (ed): *Cardiac Emergency.* Lange, Los Altos, Calif (in press), with permission.)

or ventricular fibrillation in 233 patients undergoing electrophysiologic testing.[80] Treatment consisted of drugs in 158 patients, surgery in 65 patients, implanted devices in six patients, and therapy withdrawal in four patients. After a mean followup period of 1.2 years, there were 73 cardiac deaths, 50 of which were sudden. Survival by actuarial analysis was 73 percent at 1 year, 64 percent at 2 years, and 50 percent at 3 years. Further analysis revealed that lesser severity of heart failure was most predictive of survival. This may indicate that patients with poor left ventricular function are less likely to respond to antiarrhythmic therapy, or that they have more frequent episodes of ventricular arrhythmias, or that they are less likely to survive an episode of ventricular arrhythmia. A life table analysis comparing patients treated with drugs predicted to be effective or ineffective at electrophysiologic testing is illustrated in Figure 5. Treatment directed by electrophysiologic testing was associated with a significant reduction in the incidence of sudden death. Programmed stimulation was almost as strong as severity of heart failure in predicting survival.

Therefore, therapy with antiarrhythmic drugs for lethal ventricular arrhythmias can be effective, particularly when directed by programmed stimulation testing. Success is limited in part by the severity of the patient's myocardial dysfunction and our incomplete knowledge of arrhythmia mechanisms and antiarrhythmic drug effects.

REFERENCES

1. Ruskin, JN, DiMarco, JP, and Garan, H: *Out of hospital cardiac arrest. Electrophysiologic observations and selection of long-term antiarrhythmic therapy.* N Engl J Med 303:607, 1980.

2. Mason, JW, Stinson, EB, Winkle, RA, et al: *Mechanisms of ventricular tachycardia: Wide complex ignorance.* Am Heart J 102:1083, 1981.
3. Wellens, JJ, Bar, FWHM, and Lie, KL: *The value of the electrocardiogram in the differential diagnosis of a tachycardia with a widened QRS complex.* Am J Med 64:27, 1978.
4. Velebit, V, Podrid, P, Lown, B, et al: *Aggravation and provocation of ventricular arrhythmias by antiarrhythmic drugs.* Circulation 65:886, 1982.
5. Calvert, A, Lown, B, and Gorlin, R: *Ventricular premature beats and anatomically defined coronary heart disease.* Am J Cardiol 39:627, 1977.
6. Schultze, RA, Strauss, HW, and Pitt, B: *Sudden death in the year following myocardial infarction: Relation to ventricular premature contractions in the late hospital phase and left ventricular ejection fraction.* Am J Med 62:192, 1977.
7. Josephson, ME, Horowitz, LN, Spielman, SR, et al: *Electrophysiologic and hemodynamic studies in patients resuscitated from cardiac arrest.* Am J Cardiol 46:948, 1980.
8. Hammermeister, KE, DeRouen, TA, Murray, JA, et al: *Effect of aortocoronary saphenous vein bypass grafting on death and sudden death.* Am J Cardiol 39:925, 1977.
9. Vismara, LA, Miller, RR, Price, JE, et al: *Improved longevity due to reduction of sudden death by aortocoronary bypass in coronary atherosclerosis.* Am J Cardiol 39:925, 1977.
10. Ricks, WB, Winkle, RA, Shumway, NE, et al: *Surgical management of life-threatening ventricular arrhythmias in patients with coronary artery disease.* Circulation 56:38, 1977.
11. Mason, JW, Stinson, EB, Winkle, RA, et al: *Surgery for ventricular tachyarrhythmia: Efficacy of left ventricular aneurysm resection compared to operation guided by electrical activation mapping.* Circulation 65:1148, 1982.
12. Hoffman, BF and Rosen, MR: *Cellular mechanisms for cardiac arrhythmias.* Circ Res 49:1, 1981.
13. Josephson, ME, Horwitz, LN, Farshiti, A, et al: *Recurrent sustained ventricular tachycardia. 1. Mechanisms.* Circulation 57:431, 1978.
14. Opie, LH: *Antiarrhythmic agents.* Lancet 1:861, 1980.
15. Singh, BN, Collett, JT, and Chew, CYC: *New perspectives in the pharmacologic therapy of cardiac arrhythmias.* Prog Cardiovasc Dis 22:243, 1980.
16. Zipes, DP and Troup, PJ: *New antiarrhythmic agents.* Am J Cardiol 41:1005, 1978.
17. Keefe, DLD, Kates, RE, and Harrison, DC: *New antiarrhythmic drugs: Their place in therapy.* Drugs 22:363, 1981.
18. Koch-Weser, J: *Drug therapy: Bretylium.* N Engl J Med 300:473, 1979.
19. Kayden, HJ, Brodic, BB, and Steele, JM: *Procainamide: A review.* Circulation 15:118, 1975.
20. Mason, JW: *Efficacy of verapamil in recurrent ventricular tachycardia.* Am J Cardiol 49:1015, 1982.
21. The Norwegian Multicentre Study Group: *Timolol-induced reduction in mortality and reinfarction in patients surviving acute myocardial infarction.* N Engl J Med 304:801, 1981.
22. Swerdlow, CD, Yu, JO, Jacobson, E, et al: *Safety and efficacy of intravenous quinidine.* Am J Cardiol 49:1043, 1982.
23. Strasberg, B, Palileo, E, Prechel, D, et al: *Ventricular tachycardia: Prediction of response to oral aprindine with intravenous aprindine.* Am J Cardiol 47:676, 1981.
24. Benditt, DG, Pritchett, ELC, Wallace, AG, et al: *Recurrent ventricular tachycardia in man: Evaluation of disopyramide therapy by intracardiac electrical stimulation.* Eur J Cardiol 9:255, 1979.
25. Mason, JW and Peters, FA: *Antiarrhythmic efficacy of encainide in patients with refractory recurrent ventricular tachycardia.* Circulation 63:670, 1981.
26. Cocco, GT and Strozzi, C: *Initial clinical experience of lorcainide (Ro 13-1042) a new antiarrhythmic agent.* Eur J Clin Pharmacol 14:105, 1978.
27. Campbell, RWF, Henderson, A, Bryson, LG, et al: *Intravenous flecainide—pharmacokinetics and efficacy.* Circulation 64:IV-265, 1981.
28. Vismara, LA, Mason, DT, and Amsterdam, EA: *Efficacy of disopyramide phosphate in the treatment of refractory ventricular tachycardia.* Am J Cardiol 39:1027, 1977.
29. Reddy, CP and Benes, J: *Efficacy and safety of a new intravenous dosage regimen of disopyramide in treating patients with ventricular arrhythmia.* Circulation 64:IV-265, 1981.
30. VanHamersveld, DD, Stewart, JR, Johnson, TA, et al: *Oral flecainide acetate for long-term treatment of ventricular arrhythmias in man.* Circulation 64:IV-316, 1981.
31. Winkle, RA, Gradman, AH, and Fitzgerald, JW: *Antiarrhythmic drug effect assessed from ventricular arrhythmia reduction in the ambulatory electrocardiogram and treadmill test: Comparison of propranolol, procainamide, and quinidine.* Am J Cardiol 42:473, 1978.

32. SCHWARTZ, JB, KEEFE, D, AND HARRISON, DC: *Adverse effects of antiarrhythmic drugs.* Drugs 21:23, 1981.

33. STONE, N, KLEIN, MD, AND LOWN, B: *Diphenylhydantoin in the prevention of recurrent ventricular tachycardia.* Circulation 43:420, 1971.

34. SINGH, SN, DEBIANCO, R, DAVIDOV, ME, ET AL: *Comparison of acebutolol and propranolol for treatment of chronic ventricular arrhythmia: A placebo-controlled double-blind, randomized crossover study.* Circulation 65:1356, 1982.

35. JACKMAN, WM, ZIPES, DP, NACARELLI, GV, ET AL: *Electrophysiology of oral encainide.* Am J Cardiol 49:1270, 1982.

36. WINKLE, RA, MASON, JW, AND HARRISON, DC: *Tocainide for drug resistant ventricular arrhythmias. Efficacy, side effects and lidocaine responsiveness for predicting tocainide success.* Am Heart J 100:1031, 1980.

37. ANDERSON, JL, STEWART, JR, PERRY, BA, ET AL: *Oral flecainide acetate for the treatment of ventricular arrhythmias.* N Engl J Med 305:473, 1981.

38. DUFF, HJ, RODEN, DM, MAFFUICCI, RJ, ET AL: *Suppression of resistant ventricular arrhythmias by twice daily dosing of flecainide.* Am J Cardiol 48:1133, 1981.

39. SMITH, WM AND GALLAGHER, JJ: *"Les torsades de pointes": An unusual ventricular arrhythmia.* Ann Intern Med 93:578, 1980.

40. KEREN, A, TZIVONI, D, GAVISH, D, ET AL: *Etiology, warning signs and therapy of torsade de pointes.* Circulation 64:1167, 1981.

41. ANDERSON, JL AND MASON, JW: *Successful treatment by overdrive pacing of recurrent quinidine syncope due to ventricular tachycardia.* Am J Med 64:715, 1981.

42. SCHWARTZ, PY, PERITI, M, AND MALLIANT, A: *The long QT syndrome.* Am Heart J 89:378, 1975.

43. NIXON, JV, PENNINGTON, W, RITTER, W, ET AL: *Efficacy of propranolol in the control of exercise-induced or augmented ventricular ectopic activity.* Circulation 57:115, 1978.

44. WINKLE, RA, LOPES, MG, GOODMAN, DJ, ET AL: *Propranolol for patients with mitral valve prolapse.* Am Heart J 93:422, 1978.

45. GALLAGHER, JJ, PRITCHETT, EC, SEALY, WC, ET AL: *The pre-excitation syndromes.* Prog Cardiovasc Dis 20:295, 1978.

46. AKHTAR, M, GILBERT, CJ, AND SHENASA, M: *Effects of lidocaine on atrioventricular response via the accessory pathway in patients with Wolff-Parkinson-White syndrome.* Circulation 63:435, 1981.

47. WELLENS, HJJ, BRUGADA, P, ROY, D, ET AL: *Effect of isoproterenol on the antegrade refractory period of the accessory pathway in patients with the Wolff-Parkinson-White syndrome.* Am J Cardiol 50:180, 1982.

48. DURRER, D: *Effect of amiodarone in the Wolff-Parkinson-White syndrome.* Am J Cardiol 38:189, 1976.

49. KEN, CR, PRYSTOWSKY, EN, SMITH, WM, ET AL: *Electrophysiologic effects of disopyramide phosphate in patients with Wolff-Parkinson-White syndrome.* Circulation 65:869, 1982.

50. SELLERS, TD, CAMPBELL, RWF, BASHORE, TM, ET AL: *Effects of procainamide and quinidine sulfate in the Wolff-Parkinson-White syndrome.* Circulation 55:15, 1977.

51. GULAMHUSEIN, S, KO, P, CARRUTHERS, SG, ET AL: *Acceleration of the ventricular response during atrial fibrillation in the Wolff-Parkinson-White syndrome after verapamil.* Circulation 65:348, 1982.

52. MASON, JW, SWERDLOW, CD, WINKLE, RA, ET AL: *Ventricular tachyarrhythmia induction for drug selection: Experience with 311 patients. NIH Symposium on Antiarrhythmic Drug Therapy.* Raven Press, New York (in press).

53. HOROWITZ, LN, JOSEPHSON, ME, FARSHIDI, A, ET AL: *Recurrent sustained ventricular tachycardia III. Role of the electrophysiologic study in selection of antiarrhythmic regimens.* Circulation 58:986, 1978.

54. FISHER, JC, COHEN, HL, MELMA, R, ET AL: *Cardiac pacing and pacemakers. II. Serial electrophysiologic-pharmacologic testing for control of recurrent tachyarrhythmias.* Am Heart J 93:658, 1977.

55. WELLENS, HJJ, SCHUILENBERG, RM, AND DURRER, P: *Electrical stimulation of the heart in patients with ventricular tachycardia.* Circulation 46:216, 1972.

56. LIVELLI, FD, BIGGER, JT, REIFFEL, JA, ET AL: *Response to programmed ventricular stimulation: Sensitivity, specificity and relation to heart disease.* Am J Cardiol 50:452, 1982.

57. RUSKIN, JW, DIMARCO, JP, AND GARAN, H: *Out-of-hospital cardiac arrest: Electrophysiologic observation and selection of long-term antiarrhythmic therapy.* N Engl J Med 303:607, 1980.

58. MYERBERG, RJ, CONDE, CA, SUNG, RJ, ET AL: *Clinical, electrophysiological and hemodynamic profile of patients resuscitated from prehospital cardiac arrest.* Am J Med 68:568, 1980.

59. DIMARCO, JP, GARAN, H, HARTHORNE, JW, ET AL: *Intracardiac electrophysiologic techniques in recurrent syncope of unknown cause.* Ann Intern Med 95:542, 1981.

60. MASON, JW AND WINKLE, RA: *Accuracy of the ventricular tachycardia induction study for predicting long-term efficacy and inefficacy of antiarrhythmic drugs.* N Engl J Med 303:1073, 1980.

61. Mason, JW and Winkle, RA: *Electrode-catheter arrhythmia induction in the selection and assessment of antiarrhythmic drug therapy for recurrent ventricular tachycardia.* Circulation 58:971, 1978.

62. Swerdlow, CD, Gong, G, Echt, DS, et al: *Clinical factors predicting successful electrophysiologic-pharmacologic study in patients with ventricular tachycardia.* J Am Coll Cardiol 1:409, 1983.

63. Swerdlow, CD, Blum, J, Winkle, RA, et al: *Decreased incidence of antiarrhythmic drug efficacy at electrophysiology physiology study associated with use of a third extrastimulus.* Am Heart J 104:1004, 1982.

64. Denes, P, Wu, D, Wyndham, C, et al: *Chronic long-term electrophysiologic study of paroxysmal ventricular tachycardia.* Chest 77:478, 1980.

65. Fisher, JD: *Nonsurgical treatment of ventricular tachycardia: The value of serial provocative testing.* In Narula, OS (ed): *Cardiac Arrhythmias: Electrophysiology, Diagnosis, and Management.* Williams & Wilkins, Baltimore, 1979, p 494.

66. Greene, HL, Reid, PR, and Schaeffer, AH: *The repetitive ventricular response in man: A predictor of sudden cardiac death.* N Engl Med J 299:729, 1978.

67. Swerdlow, CD, Winkle, RA, and Mason, JW: *Prognostic significance of ten and fewer induced beats during assessment of therapy for ventricular tachycardia.* Circulation (in press).

68. Hamer, AW, Finerman, WB, Peter, T, et al: *Disparity between the clinical and electrophysiologic effects of amiodarone in the treatment of recurrent ventricular tachyarrhythmias.* Am Heart J 102:992, 1981.

69. Heger, JJ, Prystowsky, EW, Jackman, WM, et al: *Amiodarone: Clinical efficacy and electrophysiology during long-term therapy for recurrent ventricular tachycardia or ventricular fibrillation.* N Engl J Med 305:539, 1981.

70. Ross, DL, Sze, DY, Keefe, DL, et al: *Antiarrhythmic drug combinations in the treatment of ventricular tachycardia: Efficacy and electrophysiologic effects.* Circulation 66:1205, 1982.

71. Bigger, JT and Giardina, EGV: *Rational use of antiarrhythmic drugs alone and in combination.* Cardiovasc Clin 6(2):103, 1974.

72. Dreifus, LS and Morganroth, J: *Antiarrhythmic agents and their use in therapy.* Clin Pharmacol Ther 9:75, 1980.

73. Winkle, RA: *Current status of ambulatory electrocardiography.* Am Heart J 102:757, 1981.

74. Winkle, RA: *Antiarrhythmic drug effect mimicked by spontaneous variability of ventricular ectopy.* Circulation 57:1116, 1978.

75. Myerburg, RJ, Kessler, KM, Kiem, I, et al: *Relationship between plasma levels of procainamide, suppression of premature ventricular complexes, and prevention of recurrent ventricular tachycardia.* Circulation 64:280, 1982.

76. Winkle, RA: *Ambulatory electrocardiography and the diagnosis, evaluation, and treatment of chronic ventricular arrhythmias.* Prog Cardiovasc Dis 23:99, 1980.

77. Ryan, M, Lown, B, and Horn, H: *Comparison of ventricular ectopic activity during 24-hour monitoring and exercise testing in patients with coronary heart disease.* N Engl J Med 292:224, 1975.

78. Sami, M, Kraemer, A, Harrison, DC, et al: *A new method for evaluating antiarrhythmic drug efficacy in individual patients.* Circulation 62:1172, 1980.

79. Lown, B and Graboys, TB; *Management of patients with malignant ventricular arrhythmias.* Am J Cardiol 39:910, 1977.

80. Swerdlow, CD, Echt, DS, Winkle, RA, et al: *Determinants of survival in patients with ventricular tachyarrhythmias.* Circulation 66:II-25, 1982.

Platelet-Suppressive Therapy in Cardiovascular Disease*

Jawahar Mehta, M.D., and Louis Roy, M.D.

It has been recognized for a long time that blood platelets play a major role in hemostasis. However, recent information on the role of platelets in the evolution of atherogenesis and the discovery of a new class of biologically active substances derived from phospholipids have generated interest in platelet–vessel wall interaction as it may relate to ischemic heart disease. These developments have also provided insights into the mechanism of action of many new and old pharmacologic agents in the management of cardiovascular disease states.

This chapter will describe platelet physiology with some discussion of arachidonic acid metabolism in relation to the development of atherosclerosis. The mechanism of certain platelet- and prostaglandin-active drugs will be reviewed. Some of these drugs that act on prostaglandin pathways may be of great value in the future.

PLATELETS

Blood platelets are derived from cytoplasmic fragmentation of megakaryocytes and circulate in the peripheral blood for 7 to 10 days before being cleared by the reticuloendothelial system. Platelets possess specific membrane receptors for (1) epinephrine (alpha-adrenergic receptors, mainly of alpha$_2$-subtype), (2) ADP, (3) thrombin, (4) collagen, (5) fibrinogen, (6) platelet-activating factor, (7) probably thromboxane A_2 (TXA_2) and prostaglandin (PG) H_2, (8) prostacyclin (PGI_2) and PGE_1, and probably for several other substances. Platelet cytoplasm contains a secretory apparatus consisting of (1) a canalicular system open to the surface and formed by invagination of the cytoplasmic membrane coming in close relation to the sarcoplasmic reticulum, and (2) a secretory system consisting mainly of alpha granules and dense bodies (Fig. 1). The alpha granules contain platelet factor 4, beta-thromboglobulin, and lysosomal enzymes. The dense bodies contain the ADP storage pool, ATP, serotonin, and calcium. Another pool of ADP is freely available within the cytoplasm.[1] Platelets also contain an enzyme, phospholipase A_2, that is involved in the release of arachidonic acid from the membrane phospholipids. Arachidonic acid is immediately transformed by the action of enzyme cyclo-oxygenase into cyclic endoperoxides, which are further converted by enzyme thromboxane synthetase to TXA_2. TXA_2 is rapidly converted to a stable inactive metabolite, TXB_2.[2] Platelets also contain an enzyme, 9-hydroxy-prostaglandin dehydrogenase, which can convert vessel wall–generated PGI_2 to a stable active metabolite, 6-keto-PGE_1.[3]

Platelets possess a cytoskeleton consisting of a microtubular system that forms a ring around the cytoplasm (see Fig. 1). This is called the equatorial plaque and gives an ovoid

*Supported in part by American Heart Association, Florida Affiliate.

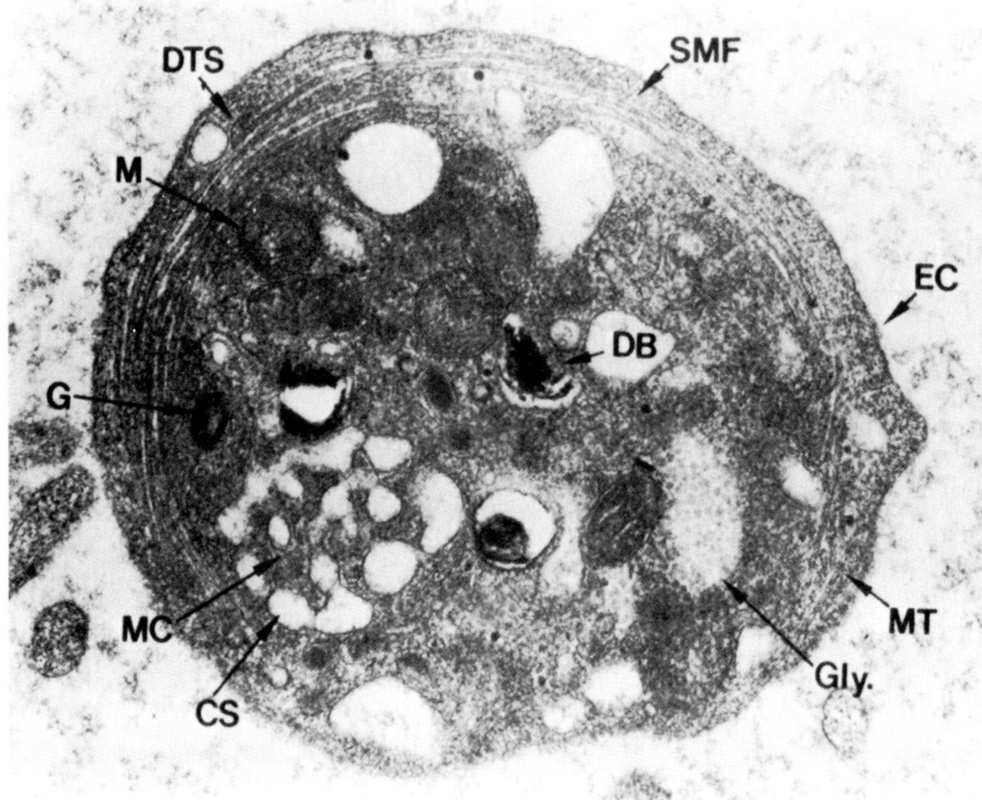

Figure 1. Discoid platelet. The ultrastructural features observed in a thin section of discoid platelet cut in the equatorial plane. Components of the peripheral zone include the exterior coat (EC), trilaminar unit membrane, and submembrane area containing specialized filaments (SMF) that form the wall of the platelet, and line channels of the surface-connected canalicular system (CS). The membrane complex (MC) is a specialized association of the dense tubular system (DTS) and CS. The matrix of the platelet interior is the solgel zone containing actin microfilaments, structural filaments, the circumferential band of microtubules (MT), and glycogen (Gly). Formed elements embedded in the solgel zone include mitochondria (M), granules (G), and dense bodies (DB). Collectively, they constitute the organelle zone. The membrane systems include the surface-connected canalicular system (CS) and the dense tubular system (DTS), which serve as the platelet sarcoplasmic reticulum. An occasional Golgi apparatus is found in some platelets. (From Mehta, P and Mehta, J: *Role of platelet and endothelum in vascular disease.* In Mehta, J and Mehta, P (eds): *Platelets and Prostaglandins in Cardiovascular Disease.* Futura, Mt Kisco NY, 1981, p 2, with permission.

shape to platelets.[1] A contractile protein closely related to actinomyosin, that is, thrombosthenin, constitutes 15 to 20 percent of platelet protein content. This contractile element, which is calcium-dependent, is responsible for platelet shape change upon platelet activation and is also implicated in the active secretory phase of platelets.

Platelet Activation

In a state of health, platelets do not adhere to the vessel wall, although they provide a substance that is essential in the maintenance of endothelial integrity. Once the endothelial continuity is disrupted, platelets play a crucial role in reparative and hemostatic functions (Fig. 2). Platelet hemostatic or thrombotic reactions are essentially the same and include adhesion, secretion, aggregation, and stabilization-retraction of the clot.

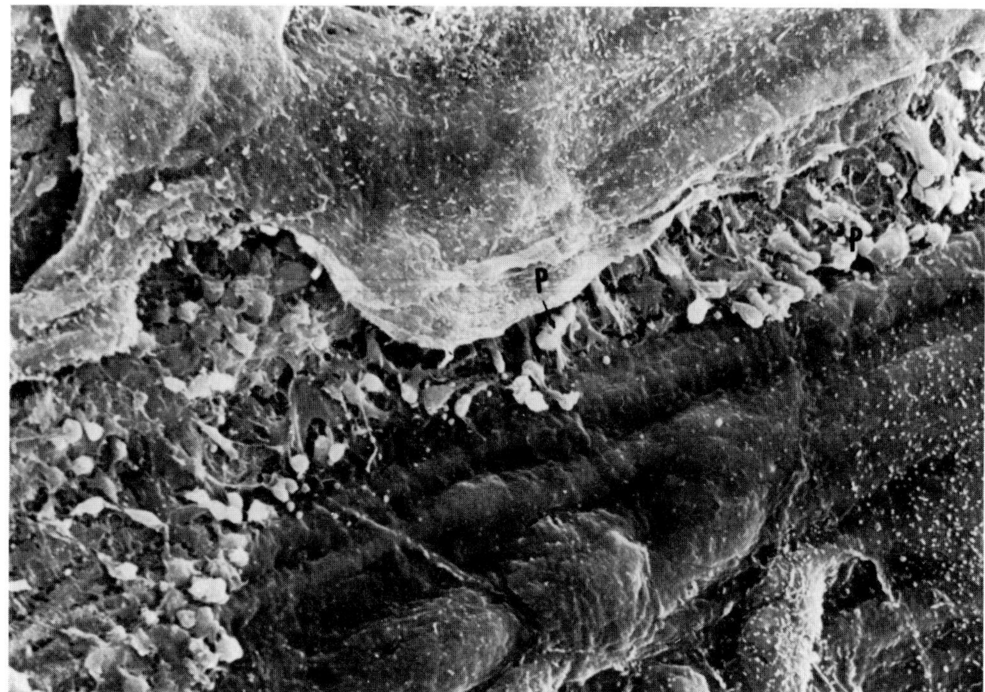

Figure 2. Adhesion of platelets (P) to the subendothelial collagen at the site of endothelial tear in human saphenous vein. (Courtesy of Don Hay, PhD.)

ADHESION. Platelets adhere to many vascular and perivascular tissues. Major stimuli for adhesion are in order of potency: collagen, microfibrils, and basement membrane. The reaction with collagen does not require the presence of calcium as the others do.

SECRETION. Adhesion or activation of platelets leads to platelet shape change and secretion or release. The so-called "release I" and "release II" reactions have been related to exocytosis of dense bodies and alpha granules, respectively. Factors like platelet factor 3 are membrane proteins that are unmasked by stoichiometric membrane rearrangement.[1] Arachidonic acid metabolites are released as their synthesis is enhanced after activation of enzyme phospholipase A_2. Release of ADP, serotonin, and other contents of platelets occurs. Some of these substances attract other platelets, whereas still other release products enter the endothelial lining. Another substance, "smooth-muscle proliferating factor," is also released from the platelets upon activation. This substance may have an important role in atherogenesis.[4]

AGGREGATION. Clumping of platelets takes place in two steps, called "primary" and "secondary" waves of aggregation. The first, or primary, wave has been attributed to platelet reaction to external stimuli, which are the same as for secretion. This active platelet secretion induces the secondary wave of aggregation. The intracellular concentration of cyclic nucleotides modulates platelet sensitivity to proaggregants.[5] An increase in cyclic adenosine monophospate (cAMP) prevents platelet secretion and aggregation, whereas a decrease enhances aggregation. Another nucleotide, cyclic guanine monophosphate (cGMP), is also believed to play a role in platelet activation, and its actions are opposite to those of cAMP.[6] Intracellular concentration of free calcium also plays a key role in arachidonate metabolism. A slight increase in calcium concentration can cause activation of contractile protein and shape change; further increase causes TXA_2 generation, which amplifies calcium mobilization leading to platelet secretion and aggregation (see Fig. 2).[5,7] Inhibitors of enzyme cyclo-oxygenase, for example, aspirin, inhibit alpha-granule release. Therefore, arachidonic acid metabolism in platelets and generation of TXA_2 are reduced and the secondary wave is inhibited. However, high concentrations of thrombin and ionophore A 23187 still can activate platelets despite cyclo-oxygenase enzyme inhibition. Both thrombin and ionophore A 23187 are believed to act by a different pathway that uses a recently described "platelet-activating factor."[8] The latter has been shown to be released by platelets and by IgE-sensitized basophils in response to antigen stimulation. This factor, not affected by aspirin, is strongly inhibited by lipid-soluble agents such as lidocaine and methylprednisolone.

PROSTAGLANDIN METABOLISM

Prostaglandins, derived from essential fatty acids with a 20-carbon structure, are of 1, 2, or 3 series based on the number of double bonds (1, 2, or 3) present in the side chain. Diet is the source of prostaglandin precursors except for oleic acid, which can be synthesized in humans (Fig. 3). Oleic, linolenic, and linoleic acids have an 18-carbon structure and can be converted to mead, eicosapentaenoic, and dihomo-γ-linolenic acids, respectively, which have a 20-carbon structure. Dihomo-γ-linolenic acid is mainly metabolized to arachidonic acid, which is the precursor of major prostaglandins in man. Prostaglandins derived from arachidonic acid metabolism are of 2 series, whereas those derived from dihomo-γ-linolenic and eicosapentaenoic acid are of 1 and 3 series, respectively. These precursor fatty acids are incorporated in the phospholipids of cell membrane. Upon activation of enzyme phospholipase A_2 of C or diglyceride lipase, these fatty acids are liberated and undergo a rapid transformation following three major biochemical pathways (Fig. 4).[9]

First, by action of cyclo-oxygenase enzyme, arachidonic acid is transformed into unstable cyclic endoperoxides, PGG_2 and PGH_2, which are further metabolized to TXA_2, PGI_2, PGD_2, PGE_2, and $PGF_{2\alpha}$. TXA_2 formed by action of TXA_2 synthetase is very unstable (half-life 30 sec) and has potent vasoconstrictor and platelet proaggregatory actions. TXA_2 is synthesized mainly by platelets and white cells. Recent data suggest synthesis of small amounts of TXA_2 by the blood vessels also.[10] PGI_2 generated by vessel walls[11] by action of PGI_2 synthetase is also unstable and has a short plasma half-life. By its potent vasodilator and platelet aggregation inhibitor properties, it counteracts the effects of TXA_2. PGI_2 has many stable metabolites, of which 6-keto-PGE_1 is active but probably not present in large amounts in humans.[12] Another major metabolite, 6-keto-$PGF_{1\alpha}$, is a hydrolysis product and is not derived by enzy-

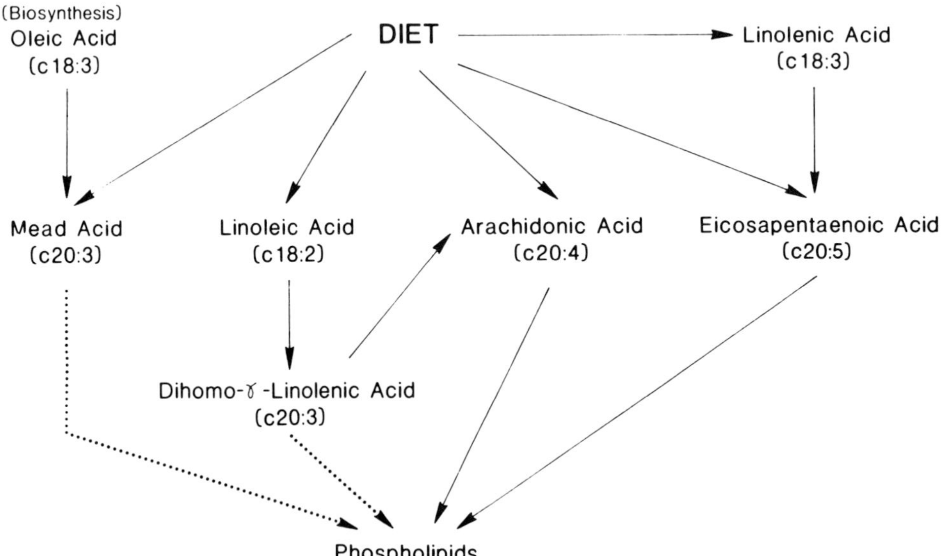

Figure 3. Source of polyunsaturated fatty acids in the phospholipids. Arachidonic acid can be obtained either directly from the diet or via desaturation and chain lengthening of linoleic acid. Oleic acid can be synthesized in the body or obtained from the diet.

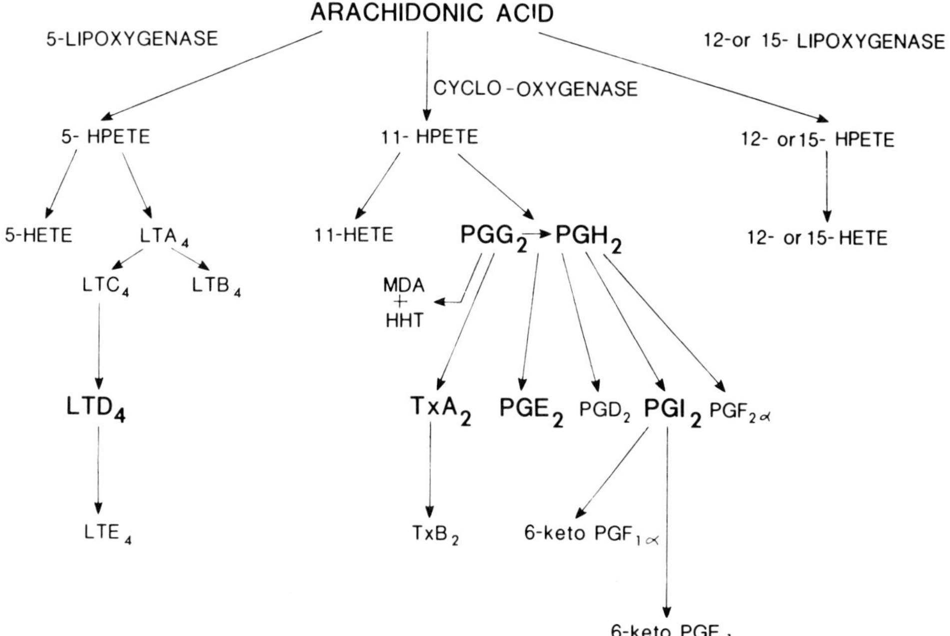

Figure 4. Diagram of the conversion of arachidonic acid into biologically active substances. The first step in each pathway is the incorporation of molecular oxygen into arachidonic acid to form a hydroperoxide intermediate: 5-hydroperoxy-eicosatetraenoic acid (5-HPETE), 11-HPETE, 12-HPETE, or 15-HPETE. These hydroperoxides can spontaneously degrade to the corresponding hydroxy-eicosatetraenoic acid (HETE), or some are converted enzymatically to leukotrienes (LT), prostaglandins (PG), thromboxane (TX), or prostacyclin (PGI_2). The cyclo-oxygenase forms PGG_2 (via the intermediate 11-HPETE). This endoperoxide is the common precursor to the prostaglandins, thromboxane, and prostacyclin. The 5-lipoxygenase forms leukotriene (LT) A_4, which is 5,6-oxido-7,9,11,14-eicosatetraenoic acid. Addition of glutathione forms LTC_4 (5-hydroxy-6-S-gluthathionyl-7,9,11, 14-eicosatetraenoic acid). Removal of the terminal amino acids in glutathione forms LTD_4 and LTE_4. LTE_4 = 5,12-dihydroxy-eicosatetraenoic acid. HHT = 12L-hydroxy-5,8,10-hepta-decatrienoic acid. MDA = malondialdehyde.

matic degradation.[9] Recent evidence would suggest that platelet-generated PGG_2 and PGH_2 can be diverted to PGE_2 and PGI_2, if enzyme TXA_2 synthesis is blocked. Prostaglandins of D, E, and F series, considered previously to be of major significance in the regulation of platelet homeostasis and blood flow, are now believed to be less important than TXA_2 and PGI_2.

Secondly, by action of 5-lipoxygenase, the 20-carbon fatty acids are transformed to another class of prostaglandins called leukotrienes, which derived their names from leukocytes from which these were first identified.[13] Arachidonic acid is metabolized to leukotrienes of 4-series. Leukotrienes C_4 and D_4 seem to be related to the slow-reacting substance of anaphylaxis (SRS-A).[14] Leukotriene B_4 is a potent stimulator of leukocyte migration and aggregation.[15]

The third pathway is related to the action of 12- or 15-lipoxygenase that results in formation of 12- or 15-hydroxy fatty acids. Although the actions of these substances are not well known, they seem to promote leukocyte migration and can interact with the enzyme PGI_2 synthetase and block PGI_2 synthesis.[16]

ATHEROGENESIS

The concept of atherogenesis is based mainly on two theories that have been debated for more than 130 years. The "incrustation theory," proposed by von Rokitansky in 1842[17] and later by Duguid,[18] stresses the atherogenic role of incorporation of mural thrombi by the arterial endothelium. The importance of an endothelial lesion as the initial event, which triggers a proliferative inflammatory reaction and a secondary intimal thickening, was emphasized by Virchow in 1856[19] and later by Haust and Mustard and their coworkers.[20,21] This last concept better accommodates the role of an elevated plasma concentration of cholesterol as an atherogenic factor and constitutes the "imbibition" or "insudation theory."

These theories have evolved into a unified concept that envisions the presence of these different mechanisms acting together or separately in time, and also takes into account important recent discoveries.

The key event in atherogenesis seems to be a multifactorial imbalance in the platelet–vessel wall integrity that leads to an initial endothelial injury. This injury induces platelet adhesion and activation and also activates blood coagulation factors that form a fibrin-platelet thrombus. Platelet secretory products play a role in expansion of the thrombus. Release of smooth-muscle proliferative factor leads to smooth muscle hypertrophy and migration. Other platelet-released substances like TXA_2 can increase vascular permeability and exhibit potent vasoconstrictor activities resulting in tissue ischemia. Thus, endothelial damage could be enhanced. After 24 to 48 hours, re-endothelization occurs, and the intimal lining progressively returns to its previous state. However, if platelet activation is persistent or if the endothelial injury continues, the physiologic healing process may become pathologic and form a nidus for an atherosclerotic lesion. This nidus leads to formation of a fibrous plaque that with time may become ulcerative and obstructive, and form in situ thrombus with downstream embolization. Arterial lipid accumulation could also be secondary to deficiency of lipid removal mechanism,[22] defective or decreased number of low-density lipoprotein receptors,[23] deficient smooth-muscle proliferative factor, or deficiency of lysosomal enzyme activity.[24] The site of the atherosclerotic lesion is usually related to an area of increased hemodynamic shear stress, such as may occur at the arterial bifurcation or downstream to an arterial stenosis.[25] At this level, the endothelial cell turnover is increased and a constant stress is present. Benditt and Benditt demonstrated that atheromatous lesions usually include endothelial cells of a monoclonal origin,[26] a finding allied to the fact that analysis of fatty streaks and fibrous plaques shows a decreased production of PGI_2.[27] It is attractive to postulate that a high cell turnover could favor the emergence of mutant cells that have defective protective mechanism. Other factors such as lipid peroxides and low-density lipoproteins seem to limit vascular production of PGI_2, which enhances platelet deposition to the vessel wall.[16]

Platelet Function in "Risk Factors" for Atherosclerosis

Epidemiologic and experimental data have identified certain risk factors in the development of atherosclerosis. However, the precise mechanism by which these factors act is not well established. High blood pressure, besides increasing the hemodynamic stress on vessel wall, is accompanied by increased platelet adhesion and release reaction.[28] Cigarette smoking has been demonstrated to increase PGI_2 release in nonsmokers, a finding that is not observed among habitual smokers.[29] In hypercholesterolemia, platelets generate increased amounts of TXA_2 and have decreased survival.[30,31] In diabetes mellitus, platelet activity is increased, as demonstrated by increased adhesion and TXA_2 generation; spontaneous aggregation; increased sensitivity to ADP, epinephrine, and collagen; increased circulating platelet aggregates; and increased plasma beta-thromboglobulin concentration.[32,33] Preliminary data indicate that high-density lipoproteins, besides being implicated in cholesterol removal, stimulate vascular synthesis of PGI_2 by providing the tissues with substrate arachidonic acid.[34] It is possible that these "risk factors" relate to atherogenesis by their effects on platelet–vessel wall interaction.

Platelet Function and Coronary Heart Disease

Various platelet function abnormalities have been described in patients with coronary heart disease (Table 1). Some investigators have shown in these patients increased platelet aggre-

Table 1. Platelet and prostaglandin abnormalities in patients with coronary heart disease

1.	Increased platelet aggregation in vitro
2.	Increased platelet aggregation in vivo
3.	Shortened platelet survival time
4.	Thrombocytosis
5.	Increase in megakaryocytes
6.	Platelet consumption in atherosclerotic vessels
7.	Increased platelet serotonin release
8.	Increased beta-thromboglobulin release at rest and with exercise
9.	Increased thromboxane A_2 synthesis at rest and with exercise
10.	Decreased prostacyclin synthesis
11.	Minimal increase in prostacyclin with exercise
12.	Decreased platelet sensitivity to prostacyclin
13.	Increased platelet sensitivity to cyclic endoperoxide

gation and megathrombocytosis, and decreased platelet survival indicating platelet "hyperactivity" and in vivo sequestration. Hampton and Gorlin[35] found increased platelet electrophoretic mobility of platelets even in relatives of patients with coronary artery disease. Other investigators, including ourselves, have not identified consistent changes in platelet function parameters in these patients at rest. However, certain platelet-released products used as markers of platelet activity, such as platelet factor 4 and beta-thromboglobulin, have been increased in some patients with stable coronary artery disease. This is particularly so during exercise-induced angina. In one study, platelet factor 4 levels were found to increase in 60 percent of patients with a positive stress test.[36] In another study, plasma beta-thromboglobulin levels were increased at rest and showed a further increase in patients with documented cor-

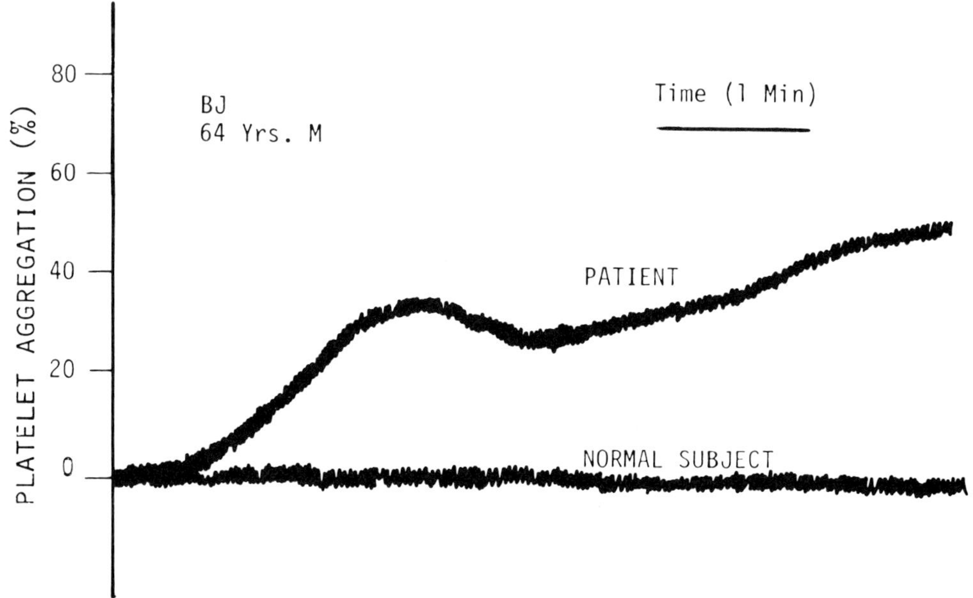

Figure 5. Spontaneous platelet aggregation in a 51-year-old man hospitalized with unstable angina pectoris. This patient developed anterior wall myocardial infarction a few hours later. Note absence of spontaneous platelet aggregation in the normal subject.

onary artery disease during exercise. These data suggest that, at least in some patients, certain platelet function parameters are abnormal, and the abnormalities of platelet function may become apparent during exercise.[37]

In patients with myocardial infarction, however, studies of platelet function have yielded more consistent information. Dreyfuss and Zahavi first described increased platelet aggregation in patients with acute myocardial infarction.[38] Although increased aggregability of platelets may not be observed in the early stages of myocardial infarction because of prior platelet activation, there is evidence for enhanced platelet activity at least in some patients either preceding or during acute myocardial infarction.[39] Spontaneous platelet aggregation occurring just prior to acute myocardial infarction also may be observed occasionally (Fig. 5).

Transcardiac Platelet Function in Coronary Artery Disease

It is evident that abnormalities of platelet function detected in the peripheral venous blood may not reflect changes occurring in an isolated vascular bed. It is important, therefore, to examine platelet function across an isolated atherosclerotic vascular bed in comparison with normal nonatherosclerotic beds. In the coronary vascular bed, wherein coronary arterial and venous blood samples can be collected by catheterization, the influence of myocardial stress states can also be examined.

In atherosclerotic coronary beds, a significant gradient in platelet count and aggregability has been observed between aortic and coronary venous blood, implying passage of biologically less active platelets.[40] During tachycardia stress, marked activation of platelets exiting in the coronary sinus is found, but no change is observed in the aortic blood.[41] These observations suggest that platelet activation takes place at the level of the atherosclerotic coronary vascular bed during myocardial stress. No such gradient at rest or activation with exercise is generally observed in subjects with normal coronary arteries. Likewise, changes are not observed in other vascular beds without significant atherosclerosis.[42]

Using this human model to study platelet function across atherosclerotic vascular beds, it has been shown that drugs like aspirin and dipyridamole eliminate the differential in platelet counts and also result in similar platelet aggregation function in aortic and coronary venous blood.[43,44] Drugs such as aspirin and propranolol also inhibit myocardial stress-related increase in platelet function in the coronary venous blood as observed before administration of these drugs.[41,42]

PROSTAGLANDINS IN CORONARY HEART DISEASE

As discussed earlier, platelet activation leads to release of TXA_2. The potent proaggregant and vasoconstrictor actions of TXA_2 are usually balanced by release from the vessel walls of PGI_2, which has potent antiaggregant and vasodilatory actions. It has been suggested that if an imbalance in TXA_2 and PGI_2 equilibrium were to exist, excess of TXA_2 may cause local or downstream spasm of the coronary vascular bed after it is released by platelets. Several studies indeed suggest enhanced generation of TXA_2 in patients with coronary heart disease. This increase in platelet prostaglandin generation is observed in patients with unstable angina,[45] during and after acute myocardial infarction,[46] with coronary vasospasm,[47] and during pacing-induced myocardial ischemia.[48] The plasma levels of PGI_2 metabolites, on the other hand, are extremely low or undetectable in patients with coronary artery disease. Furthermore, plasma levels of 6-keto-$PGF_{1\alpha}$ increase during exercise in normal volunteers. In contrast, in patients with coronary artery disease, the increase in 6-keto-$PGF_{1\alpha}$ is markedly reduced.[49] The increase in TXA_2, however, is maintained, resulting in an imbalance between PGI_2 and TXA_2 in favor of the latter. Platelets from patients with unstable angina and acute myocardial infarction have markedly decreased sensitivity to the antiaggregatory effects of PGI_2 and an increased sensitivity to the proaggregant actions of TXA_2.[45]

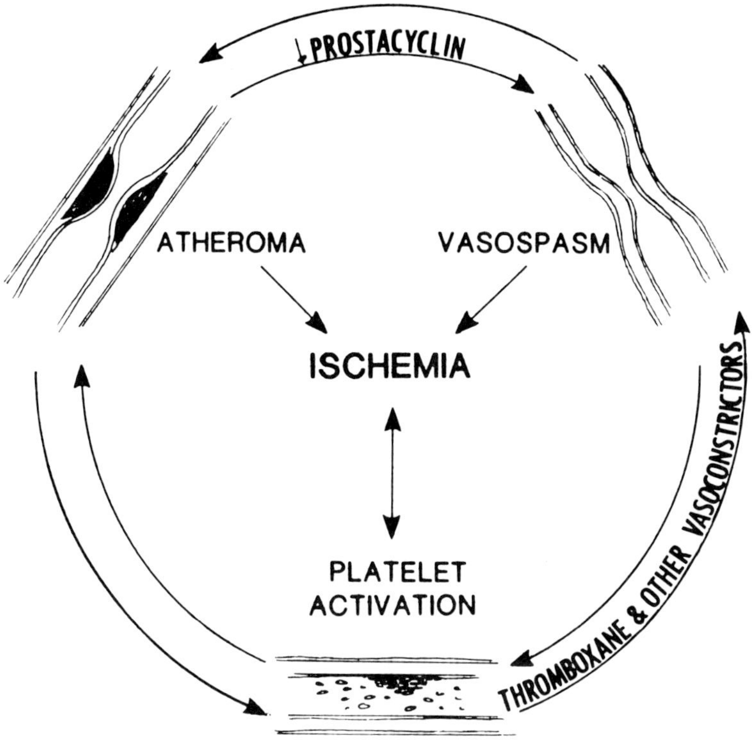

Figure 6. A proposed interrelationship among atherosclerosis, platelet activation, vasospasm, abnormalities in prostaglandin metabolism, and the evolution of myocardial ischemia.

ATHEROSCLEROSIS, PLATELETS, PROSTAGLANDINS, AND CORONARY HEART DISEASE

It is difficult to prove whether platelet dysfunction precedes myocardial ischemia or occurs secondary to the ischemic event. Some investigators have shown that coronary spasm may precede the ischemic event. Others have demonstrated absence of obliterative atherosclerotic lesions in the acute phase of myocardial infarction. Still others have documented presence of a fresh occlusive clot,[50,51] suggesting that platelets and prostaglandins may have an important primary role in causing vascular spasm and physical occlusion of the lumen of the atherosclerotic vessel.[39] On the other hand, if platelet hyperactivity and TXA_2 release are not primary phenomena, the presence of myocardial ischemia by itself may activate platelets, which in turn release large amounts of TXA_2. Release of TXA_2 and platelet hyperactivity could lead to propagation of the ischemic process. Therefore, whether platelet "hyperactivity" is a primary event or occurs after the ischemic event has taken place, platelet dysfunction may be detrimental to the entire process of tissue ischemia. It is our belief, at this time, that there is an intimate relationship among atherosclerosis, vascular spasm, and platelet aggregation (Fig. 6). Vascular spasm probably occurs on the basis of autonomic dysfunction, which also relates to platelet "hyperactivity." Abnormalities of TXA_2–PGI_2 equilibrium may also be instrumental in causing the vasospastic process.

PLATELET-ACTIVE AGENTS

Based on the interrelationship among platelets, intimal damage, and various prostaglandins in the context of cardiovascular disease, we will focus on pharmacologic means to alter this relationship. Various drugs acting on the platelet-prostaglandin axis are shown in Table 2.

Table 2. Platelet-suppressive drugs: Mechanism and site of action

A. Receptor mediated increase in cAMP
   PGI_2
   PGE_1
   PGD_2
B. Adenyl cyclase activator
   Forskolin
C. Phosphodiesterase inhibitors
   Dipyridamole and analogs
   Papaverine
   Cilostamide
   Methylxanthines
D. Phospholipase inhibitors
   Corticosteroids
   Quinacrine
E. Cyclo-oxygenase inhibitor
   Aspirin
   Nonsteroidal anti-inflammatory agents
F. Thromboxane synthetase inhibitors
   Imidazole analogs
   OKY 1581
   9,11-azoprosta 5,13-dienoic acid (U-51605)
   Nictindole
G. Thromboxane-receptor blockers
   13-azo-prostanoic acid
   N-0164
H. Blockers of receptor-mediated calcium release
   Phentolamine
   Phenoxybenzamine
   Indoramin
   Yohimbine
   Dopamine
   Cyproheptadine
   Synthetic alpha-adrenergic agonists
I. Slow-channel calcium blockers
   Verapamil
   Nifedipine
   Diltiazem
   TMB-8
J. Membrane-stabilizing effect or platelet-activating factor inhibitors
   Corticosteroids
   Lidocaine
   Beta blockers
   Imipramine
   Chlorpromazine
   Methysergide
   Reserpine
   Quinacrine
   Chloroquine
   Hydroxychloroquine
K. Decreased content of platelet arachidonic acid
   Eicosapentaenoic acid
   Clofibrate
L. Increased prostacyclin release
   Dipyridamole
   Nitrates
   Vitamin E

Table 2. Platelet-suppressive drugs: Mechanism and site of action (*Continued*)

M. Prostacyclin stabilization or prevention of PGI_2 degradation
  Nafazatrom (Bay g 6575)
N. Site unknown
  Penicillin and other antibiotics
  Amagrelide (BL-4162A)

Aspirin

Aspirin is probably the first drug recognized to have important platelet-inhibitory effects. Aspirin inhibits (1) platelet aggregation induced by collagen, arachidonic acid, and thrombin, and the secondary wave of aggregation induced by ADP, epinephrine, and ristocetin; and (2) secretion of ADP, ATP serotonin, and platelet factor 4.[1,52] Aspirin irreversibly inhibits enzyme cyclo-oxygenase[53] and thus blocks the synthesis of vasoactive substances like cyclic endoperoxides and TXA_2. Inasmuch as platelet protein-synthesizing ability is very limited, this enzymatic inactivation lasts for the entire platelet life span. This inhibition of enzyme cyclo-oxygenase is not restricted to platelets but also involves the blood vessels, so that PGI_2 synthesis is also decreased. Cyclo-oxygenase in the vessel wall is probably less sensitive to aspirin than that in the platelet.[54] This action has been the basis for advocating use of low doses of aspirin in possible prevention of atherosclerosis and its thromboembolic complications.

Other evidence in favor of this dose-dependent action of aspirin is that high dosage of aspirin may cause more atherosclerosis in experimental animals,[55] whereas small doses may be protective.[56] This differential action could also explain why low doses of aspirin increase bleeding time whereas high doses do not.[52] During coronary occlusion in dogs, aspirin has been demonstrated to decrease collateral flow but exerts antiarrhythmic effects. Aspirin eliminates periodic fluctuations in blood flow observed in narrowed coronary arteries and attributed to in situ periodic platelet thrombus formation.[57]

In patients with coronary disease, aspirin decreases the gradient in platelet counts and aggregation existing between the aorta and coronary sinus. It also prevents increase in platelet aggregation in coronary venous blood induced by tachycardia stress.[43] However, clinical studies have failed to show a difference in exercise tolerance in patients with coronary artery disease given aspirin compared with control subjects. Reports from large clinical trials with aspirin in patients with recent myocardial infarction have been fraught with methodologic problems. However, some of these studies demonstrate a trend toward decrease in longer-term mortality related to coronary heart disease, especially if patients begin treatment early after the myocardial infarction.[58]

Aspirin is also used alone or in conjunction with anticoagulant therapy in patients with prosthetic heart valves. A Japanese group showed decrease in thromboembolic events in patients with prosthetic valves when aspirin was added to warfarin. However, the Mayo Clinic group has reported an increase in frequency of bleeding episodes without modification in the frequency of thromboembolic episodes using aspirin and warfarin in patients with prosthetic valves.[59] Nevertheless, the use of low-dose aspirin has reduced the frequency of thromboembolic episodes in patients with arteriovenous shunts while on chronic hemodialysis and in patients undergoing total hip replacement.[60] Human clinical studies have demonstrated a decrease in the frequency of transient cerebral ischemic events with aspirin.[61] The latter difference has been observed only in men and not in women.

Nonsteroidal Anti-inflammatory Agents

All these different substances have aspirin-like effects, and have in common anti-inflammatory and antipyretic properties (Table 3). These agents have an ability to interfere with arachidonic acid metabolism. Some of these compounds are no longer used in clinical practice because of serious side effects; for example, aminopyrine may cause fatal bone marrow toxicity, and phenacetin may induce interstitial nephritis. Others like flurbiprofen, which is 600 times more potent in inhibiting cyclo-oxygenase enzyme than aspirin, have not been extensively studied as platelet-active drugs. Sulfinpyrazone is a competitive inhibitor of cyclo-oxygenase enzyme and also interferes with platelet adhesion to collagen, suggesting a second mode of action not shared with aspirin.[62] Sulfinpyrazone does not prolong the bleeding time but inhibits platelet aggregation induced by collagen, ADP, serotonin, epinephrine, and fibrinogen.[1] However, platelets obtained from patients taking sulfinpyrazone respond normally to collagen. In an experimental model of atherosclerosis in monkeys, sulfinpyrazone at a dose of 200 mg daily decreases the severity and the extent of coronary atherosclerosis compared with untreated animals.[63] Sulfinpyrazone corrects shortened platelet survival time observed in atherosclerosis, in experimental models of damaged endothelium, in dogs with aortic prostheses, and in patients with prosthetic heart valves.[64–66] In the Anturane Reinfarction Trial, a protective effect against sudden cardiac death was demonstrated in patients taking sulfinpyrazone.[67]

Table 3. Nonsteroidal anti-inflammatory agents

I. Pyrazoles
- Phenylbutazone
- Sulfinpyrazone
- Oxyphenbutazone

II. Carboxylic Acids
- A. Acetic Acids
  - Indomethacin
  - Sulindac
  - Tolmetin
  - Zomepirac
  - Many others
- B. Salicylates
  - Aspirin
  - Fendosal
  - Many others
- C. Propionic Acids
  - Ibuprofen
  - Fenoprofen
  - Naproxen
  - Oxaprozin
  - Many others
- D. Fenamates
  - Flufenamic acid
  - Meclofenamate
  - Mefenamic acid
  - Niflumic acid
  - Tolfenamic acid

III. Oxicams
- Piroxicam

Phosphodiesterase Inhibitors

Dipyridamole and related compounds inhibit enzyme phosphodiesterase. Papaverine, cilostamide, caffeine, theophylline, and other methylxanthines also have similar actions. This inhibition of enzyme phosphodiesterase contributes to an increase in intracellular cAMP. An increase in platelet cAMP stabilizes the storage pool of calcium by activating membrane transport.[1,52] Consequently, the availability and the amount of free cytoplasmic divalent calcium levels decrease, thereby impeding platelet activation. Most phosphodiesterase inhibitors also inhibit degradation of cGMP. Three protein fractions have been identified as responsible for platelet phosphodiesterase activity. These fractions possess different affinities for the two cyclic nucleotides, and the fraction F III seems to be the most specific for cAMP. Methylxanthines, papaverine, and adenosine are moderately selective for F III, whereas cilostamide is very selective.[68]

Dipyridamole in high concentrations (>50 μg/ml) not achieved with usual therapeutic use inhibits platelet aggregation induced by ADP, epinephrine, arachidonic acid, and collagen. In therapeutic concentrations (5 to 10 μg/ml), dipyridamole decreases platelet TXA_2 generation induced by thrombin and arachidonic acid, suggesting a direct action upon platelet cyclo-oxygenase or thromboxane synthetase enzymes.[69] It also potentiates actions of aspirin and PGI_2 platelets. In addition, dipyridamole stimulates PGI_2 production from exhausted human endothelial cells in concentrations above 50 μg/ml.[69] In rabbit tendon superfused with whole blood, dipyridamole causes disaggregation of platelets; this effect is blocked by pretreatment of the tissue with aspirin or antiserum against PGI_2.[70] These data suggest a dependency on PGI_2 for its anti-aggregatory effects in vivo.

Dipyridamole may affect progression of atherosclerosis by stimulating PGI_2 synthesis and/or decreasing the secretion of the platelet factor responsible for smooth muscle cell proliferation. Indeed, in baboons fed homocystine, dipyridamole prevents the shortening of platelet survival and the development of intimal lesions.[71] In combination with aspirin, it also decreases the severity and the extent of coronary atherosclerosis in monkeys fed high-cholesterol diets.[72] In a recent report, however, dipyridamole was found to enhance atherosclerosis in rabbits fed cholesterol-rich diets.[73] Precise explanation for these discrepancies is not known.

By influencing the platelet–vessel wall interaction, dipyridamole equalizes the platelet counts in aortic and coronary sinus blood in subjects with coronary artery disease. At the same time, the gradient in platelet aggregability between aortic and coronary sinus blood is decreased.[64] In clinical trials, dipyridamole has been shown to correct the shortened platelet survival in patients with prosthetic heart valves, coronary artery disease, and ventriculoperitoneal shunt.[74,75] Its use in combination with warfarin therapy in patients with valvular prostheses leads to decrease in thromboembolic events. However, in one study[76] there were two deaths related to hemorrhagic complications, whereas in another[59] the number of bleeding events requiring transfusion or hospitalization was not different from the group treated with warfarin alone.

Because dipyridamole also causes coronary vasodilation, its antianginal effect has been clinically evaluated, but the results are inconclusive. In some studies, dipyridamole has been shown to induce "coronary steal syndrome."[77] Some investigators have even used dipyridamole as an alternative to stress tests for inducing myocardial perfusion defects that can be detected by perfusion myocardial scintigraphy in subjects with coronary artery disease.[77–79]

In one study,[80] no significant benefit of dipyridamole compared with placebo in terms of thromboembolic events, recurrence of myocardial infarction, or death could be shown in patients with myocardial infarction. However, the study groups were small and the followup period lasted only 4 weeks. Dipyridamole administered in combination with aspirin in the Persantine Aspirin Re-Infarction Study (PARIS) did not seem to provide any additional benefit when compared with use of aspirin alone.[81] However, dipyridamole 400 mg/day for 2 days before coronary artery bypass surgery and continued at 225 mg/day with aspirin 975 mg/day after surgery may improve early and late coronary bypass graft patency.[82]

Beta-Adrenergic Blockers

Among this class of drugs, propranolol is the one that has been extensively evaluated as a platelet-active drug. It inhibits the secondary wave of platelet aggregation induced by epinephrine, ADP, and arachidonic acid in some patients. It also delays and inhibits platelet aggregation induced by collagen, thrombin, and ionophore A 23187.[83] However, these effects on platelet aggregation necessitate drug concentrations higher than those required for beta-adrenergic blockade alone (50 to 150 ng/ml). Propranolol seems to inhibit platelet aggregation by its "membrane-stabilizing" effect and by decreasing the availability of calcium which is necessary for platelet activation. Platelet generation of malondialdehyde and TXA_2 is a more sensitive index of platelet activity than platelet aggregation alone. In patients with coronary artery disease, propranolol intake reduces platelet generation of TXA_2, suggesting possible inhibition of TXA_2 synthetase enzyme.[84] In vitro propranolol stimulates PGI_2 release from guinea pig heart preparation.[85] Other beta blockers such as timolol seem to have effects on platelets similar to those of propranolol. Pick and Glick have demonstrated that monkeys fed atherogenic diets and pretreated with propranolol develop less atherosclerosis than do control monkeys.[86]

The beneficial effects of propranolol in ischemic heart disease are well known. Studies in patients with coronary artery disease indicate that propranolol may also decrease platelet aggregation in aortic and coronary sinus blood and blunt the increased sensitivity of platelets induced by tachycardia stress.[41]

In post–myocardial infarction trials, the protective effects of propranolol against further ischemic events are generally accepted.[87] Other trials using practolol,[88] alprenolol,[89] and timolol[90] have shown similar reduction in the incidence of ischemic events and subsequent mortality. Whether these protective effects are necessarily related to platelet suppressive actions is not known.

Slow-Channel Calcium Antagonists

Diltiazem, verapamil, nifedipine, and TMB-8 inhibit platelet aggregation and release induced by epinephrine, ADP, collagen, and arachidonic acid.[42] These effects can be abolished by addition of calcium to platelet-rich plasma. These compounds also seem to reduce platelet TXA_2 generation in vitro.[91] Administration of verapamil to patients with ischemic heart disease and normal subjects inhibits platelet aggregation and circulating platelet aggregates.[92] In dogs, verapamil has been shown to prevent platelet adhesion to femoral artery bypass grafts.[93] It is possible that the platelet-inhibitory effects of calcium-channel blockers contribute to their anti-ischemic activity. Some recent studies indicate that calcium metabolism is important in the development of atherosclerosis.[94] Use of calcium blockers lanthanum and nifedipine in experimental animals fed high-cholesterol diets has been shown to inhibit atherogenesis.[95] However, tissue levels of calcium measured in one study were not affected.[95] These effects of calcium blockers were not mediated through alterations in lipid metabolism. Some studies indicate blockade of $alpha_2$ platelet adrenergic receptors by verapamil, suggesting that alpha-adrenergic receptors may be linked to calcium channels.[96]

Specific Receptor Blockers

As mentioned previously, platelet membrane possesses different receptors. Yohimbine, a plant alkaloid, is considered to be an $alpha_2$ antagonist, whereas prazosin, indoramin, and phenoxybenzamine are $alpha_1$ antagonists. Phentolamine and dihydroergocryptine specifically occupy alpha$_2$ receptors and are strong inhibitors of platelet aggregation. Folts and Bonebrake have demonstrated that phentolamine abolishes cigarette smoke– or nicotine-induced cyclic flow variations seen in stenosed coronary arteries.[97] Surprisingly, synthetic alpha-adrenergic agonists like phenylephrine, methoxamine, xylometazoline, and oxymetazoline are alpha-adrenergic blockers in human platelets. TXA_2- and PGH_2-induced platelet aggregation is blocked by 13-azo-prostanoic acid and N-0164, which have no effect on cyclooxygenase and only a minor effect on TXA_2 synthesis. This finding suggests that there may indeed exist a common receptor site for TXA_2 and PGH_2, and that certain agents may act at this receptor site.[98]

Membrane-Active Drugs

Imipramine, chlorpromazine, lidocaine, methysergide, methylprednisolone, reserpine, quinacrine, chloroquine, and hydroxychloroquine exert a variety of effects upon platelet aggregation. Their mechanism of action is unknown, but they seem to share a common effect on platelet membrane lipids. Several of these lipid-soluble drugs inhibit phospholipase A_2 and platelet-activating factor.[52] These effects may account for their platelet-inhibitory actions. Lidocaine has recently been shown to stimulate PGI_2 release. Local anesthetics may influence platelet function by increasing both influx and availability within the cell of calcium ion. Thus, in addition to their separate actions, the membrane-active drugs may have an action on the so-called third pathway of platelet aggregation.

A recent preliminary report indicates that chlorpromazine inhibits thrombus formation in stenosed carotid arteries of Rhesus monkeys.[99]

Thromboxane Synthetase Inhibitors

Various TXA_2 synthetase inhibitors, mostly imidazole derivatives, are under active investigation. Imidazole selectively inhibits TXA_2 synthesis in human platelets.[100] UK-37, 248-01 is a potent orally active selective TXA_2 inhibitor.[101] It has been shown to inhibit TXA_2 formation in a dose-related manner in man. Peak inhibition is obtained at 1 hour after a 50-mg or higher dose. Six hours after a dose of 100 or 200 mg, there is still 50 percent inhibition of TXA_2 synthesis. There is presently no known toxicity except that a slight increase in BUN was noted in 3 of 12 patients 24 hours after a single dose. Synthetic prostaglandin analog 9,11-azoprosta 5,13-dienoic acid is a potent inhibitor of human platelet TXA_2 synthetase and inhibits the secondary wave of platelet aggregation induced by epinephrine and ADP. Another agent, OKY-1581, inhibits platelet aggregation and TXA_2 generation induced by arachidonic acid and ADP. In dogs, it decreases the myocardial infarct size, increases coronary blood flow to the ischemic zone, and decreases the incidence of arrhythmias from 12 to 24 hours after coronary occlusion.[102] Studies on the efficacy of these compounds in humans are underway. Drugs of this nature hold promise in the management of patients with platelet hyperactivity as a dominant feature in thrombosis.

Prostacyclin (PGI_2) and PGE_1

PGI_2 is very unstable at physiologic pH and must be kept at alkaline pH until administration. It inhibits platelet adhesion and platelet aggregation induced by ADP, epinephrine, arachidonic acid, and collagen, Its action upon platelets seems to correlate with adenylate cyclase activation and subsequent elevation of cAMP. Endogenous substances like angiotension II, bradykinin, adenosine, ceruloplasmin, histamine, and serotonin have been shown to stimulate PGI_2 release. PGI_2 infusion in animals has been shown to protect against loss of platelets and formation of microthrombi that occur during extracorporeal circulation of blood. When used with ionically bonded heparin-coated surface extracorporeal left ventricular assist device, it prevents coagulation and bleeding problems. Intracoronary PGI_2 increases coronary blood flow and decreases systemic vascular resistance.[103] In comparison with heparin, PGI_2 favorably protects Dacron grafts in baboons against platelet deposition.[103]

PGI_2 has been administered in normal subjects and in patients with a variety of disease states like primary pulmonary hypertension,[104] post–coronary artery surgery,[105] peripheral arterial disease,[106] and variant angina.[107] Typical systemic effects are related to profound vasodilation. In primary pulmonary hypertension and peripheral arterial disease, results are encouraging; but in six patients with variant angina given PGI_2, only one seemed to obtain relief. Instability of PGI_2 salt and difficulty in administration are major limitations to wider experience.

PGE_1, which shares some properties of PGI_2, has been used to improve the harvest and storage of blood platelets for therapeutic transfusion. Recent studies in patients with congestive heart failure suggest possible beneficial effects.[108]

Nafazatrom (Bay g6575) is believed to increase PGI_2 activity.[109] Its mechanism of action is still debated, but some authors have demonstrated inhibition of 15-hydroxy-prostaglandin dehydrogenase, which is responsible for catabolism of PGI_2, PGE_2, and $PGF_{2\alpha}$.[110] This substance has no effects on blood coagulation, platelet aggregation, or fibrinolysis, but upon administration with dipyridamole, it inhibits platelet aggregation.[109] Plasma obtained from volunteers after ingestion of 1.2 gm of nafazatrom stimulates release of PGI_2 from rat aorta[109] and prevents experimental thrombus formation in arteries and veins of rabbits and rats. However, in our experience, single-dose nafazatrom failed to ameliorate angina or enhance tolerance to exercise in patients with coronary disease.

Dietary Manipulation

In an attempt to modify platelet–vessel wall interaction, dietary manipulation has been examined. Eicosapentaenoic acid administration results in formation of prostaglandins with three double bonds (PGE_3, TXA_3, etc.). Unlike TXA_2, TXA_3 is biologically inactive. In contrast, PGI_3 shares the properties exhibited by PGI_2. Ten Hoor showed that cod liver oil–fed rats have a high incorporation of eicosapentaenoic acid into phospholipids of blood platelets and aortic wall at the expense of arachidonic acid with subsequent decrease in TXA_2 and PGI_2 generation, but appreciable increase in TXA_3 and PGI_3 could not be detected. However, thrombotic tendency was significantly decreased.[112] In rats, a linoleic acid–rich diet (sunflower seed oil) caused same decrease in thrombotic tendency as with an eicosapentaenoic acid–rich diet, but without decrease in PGI_2 and TXA_2 synthesis.[112]

Greenland Eskimos, who have a lower prevalence of cardiovascular disease than Western Europeans, derive their diet from cold water fish (cod fish, mackerel, etc.) and from animals that feed on these fish, which are rich in eicosapentaenoic acid. These Eskimos show inhibition of platelet aggregation, and their bleeding time is prolonged. Their platelets have a high membrane content of eicosapentaenoic acid, and platelet aggregation and release are markedly decreased. When placed on the same diet, Western Europeans develop similar changes in platelet function. Even 10 ml of 50 percent eicosapentaenoic acid ethyl ester administered daily for 3 weeks is enough to alter plasma fatty acid distribution, plasma lipids, and lipoproteins. In addition, it causes increase in platelet eicosapentaenoic acid content with decrease in platelet aggregation and TXA_2 generation, which is associated with increase in bleeding time.[113] In contrast, men fed with diets rich in ethyl arachidonate have proportionally more arachidonate in their platelet phospholipids, and this change is associated with an increase in platelet aggregation response to ADP. More studies are needed before establishing the beneficial role of eicosapentaenoic acid–rich diet.

Nitrates and Vasodilators

Nitroglycerin, isosorbide dinitrate, and inorganic nitrates have been shown to inhibit platelet aggregation induced by collagen, arachidonic acid, epinephrine, and ionophore A 23187 in vitro, but this effect is generally seen at concentrations higher than those achieved clinically.[114,115] Nitroglycerin inhibits oxygen burst and platelet malondialdehyde generation induced by arachidonic acid. Isosorbide dinitrate has been shown to decrease circulating platelet aggregates in some patients with coronary disease and high circulating platelet aggregates. Some recent data show that platelet TXA_2 generation is inhibited by nitroglycerin and isosorbide dinitrate in clinically used dosages.[116] It has been shown that nitroglycerin causes a dose-dependent increase in PGI_2 synthesis by endothelial cells.[117]

Other vasodilators such as nitroprusside, which strongly inhibits TXA_2 production,[117] exert significant inhibitory effects on platelet aggregation and adhesion in clinically achieved dosage.[118] Agents like prazosin and hydralazine inhibit platelet aggregation in high dosages.[119] Cyclo-oxygenase inhibitors attenuate vasodilatory response to hydralazine, suggesting that vasodilation may be prostaglandin-mediated.[120]

Ticlopidine

This pyridine derivative irreversibly inhibits platelet aggregation induced by several stimuli.[121] It seems to have no effect upon PGI_2 generation in rats. It is effective in prevention of thrombosis and thromboembolic events in animal models, and in this setting it is superior to aspirin and dipyridamole.[122,123] Ticlopidine is partially effective in reducing episodes of ST segment depression in patients with myocardial ischemia, especially when the ischemia occurs at slow heart rates and nocturnally.[124]

Forskolin

Forskolin is a diterpene that is extracted from a plant called Coleus forskohlii. This substance induces a marked reversible activation of adenylate cyclase activity, causing a 45-fold increase in platelet cAMP with concomitant inhibition of platelet aggregation induced by arachidonic acid, ADP, epinephrine, and collagen. At low dosage, it potentiates effects of PGE_1, PGD_2, and phosphodiesterase inhibitors.[125]

Heparin

Heparin is a glycoaminoglycan that indirectly acts on blood coagulation. Its anticoagulant actions are mediated through actions on plasma cofactor antithrombin III, which is a protease inhibitor that neutralizes kallikrein and activates factors XIIIa, XIIa, XIa, Xa, IXa, and IIa. It forms an irreversible complex with thrombin. Low concentration of heparin increases activity of antithrombin III, particularly against factor Xa and thrombin. This response is the basis for low-dose administration of heparin in prevention of thrombosis and thromboembolic events. However, patients receiving intermittent or continuous high doses of heparin have a progressive reduction in antithrombin III activity of levels approximately one third of normal, and thus the thrombotic tendency in man may paradoxically increase. Platelet factor 4 neutralizes and binds heparin, and so it may facilitate accumulation of thrombin and clot formation. Heparin causes transient mild thrombocytopenia in about 25 percent of patients and severe thrombocytopenia in a few. Mild thrombocytopenia results from heparin-induced platelet aggregation,[126] whereas severe thrombocytopenia follows formation of heparin-dependent antiplatelet antibodies. Occasionally, enhanced platelet aggregation with subsequent hemorrhage, thromboembolism, and death may occur. The mechanism of heparin-induced potentiation of platelet aggregation is being actively investigated. Early studies suggested neutralization of PGI_2 and PGE_1.[127,128] Cyclic endoperoxide analog–induced aggregation is potentiated by heparin, but this is not associated with enhanced TXA_2 synthesis.[129]

Dextran

Plasma expanders have no in vitro effect on platelet aggregation, but in vivo they decrease platelet aggregation and fibrin polymerization and increase the bleeding time. Their usefulness as antithrombotic agents in clinical situations is still to be established. A randomized double-blind trial in prevention of postoperative thromboembolic disease in surgical patients is presently underway.[130]

Clofibrate

This drug decreases plasma triglyceride levels and also decreases in vivo platelet adhesiveness and platelet aggregation induced by collagen, ADP, and epinephrine.[126] Rhesus monkeys fed atherogenic diets demonstrate a reduced severity of atherosclerotic lesions with clofibrate therapy.[63] In patients with coronary disease, clofibrate increases platelet survival time and decreases platelet aggregability; these effects correlate with increased platelet phospholipid-to-cholesterol ratio.

Prospective studies have provided conflicting results in patients at high risk of developing coronary artery disease treated with clofibrate. One study reports decrease in sudden death and overall mortality mainly in patients with angina,[131] whereas another suggests an increase in incidence of thromboembolic episodes, angina pectoris, intermittent claudication, and death rate.[132]

CONCLUSION

The mechanism for thrombus formation is complex, and platelets are involved in different stages. An understanding of the platelet–vessel wall interaction, platelet aggregation, platelet release reaction, and platelet-mediated vascular occlusion is important in determining action of pharmacologic agents. A combination of platelet-suppressive drugs may be necessary for proper treatment of thrombosis and atherosclerosis. It is important to have a predictive test for the detection of thrombotic or prethrombotic states, but no single test is yet available. Without the proper understanding of the mechanism of platelet thrombus formation and the pharmacology of the platelet-suppressive drugs, the expected results may not be obtained. This became apparent when aspirin and like drugs were investigated in patients with prior myocardial infarction. Large dosages of aspirin used in these studies may have been responsible for statistically insignificant results. Similarly, combined use of aspirin and dipyridamole was not effective, possibly because concurrent use of aspirin may have negated the beneficial effects that may be obtained with the dipyridamole.[133]

Most of the drugs considered as platelet-suppressive were initially introduced as anti-inflammatory drugs or vasodilators or for other purposes. The new generation of drugs synthesized specifically as platelet-suppressive agents is just appearing in research laboratories. Specific drugs working at specific sites may be more effective than those in use at present. The potential for modulation of platelet activation independent of arachidonic acid pathway and cAMP metabolism will offer a new system on which drugs will act. Studies of platelet-suppressive agents will also identify the site of action of the drugs, whether on platelet membrane receptor or platelet enzymes or on platelet metabolism. Until definite evidence of inhibition of thrombosis or regression of atherosclerosis can be demonstrated with the use of platelet-suppressive therapy, only very general recommendations can be made. These recommendations include the following:

1. Patients at high risk of re-infarction may be given aspirin, sulfinpyrazone, or dipyridamole.
2. Doses of these agents should be kept small, that is, aspirin 325 mg or less daily, sulfinpyrazone 200 to 400 mg daily, dipyridamole 25 to 50 mg three times daily.
3. Therapy should be initiated early after myocardial infarction.
4. Patients with valvular disease and atrial fibrillation may be given sulfinpyrazone (200 to 400 mg daily) prophylactically, especially if there is a previous history of thromboembolic episodes and routine anticoagulation is contraindicated.
5. Patients with prosthetic valves may be given aspirin (325 mg per day) plus dipyridamole (25 to 75 mg per day) if routine anticoagulant therapy is not feasible. In some patients who are on warfarin, dipyridamole may be added in order to reduce the risk of thromboembolic events, especially in patients with decreased platelet survival time or thromboembolic events despite warfarin therapy alone.
6. Patients with coronary artery bypass surgery may be given aspirin (325 mg every day or less) and dipyridamole (25 to 75 mg three times daily). Recent data suggest that if the therapy is started early after surgery or even before surgery (dipyridamole 400 mg per day beginning 2 days before surgery), the results may be rewarding.

REFERENCES

1. Jobin, F: *Plaquettes et maladies cardiovasculaires, Parts I to IV.* L'Union Medicale du Canada 105:231, 235, 756, 1159, 1976.
2. Hamberg, M, Svensson, J, and Samuelsson, B: *Thromboxanes. A new group of biologically active compounds derived from prostaglandin endoperoxides.* Proc Natl Acad Sci USA 72:2994, 1975.
3. Wong, PYK, Lee, WH, Chao, PHW, et al: *Metabolism of prostacyclin by 9-hydroxy prostaglandin dehydrogenase in human platelets.* J Biol Chem 255:9021, 1980.
4. Ross, R, Glomset, J, Kariya, B, et al: *A platelet-dependent serum factor that stimulates the proliferation of arterial smooth muscle cells in vitro.* Proc Natl Acad Sci USA 71:1207, 1974.
5. Gerrard, JM, Peller, JD, Krick, TP, et al: *Cyclic AMP and platelet prostaglandin synthesis.* Prostaglandins 14:39, 1977.
6. Haslam, RJ and McClenaghan, MD: *Effects of collagen and of aspirin on the concentration of guanosine 3',5'-cyclic monophosphate in human blood platelets: Measurement by a prelabelling technique.* Biochem J 138:317, 1974.
7. Vermylen, J and Carreras, LO: *The process of hemostasis.* In Herman, AG, Vanhoutte, PM, Denolin, H, et al (eds): *Cardiovascular Pharmacology of the Prostaglandins.* Raven Press, New York, 1982.
8. Chignard, M, Le Couedic, JP, Vargaftig, BB, et al: *Platelet activating factor (PAF) secretion from platelets: Effect of aggregating agents.* Br J Haematol 46:455, 1980.
9. Aiken, JW: *Arachidonic acid metabolism and the cardiovascular system.* In Mehta, J and Mehta, P (eds): *Platelets and Prostaglandins in Cardiovascular Disease.* Futura, New York, 1981, p 23.
10. Mehta, P, Mehta, J, and Roberts, A: *Synthesis of thromboxane A_2 and prostacyclin by newborn and adult human vascular tissue.* Clin Res 29:863A, 1981.
11. Moncada, S, Gryglewski, R, Bunting, S, etal: *An enzyme isolated from arteries transforms prostaglandin endoperoxides to an unstable substance that inhibits platelet aggregation.* Nature 263:663, 1976.
12. Jackson, EK, Goodman, RP, FitzGerald, GA, et al: *Evaluation of the in vivo production of 6-keto-PGE_1, an active metabolite of prostacyclin.* Circulation 64(Suppl IV):283, 1981.
13. Borgeat, P and Samuelsson, B: *Arachidonic acid metabolites in polymorphonuclear leukocytes: Effects of ionophore A 23187.* Proc Natl Acad Sci USA 76:2148, 1979.
14. Murphy, RC, Hammarstrom, S, and Samuelsson, B: *Leukotriene C: A slow reacting substance from murine mastocytoma cells.* Proc Natl Acad Sci USA 76:4275, 1979.
15. Ford-Hutchinson, AW, Bray, MA, Doig, MV, et al: *Leukotriene B: A potent chemokinetic and aggregating substance released from ploymorphonuclear leukocytes.* Nature 286:264, 1980.
16. Moncada, S, Gryglewski, R, Bunting, S, et al: *A lipid peroxide inhibits the enzyme in blood vessel microsome that generates from prostaglandin endoperoxides that substance (prostaglandin X) which prevents platelet aggregation.* Prostaglandins 12:715, 1976.

17. VON ROKITANSKY, C: *A manual of pathological anatomy* (translated by Day, GE), Vol 4. Sydenham Society, London, 1852.
18. DUGUID, JB: *Thrombosis as a factor in the pathogenesis of coronary atherosclerosis.* J Pathol Bacteriol 58:207, 1946.
19. VIRCHOW, R: *Cellular Pathology: As Based upon Physiologic and Pathological Histology* (translated by Chance, F). Dover, New York, 1971.
20. HAUST, MD AND MORE, RJ: *Significance of the smooth muscle cells in atherogenesis.* In JONES, RD (ED): *Evolution of the Atherosclerotic Plaque.* University of Chicago Press, Chicago, 1963.
21. MUSTARD, JF, PACKHAM, MA, ROWSELL, HC, ET AL: *The role of thrombogenic factors in atherosclerosis.* Ann NY Acad Sci 149:848, 1968.
22. STEIN, Y AND STEIN, O: *Interaction between serum lipoproteins and cellular components of the arterial wall.* In SCANU, AM, WISSLER, RW, AND GETZ, GS (EDS): *The Biochemistry of Atherosclerosis.* Marcel Dekker, New York, 1979.
23. BROWN, MS AND GOLDSTEIN, JL: *Receptor-mediated control of cholesterol metabolism.* Science 191:150, 1976.
24. DEDUVE, C: *The participation of lysosomes in the transformation of smooth muscle cells to foamy cells in the aorta of cholesterol-fed rabbits.* Acta Cardiol 20(Suppl):9, 1974.
25. GLAGOV, S: *Hemodynamic Risk Factors: Mechanical Stress, Mural Architecture, Medial Nutrition and the Vulnerability to Atherosclerosis.* Williams & Wilkins, Baltimore, 1972.
26. BENDITT, EP AND BENDITT, JM: *Evidence for a monoclonal origin of human atherosclerotic plaques.* Proc Natl Acad Sci USA 70:1753, 1973.
27. D'ANGELO, V, VILLA, S, MYSLEWIEC, M, ET AL: *Defective fibrinolytic and prostacyclin-like activity of human atheromatous plaques.* Thrombosis Haemostasis 39:535, 1978.
28. MEHTA, J AND MEHTA, P: *Platelet function in hypertension: Effect of therapy.* Am J Cardiol 47:331, 1981.
29. MEHTA, P AND MEHTA, J: *Effect of smoking and nicotine on platelet-endothelial cell activity.* In MEHTA, J AND MEHTA, P (EDS): *Platelets and Prostaglandins in Cardiovascular Disease.* Futura, New York, 1981.
30. CARVALHO, AC, COLMAN, RW, AND LEES, RS: *Platelet function in hyperlipoproteinemia.* N Engl J Med 290:434, 1974.
31. STUART, MJ, GERRARD, JM, AND WHITE, JG: *Effect of cholesterol on production of thromboxane B_2 by platelets in vitro.* N Engl J Med 302:6, 1980.
32. BURROWS, AW, CHANIN, SI, AND HOCKADAY, TDR: *Plasma thromboglobulin concentrations in diabetes mellitus.* Lancet 1:235, 1978.
33. HALUSHKA, PV, ROGERS, RC, LOADHOLT, CB, ET AL: *Increased platelet thromboxane synthesis in diabetes mellitus.* J Lab Clin Med 97:87, 1981.
34. FLEISCHER, LN, TALL, AR, WITTE, LD, ET AL: *Stimulation of arterial endothelial cell prostacyclin synthesis by high density lipoprotein.* Circulation 64(Suppl IV):216, 1981.
35. HAMPTON, JR AND GORLIN, R: *Platelet studies in patients with coronary artery disease.* Br Heart J 34:465, 1972.
36. GREEN, LH, SEROPPIAN, E, AND HANDIN, RI: *Platelet activation during exercise-induced myocardial ischemia.* N Engl J Med 302:193, 1980.
37. MEHTA, J AND MEHTA, P: *Comparison of platelet function during exercise in normal subjects and coronary artery disease patients: Potential role of platelet activation in myocardial ischemia.* Am Heart J 103:49, 1982.
38. DREYFUSS, F AND ZAHAVI, J: *Adenosine diphosphate–induced platelet aggregation in myocardial infarction and ischemic heart disease.* Atherosclerosis 17:107, 1973.
39. MEHTA, J AND MEHTA, P: *Role of blood platelets and prostaglandins in coronary artery disease.* Am J Cardiol 48:366, 1981.
40. MEHTA, P, MEHTA, J, AND PEPINE, CJ: *Platelet aggregation across the myocardial vascular bed in man: I. Normal versus diseased coronary arteries.* Thromb Res 14:423, 1979.
41. MEHTA, J, MEHTA, P, AND PEPINE, CJ: *Platelet aggregation in aortic and coronary venous blood in patients with and without coronary disease. 3. Role of tachycardia stress and propranolol.* Circulation 58:881, 1978.
42. MEHTA, P, MEHTA, J, AND PEPINE, CJ: *Influence of the normal human forearm vascular bed on platelet aggregation, counts and size.* Microvasc Res 21:229, 1981.
43. MEHTA, J, MEHTA, P, AND PEPINE, CJ: *Platelet function studies in coronary artery disease: VII. Effects of aspirin and tachycardia stress on aortic and coronary venous blood.* Am J Cardiol 45:945, 1980.
44. MEHTA, J, MEHTA, P, PEPINE, CJ, ET AL: *Platelet function studies in coronary artery disease. X. Effect of dipyridamole.* Am J Cardiol 47:1111, 1981.

45. MEHTA, J, MEHTA, P, AND CONTI, CR: *Platelet function studies in coronary heart disease. IX. Increased platelet prostaglandin generation and abnormal platelet sensitivity to prostacyclin and endoperoxide analog in angina pectoris.* Am J Cardiol 46:943, 1980.

46. SZCZEKLIK, A, GRYGLEWSKI, RJ, MUSIAL, J, ET AL: *Thromboxane generation of platelet aggregation in survivors of myocardial infarction.* Thrombosis Haemostasis 40:66, 1978.

47. ROBERTSON, RM, ROBERTSON, D, ROBERTS, LJ, ET AL: *Thromboxane A_2 in vasotonic angina pectoris.* N Engl J Med 304:998, 1981.

48. TADA, M, KUZUYA, T, INOUE, M, ET AL: *Elevation of thromboxane B_2 levels in patients with classic and variant angina pectoris.* Circulation 64:1107, 1981.

49. MEHTA, J, MEHTA, P, AND HORALEK, C: *The significance of platelet–vessel wall prostaglandin equilibrium during exercise-induced stress.* Am Heart J 105:895, 1983.

50. DEWOOD, MA, SPORES, J, NOTSKE, R, ET AL: *Prevalence of total coronary occlusion during the early hours of transmural myocardial infarction.* N Engl J Med 303:897, 1980.

51. GANZ, W, BUCHBINDER, N, MARCUS, H, ET AL: *Intracoronary thrombolysis in evolving myocardial infarction.* Am Heart J 101:4, 1981.

52. BISHOPRIC, N, MEHTA, J, AND MEHTA, P: *Platelet activation and platelet suppressive drugs.* In MEHTA, J AND MEHTA, P (EDS): *Platelets and Prostaglandins in Cardiovascular Disease.* Futura, New York, 1981.

53. ROTH, GJ, STANFORD, N, AND MAJERUS, P: *Acetylation of prostaglandin synthetase by aspirin.* Proc Natl Acad Sci USA 72:3073, 1975.

54. MASOTTI, G, POGGESI, L, GALANTI, G, ET AL: *Differential inhibition of prostacyclin production and platelet aggregation by aspirin.* Lancet 2:1213, 1979.

55. KELTON, JG, HIRSH, J, AND CARTER, CJ: *Thrombogenic effect of high dose aspirin in rabbits. Relationship to inhibition of vessel wall synthesis of prostaglandin I_2-like activity.* J Clin Invest 62:892, 1978.

56. PICK, R, CHEDIAK, J, AND GLICK, G: *Aspirin inhibits development of coronary atherosclerosis in cynomolgus monkeys (Macaca fascicularis) fed an atherogenic diet.* J Clin Invest 63:158, 1979.

57. FOLTS, JD, CROWELL, EB, AND ROWE, GG: *Platelet aggregation in partially obstructed vessels and its elimination with aspirin.* Circulation 54:365, 1976.

58. GENT, M AND CAIRNS, J: *The clinical evaluation of platelet-suppressive drugs in post myocardial infarction patients.* In MEHTA, J AND MEHTA, P (EDS): *Platelets and Prostaglandins in Cardiovascular Disease.* Futura, New York, 1981.

59. CHESEBRO, JH, FUSTER, V, PUMPHREY, CW, ET AL: *Combined warfarin–platelet inhibitor anti-thrombotic therapy in prosthetic heart valve replacement.* Circulation 64(Suppl IV):76, 1981.

60. HARTER, HR, BURCH, JW, MAJERUS, PW, ET AL: *Prevention of thrombosis in patients on hemodialysis by low dose aspirin.* N Engl J Med 301:577, 1979.

61. THE CANADIAN COOPERATIVE STUDY GROUP: *A randomized trial of aspirin and sulfinpyrazone in threatened stroke.* N Engl J Med 299:53, 1978.

62. PACKHAM, MA, WARRIOR, ES, GLYNN, MF, ET AL: *Alteration of the response of platelets to surface stimuli by pyrazole compounds.* J Exp Med 126:171, 1967.

63. PICK, R: *Experimental atherosclerosis and its inhibition by platelet active drugs.* In MEHTA, J AND MEHTA, P (EDS): *Platelets and Prostaglandins in Cardiovascular Disease.* Futura, New York, 1981, p 149.

64. STEELS, P, BATTOCK, D, AND GENTON, E: *Effect of clofibrate and sulfinpyrazone on platelet survival time in coronary artery disease.* Circulation 52:473, 1975.

65. WILKINSON, AL, HAWKER, RJ, AND HAWKER, LM: *The influence of antiplatelet drugs on platelet survival after aortic damage or implantation of a Dacron arterial prosthesis.* Thromb Res 15:181, 1979.

66. WEILY, HS AND GENTON, E: *Altered platelet function in patients with prosthetic mitral valves. Effect of sulfinpyrazone therapy.* Circulation 42:967, 1970.

67. THE ANTURANE REINFARCTION TRIAL RESEARCH GROUP: *Sulfinpyrazone in the prevention of cardiac death after myocardial infarction.* N Engl J Med 298:289. 1978.

68. ASANO, T, OCHIAI, Y, AND HIDAKA, H: *Selective inhibition of separated forms of human platelet cyclic nucleotide phosphodiesterase by platelet aggregation inhibitors.* Mol Pharmacol 13:400, 1977.

69. MEHTA, P, MEHTA, J, AND HORALEK, C: *Dipyridamole inhibits thromboxane generation and promotes prostacyclin release.* Circulation 64(Suppl IV):284, 1981.

70. MONCADA, S AND KORBUT, R: *Dipyridamole and other phosphodiesterase inhibitors act as antithrombotic agents by potentiating endogenous prostacyclin.* Lancet 1:1286, 1978.

71. HARKER, LA, ROSS, R, SLICHTER, SJ, ET AL: *Homocystine induced arteriosclerosis. The role of endothelial cell injury and platelet response in its genesis.* J Clin Invest 58:731, 1976.

72. Hollander, W, Kirpatrick, B, Paddock, J, et al: *Studies on the progression and regression of coronary and peripheral atherosclerosis in the cynomolgus monkey. I. Effects of dipyridamole and aspirin.* Exp Mol Pathol 30:55, 1979.
73. Dembinska-Kiec, A, Rucker, W, and Schonhofer, PS: *Effects of dipyridamole in experimental atherosclerosis. Actions on PGI_2, platelet aggregation and atherosclerotic plaque formation.* Atherosclerosis 33:315, 1979.
74. Harker, LA and Slichter, SJ: *Studies of platelet and fibrinogen kinetics in patients with prosthetic heart valves.* N Engl J Med 283:1302, 1970.
75. Stuart, M, Stockman, J, Murphy, S, et al: *Shortened platelet life span in patients with hydrocephalus and ventriculojugular shunts: Results of preliminary attempts at correction.* J Pediatr 80:21, 1972.
76. Sullivan, JM, Harken, DE, and Gorlin, RG: *Pharmacologic control of thrombo-embolic complications of cardiac valve replacement.* N Engl J Med 284:1391, 1971.
77. Editorial: *Dipyridamole in myocardial scintigraphy.* Lancet 2:1346, 1980.
78. Gould, KL: *Non-invasive assessment of coronary stenoses by myocardial perfusion imaging during pharmacologic coronary vasodilatation. I. Physiologic basis and experimental validation.* Am J Cardiol 41:267, 1978.
79. Gould, KL, Schelbert, HR, Phelps, MD, et al: *Noninvasive assessment of coronary stenoses with myocardial perfusion imaging during pharmacologic coronary vasodilatation. V. Detection of 47 percent diameter coronary stenosis with intravenous nitrogen-13 ammonia and emission-computed tomography in intact dogs.* Am J Cardiol 43:200, 1979.
80. Gent, AE, Brook, CGD, Foley, TH, et al: *Dipyridamole: A controlled trial of its effects in acute myocardial infarction.* Br Med J 4:366, 1968.
81. The Persantine Aspirin Reinfarction Study Research Group: *Persantine and aspirin in coronary heart disease.* Circulation 62:449, 1980.
82. Chesebro, JM, Clements, IP, Fuster, V, et al: *A platelet inhibitor-drug trial in coronary bypass operation: Benefit of perioperative dipyridamole and aspirin therapy on early postoperative vein-graft patency.* N Engl J Med 307:73, 1982.
83. Weksler, BB, Gillick, M, and Pink, J: *Effect of propranolol on platelet function.* Blood 49:185, 1977.
84. Mehta, J, Mehta, P, Horalek, C, et al: *Effect of propranolol therapy on platelet release and prostaglandin generation in patients with coronary heart disease.* Circulation 66:1294, 1982.
85. Förster, W: *Effect of various agents in prostaglandin biosynthesis and the anti-aggregatory effect.* Acta Med Scand 642(Suppl):35, 1980.
86. Pick, R and Glick, G: *Effects of propranolol, minoxidil and clofibrate on cholesterol-induced atherosclerosis in stump tail macaques (Macaca arctiodes).* Atherosclerosis 27:71, 1977.
87. Beta-Blocker Heart Attack Study Group: *The β-blocker heart attack trial.* JAMA 246:20, 1981.
88. Multicenter International Study: *Improvement in prognosis of myocardial infarction by long-term beta adrenoreceptor blockade using practolol: A multicenter international study.* Br Med J 3:735, 1975.
89. Anderson, MP, Frederiksen, J, Jürgensen, HJ, et al: *Effect of alprenolol on mortality among patients with definite or suspected acute myocardial infarction.* Lancet 2:865, 1979.
90. The Norwegian Multicenter Study Group: *Timolol-induced reduction in mortality and reinfarction in patients surviving acute myocardial infarction.* N Engl J Med 304:801, 1981.
91. Mehta, J, Mehta, P, Ostrowski, N, et al: *Effects of verapamil on platelet aggregation, ATP release and thromboxane A_2 generation.* Thromb Res (in press).
92. Chierchia, S, Crea, F, Bernini, W, et al: *Antiplatelet effects of verapamil in man.* Am J Cardiol 47:399, 1981.
93. Pumphrey, CW, Fuster, V, Dewanjee, M, et al: *Verapamil is an effective in vivo inhibitor of platelet activation in peripheral vascular grafts in dogs.* Circulation 64(Suppl IV):56, 1981.
94. Kramsch, DM, Aspen, AJ, and Apstein, CS: *Suppression of experimental atherosclerosis by the calcium antagonist lanthanum.* J Clin Invest 65:967, 1980.
95. Henry, PD and Bentley, KI: *Suppression of atherogenesis in cholesterol-fed rabbits treated with nifedipine.* J Clin Invest 68:1366, 1981.
96. Barneton, E, Addonzio, P, and Shatti, S: *Interaction of verapamil with human platelet α-adrenergic receptors.* Am J Physiol 242:H19, 1982.
97. Folts, JD and Bonebrake, FC: *The effects of cigarette smoke and nicotine on platelet thrombus formation in stenosed dog coronary arteries: Inhibition with phentolamine.* Circulation 65:465, 1982.
98. Gryglewski, RJ: *Prostaglandins, platelets, and atherosclerosis.* CRC Crit Rev Biochem 7:291, 1980.
99. Folts, JD, Bertha, BG, and Lambrecht, LK: *Periodic platelet thrombus formation in stenosed carotid arteries of Rhesus monkeys.* Circulation 64(Suppl IV):57, 1981.

100. NEEDLEMAN, P, RAZ, A, FERRENDELLI, JA, ET AL: *Application of imidazole as a selective inhibitor of thromboxane synthetase in human platelets.* Proc Natl Acad Sci USA 74:1716, 1977.

101. TYLER, HM, SAXTON, CAPD, AND TAYLOR, DJE: *Administration to man of UK-37, 248-01. A selective inhibitor of thromboxane synthetase.* Lancet 1:629, 1981.

102. SHEA, MJ, DRISCOLL, EM, ROMSON, JR, ET AL: *Effect of OKY-1581, a thromboxane synthetase inhibitor, on coronary thrombosis in the conscious canine.* Circulation 64(Suppl IV):281, 1981.

103. MEHTA, J, NICHOLS, WW, MEHTA, P, ET AL: *Effects of prostacyclin on systemic and coronary hemodynamics in dog.* Am Heart J 105:835, 1981.

104. GROVES, BM, RUBIN, LJ, REEVES, JT, ET AL: *Comparable hemodynamic effects of prostacyclin and hydralazine in primary pulmonary hypertension.* Circulation 64(Suppl IV):297, 1981.

105. CHELLY, J, FABIANI, JM, CHANINE, R, ET AL: *Prostacyclin after coronary surgery.* Circulation 64(Suppl IV):202, 1981.

106. SZCZEKLIK, A, NIZANKOWSKY, R, SKAWINSKY, S, ET AL: *Successful therapy of advanced arteriosclerosis obliterans with prostacyclin.* Lancet 1:1111, 1979.

107. CHIERCHIA, S, PATRONO, C, CREA, F, ET AL: *Effects of intravenous prostacyclin in variant angina.* Circulation 65:470, 1982.

108. POPAT, KD AND PITT, B: *Hemodynamic effects of prostaglandin E_1 infustion in patients with acute myocardial infarction and left ventricular failure.* Am Heart J 103:485, 1982.

109. VERMYLEN, J, CHAMONE, DAF, AND VERSTRAETE, M: *Stimulation of prostacyclin release from vessel wall by Bay G 6575, an antithrombotic compound.* Lancet 1:518, 1979.

110. WONG, PYK AND MCGIFF, JC: *Bay G 6575, an anti-thrombotic agent, inhibits metabolism of prostacyclin (PGI_2).* Circulation 64(Suppl IV):55, 1981.

111. NEEDLEMAN, P, RAZ, A, MINKES, MS, ET AL: *Triene prostaglandins: Prostacyclin and thromboxane biosynthesis and unique biological properties.* Proc Natl Acad Sci USA 76:944, 1979.

112. TEN HOOR, F: *Dietary manipulation of prostaglandins: Feeding fish oil does not result in the production of thromboxane A_3 and PGI_3 and strongly inhibits thromboxane A_2 and PGI_2 formation in rat blood platelets and aorta.* In HERMAN, AG, VANHOUTTE, PM, DENOLIN, H, ET AL (EDS): *Cardiovascular Pharmacology of the Prostaglandins.* Raven Press, New York, 1982.

113. DYERBERG, J: *Dietary manipulation of prostaglandin synthesis: Beneficial or detrimental.* In HERMAN, AG, VANHOUTTE, PM, DENOLIN, M, ET AL (EDS): *Cardiovascular Pharmacology of the Prostaglandins.* Raven Press, New York, 1982.

114. SCHAFER, AI, ALEXANDER, RW, AND HANDIN, RI: *Inhibition of platelet function by organic nitrate vasodilators.* Blood 55:649, 1980.

115. MEHTA, J AND MEHTA, P: *Comparative effects of nitroprusside and nitroglycerin on platelet aggregation in patients with heart failure.* J Cardiovasc Pharmacol 2:25, 1982.

116. MEHTA, J, MEHTA, P, FELDMAN, R, ET AL: *Influence of tachycardia stress and nitroglycerin on thromboxane levels in coronary disease.* Am J Cardiol 49:902, 1982.

117. WEKSLER, BB, ELDOR, A, FALCONE, D, ET AL: *Prostaglandins and vascular endothelium.* In HERMAN, AG, VANHOUTTE, PM, DENOLIN, H, ET AL (EDS): *Cardiovascular Pharmacology of the Prostaglandins.* Raven Press, New York, 1982.

118. MEHTA, J AND MEHTA, P: *Platelet function studies in heart disease. VI. Enhanced platelet aggregate formation activity in congestive heart failure. Inhibition by sodium nitroprusside.* Circulation 60:497, 1979.

119. GREENWALD, JE, WONG, LK, RAO, M, ET AL: *A study of three vasodilating agents as selective inhibitors of thromboxane A_2 biosynthesis.* Biochem Biophys Res Commun 84:1112, 1978.

120. RUBIN, LJ AND LAZAR, MD: *Influence of prostaglandin synthesis inhibitors on pulmonary vasodilator effects of hydralazine in dogs with hypoxic pulmonary vasoconstriction.* J Clin Invest 67:193, 1981.

121. THIBAULT, JJ, BLATRIX, CE, BLANCHARD, JF, ET AL: *Effect of ticlopidine, a new platelet aggregation inhibitor in man.* Clin Pharmacol Ther 18:485, 1975.

122. ASHIDA, SI AND ABIKO, Y: *Effect of ticlopidine and acetylsalicyclic acid on generation of prostaglandin I_2–like substance in rat arterial tissue.* Thromb Res 13:901, 1978.

123. TOMIKAWA, M, ASHIDA, SI, KAKIHATA, ET AL: *Anti-thrombotic action of ticlopidine, a new platelet aggregation inhibitor.* Thromb Res 12:1157, 1978.

124. SELWYN, A, JONATHAN, A, AND FOX, K: *The effects of antiplatelet drug on myocardial ischemia in patients with coronary artery disease.* Am J Cardiol 45:424, 1980.

125. SIEGL, AM AND DALY, JW: *Forskolin: A potent new inhibitor of platelet aggregation.* Circulation 64(Suppl IV):284, 1981.

126. O'REILLY, R: *Anticoagulant, antithrombotic, and thrombolytic drugs.* In GOODMAN, LS AND GILMAN, A (EDS): *The Pharmacological Basis of Therapeutics.* Macmillan, New York, 1980.

127. Reches, A, Eldor, A, and Salomon, Y: *Heparin inhibits PGE_1-sensitive adenylate cyclase and antagonizes PGE_1 antiaggregating effect in human platelets.* J Lab Clin Med 93:638, 1979.

128. Saba, HI, Saba, SR, Blackburn, CA, et al: *Heparin neutralization of PGI_2: Effect upon platelets.* Science 205:499, 1979.

129. Mehta, P and Mehta, J: *Potentiation of endoperoxide analog-induced platelet aggregation by heparin.* Thromb Res 25:91, 1982.

130. Davies, WT: *Dextran or heparin?* Lancet 2:732, 1978.

131. Physicians of the Newcastle Upon Tyne Region: *Trial of clofibrate in the treatment of ischemic heart disease.* Br Med J 4:767, 1971.

132. Coronary Drug Project Research Group: *Clofibrate and niacin in coronary heart disease.* JAMA 231:360, 1975.

133. Mehta, J and Mehta, P: *Dipyridamole and aspirin in relation to platelet aggregation and vessel wall prostaglandin generation.* J Cardiovasc Pharmacol 4:688, 1982.

Regional and Systemic Thrombolytic Therapy in Acute Myocardial Infarction

Andrea Hastillo, M.D., and Michael J. Cowley, M.D.

Acute myocardial infarction is estimated to occur in more than 1 million Americans each year. In addition to a hospital mortality of 10 to 15 percent, a substantial percentage of survivors develop significant cardiac functional loss resulting in inability to return to usual employment, restricted physical activity, and recurrent hospitalization. Myocardial ischemia is due to an imbalance of oxygen supply and demand, and infarction occurs when ischemia is severe and prolonged. Early attempts to reduce the extent of necrosis with infarction have focused on decreasing oxygen demand, and demonstration of beneficial effects has been difficult to establish.[1,2] More recently, methods to directly increase myocardial oxygen supply by reperfusion have been evaluated.[3–5] Nonsurgical reperfusion by pharmacologic lysis of coronary thrombosis using intracoronary streptokinase[6–33] and, more recently, intravenous streptokinase[14] has shown promising results and is now undergoing widespread and increasing clinical application. The current status of regional and systemic thrombolytic therapy in acute myocardial infarction is the subject of this review.

RATIONALE

Studies of experimental models of infarction have clarified the pathophysiology and evolution of infarction, characterized factors influencing progression of ischemia to irreversible injury, and established the concept of preservation of ischemic myocardium and limitation of infarct size.[1,15,16] Myocardial infarction is a dynamic event with progression to irreversible ischemic change over a period of hours. Necrosis begins in the subendocardial region and progresses outward as a wavefront to the subepicardium within the ischemic zone.[15] The eventual extent of necrosis is primarily dependent on the duration of severe ischemia, the size of the ischemic vascular bed, and the presence and extent of collateral flow.[16] The time course for completed necrosis is variable in different experimental models, but most animal studies indicate that necrosis is nearly complete after 6 hours of severe ischemia.[15–17]

The initiating factor in myocardial infarction has been studied for years with no final resolution. Platelet aggregation, coronary artery spasm, intraluminal plaque hemorrhage, and thrombus formation have each been implicated.[18] Although thrombosis is not universally present at the time of necropsy studies after acute infarction, recent studies employing acute angiography have clearly established that thrombotic coronary occlusion is usually present in the early hours of evolving transmural infartion.[19,20] Experimental animal studies have demonstrated that infusion of a thrombolytic agent can lyse experimentally induced thrombi and that early infusion and regional infusion near the thrombus produce the highest incidence of successful recanalization.[21–23] Early reperfusion has been consistently associated with reduction of experimental infarct size.[15–17,24,25] Although reperfusion has been associated with hemorrhagic infarction and caused initial concern of possible infarct extension, subsequent studies have demonstrated that myocyte injury antecedes microvascular damage and that reperfusion hemorrhage is confined to areas that have already undergone necrosis.[26,27] Of available interventions to reduce infarct size, reperfusion alone directly addresses the primary abnormality of insufficient coronary flow and appears to offer the greatest potential for substantial myocardial salvage. Reperfusion by lysis of occluding thrombus seems an attractive potential means to interrupt continued ischemia and to decrease infarct size in patients.

Clinical application of thrombolytic therapy in acute myocardial infarction was first reported in 1957 by Moser.[28] Fletcher and colleagues[29] reported the first series of patients treated with intravenous streptokinase and demonstrated that a sustained thrombolytic state was well tolerated and could be safely achieved. Since that time, approximately 20 large-scale prospective studies have been performed, mostly in Europe, to evaluate the usefulness of intravenous thrombolytic therapy in patients with acute infarction. These studies have shown conflicting results and are difficult to compare because of major differences in study design, patient selection, duration of treatment, adjunctive therapy, and methods used to evaluate response. Many of these studies were poorly designed, and the difficulties with their interpretation have been reviewed by Duckert.[30] Although several studies suggested improved survival or reduced frequency of congestive heart failure in treated patients, others showed no apparent benefit, and most of these studies were associated with a significant incidence of bleeding complications in the treated patients.[31,32] For these reasons, intravenous thrombolytic therapy was never widely used. The current renewed interest in this approach is due to the introduction of selective techniques for intracoronary thrombolytic administration, which has been demonstrated to achieve thrombolysis and reperfusion in a high percentage of patients with acute coronary occlusion, and to an awareness that cardiac catheterization during evolving myocardial infarction can be safely performed.[4–13,20]

THROMBOLYTIC AGENTS

Streptokinase and urokinase are the two currently available thrombolytic drugs. Both produce activation of the fibrinolytic system, which is an important component of the vascular repair response. Streptokinase, an antigenic protein from group C beta-hemolytic streptococci, activates fibrinolysis indirectly by forming an activator complex with plasminogen, which then converts additional plasminogen to plasmin. Plasmin, a proteolytic enzyme with relatively broad specificity, degrades fibrin thrombi to soluble complexes. In contrast to streptokinase, urokinase is a direct activator of fibrinolysis and is nonantigenic. Although urokinase has theoretical advantages over streptokinase, owing to its more predictable dose-effect relationship, it is considerably more expensive and has been less widely used than streptokinase. Under physiologic conditions, lysis of fibrin occurs as a local process owing to preferential "fibrin-specific" binding and activation and the presence of circulating inhibitors that prevent a generalized lytic state. There is considerable evidence that thrombolytic agents produce lysis of pathologic thrombosis also predominantly by local activation of plasminogen bound to the thrombus and that circulating free plasmin plays only a minor role.[33] Intravenous administration of these agents requires sufficient dosage to neutralize inhibitory systems in order to achieve high levels of activator and is associated with production of a generalized lytic state with degradation of fibrinogen and production of fibrinogen degradation products, whether or not clot lysis occurs. In contrast, regional infusion of streptokinase or urokinase may produce effective local activator levels and clot lysis without induction of systemic fibrinolytic effects.

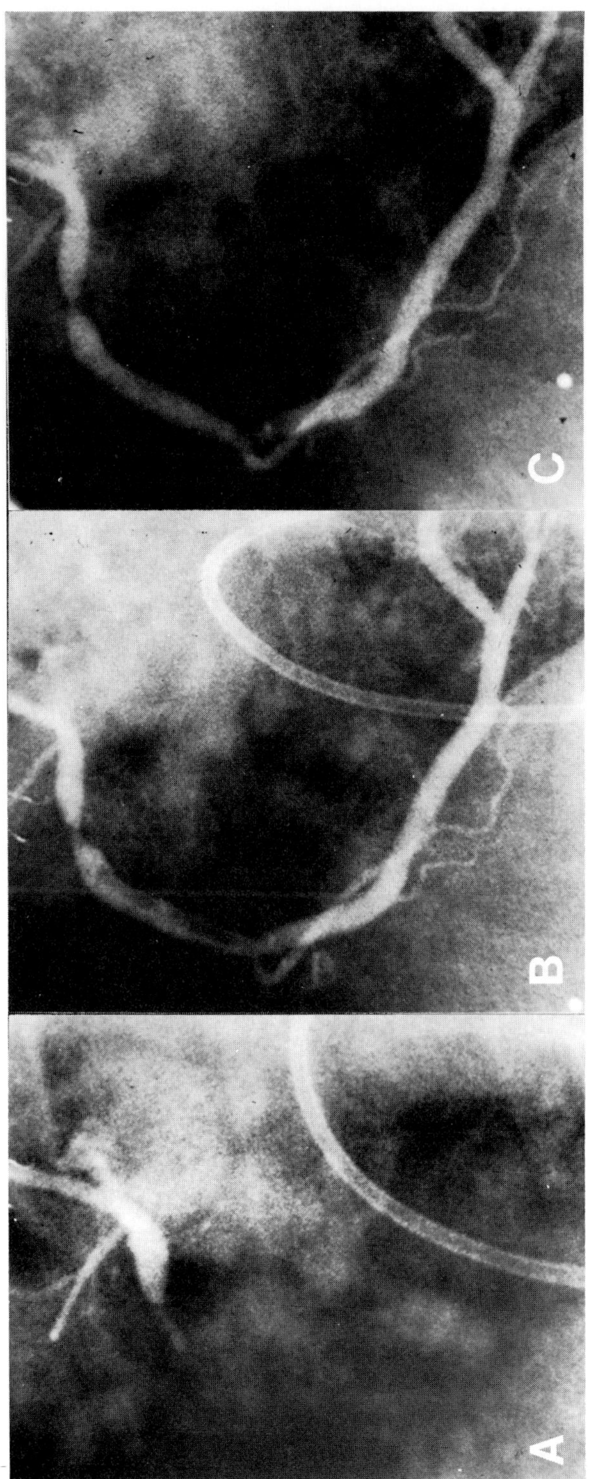

Figure 1. Right coronary angiogram (left anterior oblique view) in a patient with acute inferior infarction. *A*, Total occlusion of proximal right coronary artery (RCA). *B*, After initial restoration of patency, extensive thrombus is present in the proximal and mid-RCA. *C*, After 150,000 IU of streptokinase, filling defect representing thrombus has resolved, and there is severe residual proximal RCA stenosis.

TECHNIQUE OF INTRACORONARY THROMBOLYTIC ADMINISTRATION

Routine right and left heart catheterization is performed with heparin given at the time of arterial cannulation. Either the percutaneous femoral or the brachial approach may be used. Patients are usually premedicated with an antihistamine and/or steroids to minimize the likelihood of an allergic reaction. Baseline angiography is performed to identify the site of occlusion, and intracoronary nitroglycerin is usually given to rule out reversible spasm as a contributing factor in the occlusion. Thrombolytic infusion is then begun. Streptokinase may be infused into the ostium of the infarct-related vessel or subselectively through a small 2 to 3 French catheter that is positioned at the occlusion site. The infusion may be initiated with a bolus injection of 10,000 to 20,000 IU. Continuous infusion is then given at 2,000 to 5,000 IU/min. Repeat angiography is usually performed at 15-minute intervals during the infusion to determine if reperfusion has occurred. Once recanalization occurs, the thrombolytic agent is usually continued for 30 to 60 minutes or until residual clot is no longer apparent, or until maximal luminal diameter appears to have been achieved (Fig. 1). The total dosage and duration of infusion are individualized to achieve satisfactory reperfusion within the limits of patient tolerance and predetermined endpoints. Mean dosage in reported studies has varied between 120,000 and 350,000 IU given over 60 to 120 minutes.[6–13]

After completion of the procedure, conventional postinfarction monitoring is continued in the coronary care unit. Coagulation studies are obtained to establish whether a systemic fibrinolytic effect has occurred and to guide removal of catheters and institution of heparin. Catheter removal is usually delayed for 12 to 24 hours after the procedure if a systemic fibrinolytic state has occurred. This provides local hemostasis until the coagulopathy has resolved, and these sites may also be used for blood sampling or for access should a temporary pacemaker, Swan-Ganz catheter, arterial pressure monitoring, or early repeat angiography be necessary. When reperfusion has been achieved, additional therapy is important to maintain patency of the vessel. Nitrates and calcium antagonists are given to achieve maximal vasodilation. To prevent rethrombosis, heparinization is begun when anticoagulation parameters are approaching normal (activated PTT $\leq$ two times control). Heparinization is continued at therapeutic levels for a variable period depending on the clinical course of the patient. If the patient is stable, heparin is given for 7 to 10 days, and then warfarin or a combination of aspirin and dipyridamole is begun and continued for 3 to 6 months. If recurrent ischemia occurs early in the hospital course, coronary artery bypass surgery or percutaneous transluminal angioplasty may be necessary, and heparin is continued until revascularization or stabilization. In addition, most patients are treated with beta blockers unless contraindicated.

RESULTS OF INTRACORONARY THROMBOLYSIS

Based on current reports, successful thrombolysis has been achieved in approximately 75 to 80 percent of patients[6–13,34,35] (Table 1). Total occlusion of the infarct-related vessel has been present in 80 to 90 percent of patients in these studies. Occasionally, reperfusion occurred following injection of contrast agent. Few totally occluded vessels have responded to intracoronary nitroglycerin administration, and patency when achieved was usually transient. Reperfusion by mechanical recanalization using a flexible guide wire or small catheter has been achieved in a small percentage of patients, but this approach has generally been unsatisfactory in establishing effective flow and is not widely used. In most patients, reperfusion was achieved only after streptokinase administration. The average streptokinase dose at which vessel patency was initially restored has been 60,000 to 70,000 IU, and the average duration of infusion to patency has ranged from 20 to 35 minutes.[35] Although a composite reperfusion rate of 75 to 80 percent has been achieved, results have varied considerably at individual centers, which may be due to differences in patient selection criteria and to differences in technique. The frequency of thrombus and the response rate to streptokinase in patients with

Table 1. Reperfusion rates with intracoronary thrombolysis

	Patients	*Reperfusion*	*% Success*
Rentrop[6]	29	22	76
Ganz[7]	29	27	93
Mathey[8]	41	30	73
Reduto[9]	30	21	70
Gold[10]	30	21	70
Cowley[11]	36	31	86
Schwartz[34]	27	18	67
Total	222	170	77

subtotal occlusion have also varied considerably but appear to be lower than encountered with total occlusion.[35] An analysis of other factors that may influence reperfusion rates suggests that within the range of infusion rate and total dosage employed with intracoronary streptokinase administration, higher infusion rates and higher total dosage are associated with higher reperfusion rates. In addition, subselective infusion appears to be associated with improved results compared with ostial infusion.[36] Reperfusion rate may also depend on which coronary artery is involved. Circumflex coronary artery occlusion appears to require longer infusion times to restore patency and has a lower success rate compared with left anterior descending and right coronary artery occlusions.[13] In addition, several studies have reported an inverse relationship between duration of symptoms and the rapidity and frequency of thrombolysis, suggesting that thrombus age also influences response.[12,13]

ASSESSMENT OF BENEFICIAL EFFECTS

Although infarct size cannot be directly measured in patients, a number of parameters may be used to evaluate the effects of therapeutic intervention. Successful reperfusion has been associated with relatively prompt resolution of residual chest pain in most patients with ongoing pain and is usually associated electrocardiographically with reduction of ST segment elevation shortly after restoration of effective antegrade flow, suggesting interruption of ischemia.[6–13] The effect of reperfusion on left ventricular function represents an important endpoint and has been evaluated by determination of changes in ejection fraction using contrast or radionuclide ventriculography obtained before or immediately after intervention and at restudy 1 to 2 weeks later (Table 2). These studies indicate significant improvement of ejection fraction after successful recanalization. In contrast to the improvement from early to late study with successful reperfusion, ejection fraction did not change or else decreased in patients with unsuccessful reperfusion or in patients who had no intervention and served as controls[8,9,11] (Fig. 2). The time limit for beneficial effects of reperfusion in patients is unknown, and significant improvement of ejection fraction has occurred over a wide period

Table 2. Change in left ventricular ejection fraction with successful reperfusion

	Patients	*Early EF*	*Late EF*	*p Value**	*Time of Restudy*	*Method*
Rentrop[6]	14	50.5 ± 12	56.6 ± 12.4	<0.01	16 days	Angiogram
Mathey[8]	11	37 ± 5	47 ± 4	<0.0025	7–21 days	Angiogram
Reduto[9]	20	46 ± 15	55 ± 10	0.002	10 days	RNV**
Cowley[11]	8	42 ± 5	52 ± 5	<0.01	23 days	Angiogram

EF = ejection fraction
*p value = difference between early and late study
**RNV = radionuclide ventriculogram

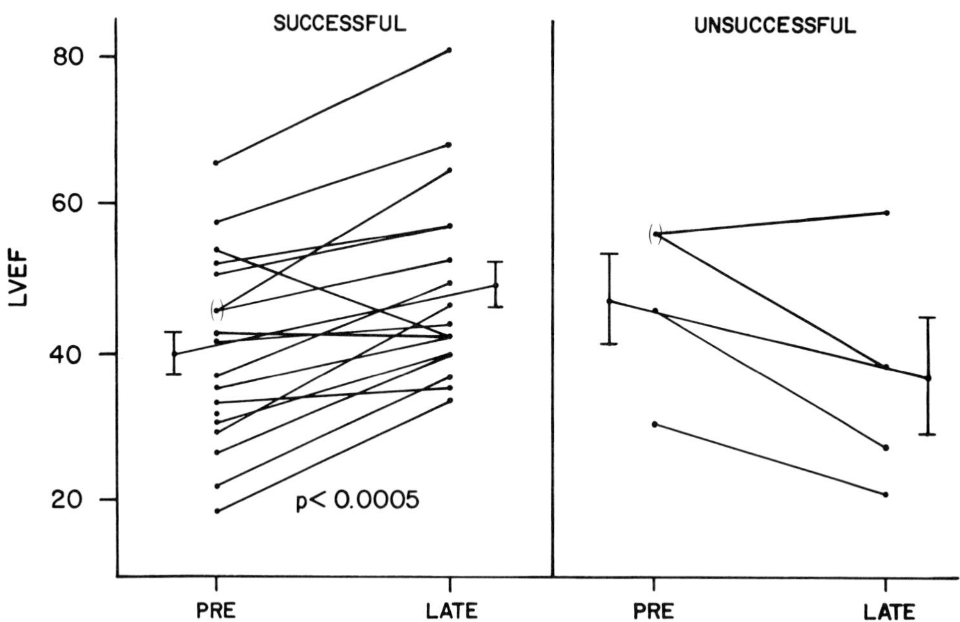

Figure 2. Left ventricular ejection fraction (LVEF) early (before streptokinase) and at late restudy (mean 18 days) in 24 patients treated with intracoronary thrombolysis. In patients with successful reperfusion (n = 20, 83%), LVEF increased from 40 ± 3% to 49 ± 3%, $p < 0.0005$. In patients with unsuccessful reperfusion (n = 4), LVEF decreased from 48 ± 6 to 38 ± 8 from early to late study.

of time following the onset of symptoms. Several studies suggest not only that early reperfusion (within 3 to 4 hours) is associated with myocardial salvage as judged by improved ejection fraction, but that reperfusion beyond 6 hours may also be associated with similar late improvement of left ventricular function, particularly if collateral vessels to the ischemic zone are present.[37,38] Evidence of myocardial salvage associated with successful thrombolysis has also been demonstrated in several studies using thallium-201 myocardial perfusion imaging.[38–41] Studies using both intravenous and intracoronary administration of thallium have demonstrated improvement in regional myocardial activity and reduction of perfusion defects in patients with successful reperfusion, in contrast to no change in defect size occurring in patients with unsuccessful reperfusion.[38,41] The importance of collaterals in salvage of myocardium is also supported by studies using thallium imaging. In the study by Schuler and colleagues[41] in which patients were reperfused within 4 hours of onset of symptoms, the greatest reduction in thallium defect size occurred in patients in whom residual coronary flow was present due either to subtotal occlusion at the start of treatment or to significant collateralization to the area supplied by the infarct vessel.

Information regarding the effects of reperfusion on hospital mortality is limited at this time. A multicenter West German study of 204 patients suggests mortality is favorably affected by successful thrombolysis.[42] Hospital mortality in successfully recanalized patients was 7 percent and cardiac mortality 5.4 percent. However, mortality in the unsuccessfully reperfused group was 24 percent, and six patients expired in the catheterization laboratory. Cardiac mortality in unsuccessfully recanalized patients who survived the procedure was 9.7 percent. In a recent preliminary report, Weinstein and colleagues analyzed outcome in a high-risk subgroup of patients with low ejection fraction enrolled in a multicenter registry for streptokinase.[43] Twenty-three patients with a baseline ejection fraction of less than 35 percent (mean 29 percent) who had successful thrombolysis were compared with 28 patients with similarly low ejection fractions (mean 24 percent) who were treated conventionally for evolving transmural infarction. Hospital mortality in the reperfused group was 4.3 percent compared with the control group mortality of 39 percent. Ejection fraction increased in 18 of 23 reperfused patients but decreased in 7 of 12 controls who survived and had restudy. Although these results are suggestive, improved survival following successful thrombolysis has not been clearly established.

Following reperfusion, significant residual stenosis is present in most patients. Rutsch and colleagues[13] have reported residual subtotal stenosis in 27 percent of patients, 75 to 90 percent stenosis in 49 percent of patients, 50 to 75 percent residual narrowing in 18 percent, and less than 50 percent residual stenosis in only 6 percent of patients following reperfusion. Reocclusion or reinfarction following thrombolysis has been reported to occur in 20 to 35 percent of patients,[10,42] usually early in the hospital course. Although reocclusion is usually associated with reinfarction, silent reocclusion in patients with well-developed collaterals has occurred in 5 to 10 percent of patients.[11,42] The presence of high-grade residual stenosis and insufficient anticoagulation appear to be important factors increasing the likelihood of reocclusion.[35,42] Recurrent ischemia following reperfusion is not uncommon, and early coronary artery bypass surgery or coronary angioplasty has been necessary in a significant percentage of patients due to an unstable course after thrombolysis.[35,44] These data indicate that intracoronary thrombolysis often does not represent definitive therapy, and additional intervention may be necessary to achieve lasting myocardial salvage. The usual indications for myocardial revascularization should apply after thrombolysis, with the decision based on the patient's hospital course, coronary anatomy, estimated extent of salvaged and jeopardized myocardium, and ventricular function. Early coronary bypass surgery after thrombolysis has been performed safely.[35,44]

SYSTEMIC THROMBOLYSIS

Intracoronary thrombolysis requires a major commitment of catheterization personnel and hospital resources and delays initiation of therapy. Intravenous infusion offers much wider potential application than intracoronary infusion because it does not require catheterization and could be used in most community hospitals. Several preliminary studies of short-course, high-dose intravenous streptokinase have employed angiography to determine reperfusion.[14,45–47] In a study by Schroder and colleagues[14] involving 19 patients who underwent catheterization within 3 hours of onset of infarction, systemic thrombolysis was attempted in 12 patients. Using a dosage of 500,000 units of streptokinase infused over 30 minutes, 5 of 12 patients (42 percent) with total occlusion achieved patency within 60 minutes. Two additional patients without patency at 60 minutes had patency demonstrated at restudy 24 hours later. In other preliminary reports of intravenous streptokinase, Neuhaus and colleagues[46] achieved reperfusion in 18 of 27 patients (67 percent) with an average dose of 1.5 million units of streptokinase infused over 60 minutes, and Huhmann and colleagues[47] achieved reperfusion of total occlusion in 6 of 15 patients (40 percent) within 2 to 4 hours after intravenous streptokinase in a dose of 500,000 units infused over 30 minutes. Reperfusion in these intravenous studies was associated with similar significant improvement in global and regional left ventricular ejection fraction as achieved with intracoronary infusion.[45,46] Although the response rate with intravenous thrombolysis appears to be lower than with intracoronary infusion, these encouraging preliminary results with intravenous infusion suggest that reperfusion may be achievable with this approach in a sufficiently high percentage of patients to make selective intracoronary infusion unnecessary in many patients.

PATIENT SELECTION

Patients considered for thrombolytic therapy should have clinical evidence of evolving acute transmural infarction as manifested by prolonged chest pain unrelieved with nitroglycerin and significant ST segment elevation with reciprocal depression. These criteria have proven highly specific as early markers of transmural infarction and correlate with a high incidence of thrombotic coronary occlusion at angiography. Patients presenting within the first few hours of symptom onset are the best candidates because the evolution of infarction is time-dependent and early reperfusion offers the greatest potential for substantial myocardial salvage. The time limit for completed infarction in patients is unclear and depends on a number of factors including the completeness of occlusion, presence and degree of collateral supply, and factors influencing myocardial oxygen demand. Although there appears to be considerable variability among individual patients and beneficial effects have been reported in patients treated beyond 8 to 12 hours after onset of symptoms, it is likely that the process of infarction is nearly complete within 4 to 6 hours in many patients. Patients should also have no contraindications to either thrombolytic therapy or anticoagulation because patients are maintained on long-term anticoagulation after reperfusion in order to minimize the likelihood of rethrombosis.

Contraindications to systemic thrombolytic therapy have recently been reviewed.[48] Absolute contraindications are active internal bleeding and an active intracranial process including recent cerebrovascular accident. Important relative contraindications include recent major surgery (within 10 days), recent puncture of noncompressible vessels, severe uncontrolled hypertension, recent trauma including cardiopulmonary resuscitation, recent gastrointestinal bleeding, significant anemia, and hematologic disorders associated with increased risk of bleeding. These contraindications should apply to both regional and systemic thrombolytic therapy because recent studies indicate that systemic fibrinolytic effects occur in a high percentage of patients treated with low-dose intracoronary streptokinase infusion.[11,49]

COMPLICATIONS

Bleeding is the most frequent complication associated with thrombolytic therapy. Although the majority of bleeding episodes have been minor and have occurred at catheterization or other puncture sites, significant blood loss requiring transfusion has occurred in 4 to 7 percent of patients.[12,13,42] Major gastrointestinal and cerebrovascular bleeding has occurred. In addition, use of streptokinase for early graft occlusion following coronary bypass surgery appears to be associated with a significant risk of mediastinal bleeding.[50] The frequency of bleeding complications appears to correlate with reduction of fibrinogen levels to less than 100 mg/100 ml and with total streptokinase dosage of more than 200,000 IU.[42] Although bleeding has been reported to occur more frequently when the percutaneous femoral approach is used, the incidence has been reduced when coagulation parameters are monitored and catheter removal is delayed if a systemic fibrinolytic state is present.

Arrhythmias have occurred frequently in association with reperfusion. The most common reperfusion arrhythmias are accelerated idioventricular rhythm and premature ventricular complexes.[35] These arrhythmias are usually transient and resolve spontaneously. Ventricular tachycardia and fibrillation have occurred infrequently and usually respond promptly to DC cardioversion. Occasionally, significant bradycardia and hypotension develop, particularly with inferior infarction, and temporary pacemaker placement may be required.[11,12,51] Allergic reactions to streptokinase have been rare.

SUMMARY

Thrombolytic therapy has emerged as a promising approach in the management of patients with acute myocardial infarction. Intracoronary infusion can achieve patency in a high percentage of patients with evolving transmural infarction, and recent preliminary evidence indicates that reperfusion may also be achieved in a substantial but lower percentage of patients with intravenous administration. The relative safety and the efficacy in restoring flow in selected patients seem established, and there is considerable evidence that successful thrombolysis with early reperfusion is associated with salvage of ischemic myocardium as determined by improvement in left ventricular function and by myocardial perfusion imaging. However, a number of important issues remain unresolved. The technique of intracoronary administration is not standardized, and optimal methodology is unknown. The most appropriate dosages for both regional and systemic infusion that will provide maximal reperfusion rates with minimal complications are undefined. Guidelines for patient selection need refinement as the time limits for beneficial effects are unclear, and current usage has been restricted to patients with transmural infarction. Improved survival following intervention has not been clearly established, and further evaluation of long-term effects is needed. Early reocclusion and reinfarction are not uncommon after thrombolysis and indicate that this approach does not represent definitive therapy in a significant percentage of patients and that additional intervention may be necessary to achieve permanent myocardial salvage. The sequence and timing of adjunctive therapy to prevent reocclusion have not been clearly determined. In addition, the relative efficacy of systemic and regional administration requires further evaluation. A number of prospective randomized controlled studies that are currently underway or planned address many of these unresolved issues and should more clearly define the role of thrombolytic therapy in the management of patients with acute myocardial infarction.

REFERENCES

1. Maroko, PR, Kjekshus, JK, Sobel, BE, et al: *Factors influencing infarct size following experimental coronary artery occlusions.* Circulation 43:67, 1971.
2. Rude, RE, Muller, JE, and Braunwald, E: *Efforts to limit the size of myocardial infarcts.* Ann Intern Med 95:736, 1981.
3. Berg, R Jr, Kendall, RW, DuVoisin, GE, et al: *Acute myocardial infarction—A surgical emergency.* J Thorac Cardiovasc Surg 70:432, 1975.
4. Rentrop, KP, Blanke, H, Karsch, KR, et al: *Initial experience with transluminal recanalization of the recently occluded infarct-related coronary artery in acute myocardial infarction—Comparison with conventionally treated patients.* Clin Cardiol 2:92, 1979.
5. Rentrop, KP, Blanke, H, Karsch, KR, et al, *Acute myocardial infarction: Intracoronary application of nitroglycerin and streptokinase.* Clin Cardiol 3:354, 1979.
6. Rentrop, P, Blanke, H, Karsch, KR, et al: *Selective intracoronary thrombolysis in acute myocardial infarction and unstable angina pectoris.* Circulation 63:307, 1981.
7. Ganz, W, Buchbinder, N, Marcus, H, et al: *Intracoronary thrombolysis in evolving myocardial infarction.* Am Heart J 101:4, 1981.
8. Mathey, DG, Kuck, KH, Tilsner, V, et al: *Nonsurgical coronary artery recanalization in acute transmural myocardial infarction.* Circulation 63:489, 1981.
9. Reduto, LA, Smalling, RW, Freund, GC, et al: *Intracoronary infusion of streptokinase in patients with acute myocardial infarction: Effects of reperfusion on left ventricular performance.* Am J Cardiol 48:403, 1981.
10. Gold, H, Leinbach, RC, Buckley, MJ, et al: *Intracoronary streptokinase in evolving infarction.* Hospital Practice 16:105, 1981.
11. Cowley, MJ, Hastillo, A, Vetrovec, GW, et al: *Effects of intracoronary streptokinase in acute myocardial infarction* Am Heart J 102:1149, 1981.
12. Lee, G, Amsterdam, EA, Low, R, et al: *Efficacy of percutaneous transluminal coronary recanalization utilizing streptokinase thrombolysis in patients with acute myocardial infarction.* Am Heart J 102:1159, 1981.
13. Rutsch, W, Schartl, M, Mathey, D, et al: *Percutaneous transluminal coronary recanalization: Procedure, results and acute complications.* Am Heart J 102:1178, 1981.
14. Schroder, R, Biamino, G, von Leitner, ER, et al: *Comparison of the effects of intracoronary and systemic streptokinase infusion in acute myocardial infarction: Preliminary results.* In Mason, DT and Collins, JJ Jr (eds): *Myocardial Revascularization: Medical and Surgical Advances in Coronary Disease.* Yorke Medical Books, New York, 1981.
15. Reimer, KA, Lowe, JE, Rasmussen, MM, et al: *The wavefront phenomenon of ischemic cell death. I. Myocardial infarct size versus duration of coronary occlusion in dogs.* Circulation 56:786, 1977.

16. Reimer, KA and Jennings, RB: *The wavefront phenomenon of myocardial ischemic cell death. II. Transmural progression of necrosis within the framework of ischemic bed size (myocardium at risk) and collateral flow.* Lab Invest 40:633, 1979.

17. Geary, GG, Smith, GT, and McNamara, J: *Quantitative effect of early coronary artery reperfusion in baboons—Extent of salvage of the perfusion bed of an occluded artery.* Circulation 66:391, 1982.

18. Willerson, JT and Buja, LM: *Cause and course of acute myocardial infarction.* Am J Med 69:903, 1980.

19. Chandler, AB, Chapman, I, Erhardt, LR, et al: *Coronary thrombosis in myocardial infarction. Report of a workshop on the role of coronary thrombosis in the pathogenesis of acute myocardial infarction.* Am J Cardiol 34:823, 1974.

20. DeWood, MA, Spores, J, Notske, R, et al: *Prevalence of total coronary occlusion during the early hours of transmural myocardial infarction.* N Engl J Med 303:897, 1980.

21. Boyles, PW, Meyer, WH, Graff, J, et al: *Comparative effectiveness of intravenous and intra-arterial fibrinolysin therapy.* Am J Cardiol 6:439, 1960.

22. Moschos, CB, Burke, WM, Lehan, PG, et al: *Thrombolytic agents and lysis of coronary artery thrombosis.* Cardiovasc Res 4:228, 1970.

23. Kordenat, R, Kezdi, P, and Powley, D: *Experimental intracoronary thrombosis and selective in situ lysis by catheter technique.* Am J Cardiol 30:640, 1972.

24. Ginks, WR, Sybers, HD, Maroko, PR, et al: *Coronary artery reperfusion: II. Reduction of myocardial infarct size at one week after coronary occlusion.* J Clin Invest 51:2717, 1972.

25. Costantini, C, Corday, E, Lang, TW, et al: *Revascularization after 3 hours of coronary arterial occlusion: Effects on regional cardiac metabolic function and infarct size.* Am J Cardiol 36:368, 1975.

26. Kloner, RA, Rude, RE, Carlson, N, et al: *Ultrastructural evidence of microvascular damage and myocardial cell injury after coronary artery occlusion: Which comes first?* Circulation 62:945, 1980.

27. Fishbein, MD, Y-Rit, J, Lando, U, et al: *The relationship of vascular injury and myocardial hemorrhage to necrosis after reperfusion.* Circulation 62:1274, 1980.

28. Moser, KM: *Thrombolysis with fibrinolysin (plasmin)—New therapeutic approach to thromboembolism.* JAMA 167:1997, 1958.

29. Fletcher, AP, Sherry, S, Alkjaersig, N, et al: *The maintenance of a sustained thrombolytic state in man. II. Clinical observations on patients with myocardial infarction and other thromboembolic disorders.* J Clin Invest 38:1111, 1959.

30. Duckert, F: *Thrombolytic therapy in myocardial infarction.* Prog Cardiovasc Dis 21:342, 1979.

31. Simon, TL, Ware, JH, and Stengle, JM: *Clinical trials of thrombolytic agents in myocardial infarction.* Ann Intern Med 79:712, 1973.

32. European Study Group for Streptokinase Therapy in Acute Myocardial Infarction: *Streptokinase in acute myocardial infarction.* N Engl J Med 301:797, 1979.

33. Alkjaersig, N, Fletcher, AP, and Sherry, S: *The mechanism of clot dissolution by plasmin.* J Clin Invest 38:1086, 1959.

34. Schwarz, F, Schuler, G, Katus, H, et al: *Intracoronary thrombolysis in acute myocardial infarction: Correlations among serum enzyme, scintigraphic and hemodynamic findings.* Am J Cardiol 50:32, 1982.

35. Cowley, MJ and Gold, HK: *Use of intracoronary streptokinase in acute myocardial infarction.* Mod Concepts Cardiovasc Dis 51:97, 1982.

36. Cowley, MJ: *Intracoronary streptokinase: Dosage and technology.* Vasc Med (in press).

37. Rentrop, P, Blanke, H, Karsch, KR, et al: *Changes in left ventricular function after intracoronary streptokinase infusion in clinically evolving myocardial infarction.* Am Heart J 102:1188, 1981.

38. Reduto, LA, Freund, CG, Gaeta, JM, et al: *Coronary artery reperfusion in acute myocardial infarction: Beneficial effects of intracoronary streptokinase on left ventricular salvage and performance.* Am Heart J 102:1168, 1981.

39. Maddahi, J, Ganz, W, Ninomiya, K, et al: *Myocardial salvage by intracoronary thrombolysis in evolving acute myocardial infarction: Evaluation using intracoronary injection of thallium-201.* Am Heart J 102:664. 1981.

40. Markis, JE, Malagold, M, Parker, JA, et al: *Myocardial salvage after intracoronary thrombolysis with streptokinase in acute myocardial infarction. Assessment by intracoronary thallium-201.* N Engl J Med 305:777, 1981.

41. Schuler, G, Schwarz, F, Hofmann, M, et al: *Thrombolysis in acute myocardial infarction using intracoronary streptokinase: Assessment by thallium-201 scintigraphy.* Circulation 66:658, 1982.

42. Merz, W, Dorr, R, Rentrop, P, et al: *Evaluation of the effectiveness of intracoronary streptokinase infusion in acute myocardial infarction: Post procedure management and hospital course in 204 patients.* Am Heart J 102:1181, 1981.

43. Weinstein, J, Sonnenblick, EH, Cowley, MJ, et al: *Improved left ventricular function and reduced hospital mortality following intracoronary thrombolysis in myocardial infarction with diminished ejection fraction.* Am J Cardiol 49:961, 1982.

44. Mathey, DG, Rodewald, G, Rentrop, P, et al: *Intracoronary streptokinase thrombolytic recanalization and subsequent surgical bypass of remaining atherosclerotic stenosis in acute myocardial infarction: Complementary combined approach effecting reduced infarct size, preventing reinfarction, and improving left ventricular function.* Am Heart J 102:1194, 1981.

45. Schroder, R, Biamino, G, and von Leitner, ER: *Intravenous short-time thrombolysis in acute myocardial infarction.* Circulation 64(Suppl IV):IV-10, 1981.

46. Neuhaus, KL, Tebbe, U, Sauer, G, et al: *Determinanten der Fruh-Rekanalisation durch intravenose Streptokinase (SK)—Infusion beim akuten Myokardinfarkt.* Z Kardiol 71:149, 1982.

47. Huhmann, W, Nieth, H, Muller, W, et al: *Vergleich IC und IV Streptokinase—Behandlung Beim Frischen Herzinfarkt.* Z Kardiol 71:148, 1982.

48. National Institutes of Health Consensus Development Conference: *Thrombolytic therapy in thrombosis.* Ann Intern Med 93:141, 1980.

49. Cowley, MJ, Hastillo, A, Vetrovec, GW, et al: *Fibrinolytic effects of low dose intracoronary streptokinase administration in acute myocardial infarction.* Circulation 64(Suppl IV):IV-10, 1981.

50. Rentrop, KP, Driesman, M, Blanke, H, et al: *Nonsurgical recanalization of early and late bypass occlusion.* Circulation 64(Suppl IV):IV-246, 1981.

51. van den Brand, M, Smissen, H vd, Serruys PW, et al: *Potential risks of intracoronary streptokinase during acute myocardial infarction.* Circulation 64(Suppl IV):IV-246, 1981.

Anticoagulation in Valvular Heart Disease Preoperatively and Postoperatively

Andrew G. Bodnar, M.D., and Adolph M. Hutter, Jr., M.D.

NATIVE HEART VALVES

Rheumatic Mitral Valve Disease

Systemic embolism has long been recognized as one of the most frequent and devastating complications of rheumatic mitral valve disease.[1] Retrospective reporting rates of a history of embolism in patients being evaluated for surgery for mitral stenosis range from 9.6 to 21 percent, with the majority of clinically recognized embolic events involving the central nervous system.[2,3] Autopsy studies, such as that of Mahapatra and coworkers,[4] indicate a high frequency of clinically unrecognized embolism in patients with rheumatic heart disease, suggesting that data derived from clinical reporting may underestimate the true frequency of systemic embolism.

Patients with rheumatic heart disease who suffer predominant mitral regurgitation bear a risk of embolism similar to that borne by patients whose predominant lesion is mitral stenosis.[5] There is no correlation between the clinical severity of the valvular disease and the risk of embolism.[1,2,5]

Although it is frequently stated that prior embolism, the size of the left atrium, and the presence of left atrial clot are important predisposing factors, only the presence of atrial fibrillation has consistently proven to be a reliable predictor of those patients at highest risk. In the large series of Coulshed and associates,[5] which included 839 patients with rheumatic mitral valve disease, 8 percent of those with predominant mitral stenosis and normal sinus rhythm had emboli compared with 31.5 percent of those whose rhythm was atrial fibrillation. Similarly, in the group who suffered primarily from mitral regurgitation, 2.7 percent of patients in sinus rhythm and 22 percent of those in atrial fibrillation had emboli.

The Benefits of Anticoagulation

Despite the clear relationship between rheumatic mitral valvular disease and systemic embolization, few studies have demonstrated rigorously the efficacy of anticoagulant therapy in reducing embolus-related mortality and morbidity. Drawing on one of the largest published series of patients with rheumatic heart disease, Szekely[6] reported two and one-half times fewer recurrences among a group of patients started on anticoagulants after an initial embolic episode. In the same series, among a subgroup of patients with atrial fibrillation and no prior embolism, 2 of 30 patients on anticoagulants had a total of two embolic episodes, compared with 29 of 98 patients not on anticoagulants who suffered 34 embolic episodes. In another large, uncontrolled series, Fleming and Bailey[7] reported a dramatic decrease in the incidence of embolization in patients with rheumatic mitral valve disease on anticoagulants when compared with historical control rates. On the basis of their findings, the authors concluded that all patients with more than trivial mitral valve disease should be considered candidates for long-term warfarin therapy, regardless of such variables as age, rhythm, or left atrial size. The authors of still another study of an uncontrolled retrospective series of patients with mitral stenosis and cerebral embolism concluded that oral anticoagulants begun immediately after the first embolus appear to decrease mortality during the ensuing 6 months, but they were unable to show longer-term benefits.[8] These findings led to the suggestion that anticoagulation might be discontinued at the end of 1 year.

Whereas the early studies of the efficacy of anticoagulation predominantly involved warfarin or its equivalent, recent attention has focused on a possible role for antiplatelet therapy. Platelet survival has been found to be shortened in some groups of patients with rheumatic heart disease, and evidence has been adduced to support the hypothesis that those patients with significantly shortened platelet survival may more frequently experience systemic embolization.[9] Treatment with sulfinpyrazone, a platelet inhibitor, enhances platelet survival in patients with abnormal heart valves and shortened platelet survival.[9,10] On the basis of these findings, Steele and Rainwater[11] conducted a prospective, double-blind study of the efficacy of sulfinpyrazone as compared with placebo in prolonging platelet survival and diminishing the incidence of embolization in a cohort of patients with rheumatic heart disease and shortened platelet survival. The study demonstrated an impressive decrease in the frequency of embolization accompanied by a significant increase in platelet life span in the treated group. Though many questions remain to be answered in this emerging area,[12] antiplatelet therapy is likely to become an important substitute for or addition to warfarin anticoagulation in appropriately selected patients.

The Risks of Anticoagulation

The available figures, inexact though they may be, regarding the benefits that may result from the administration of anticoagulants to patients with rheumatic heart disease or with the other abnormalities we will discuss must be balanced against the risk of treatment. Though reports abound in the literature, variations in definitions of complications, followup techniques, patient population, desired range of anticoagulation, methods of measurement of anticoagulant effect, and modes of statistical analysis make comparisons among studies difficult.

Forfar[13] followed 501 patients receiving anticoagulants for up to 7 years and found hemorrhagic complications sufficient to require medical advice and treatment in 8.2 percent and 4.3 percent per patient-treatment year. Nearly half of the bleeding episodes were considered potentially life-threatening; but in 96 percent of these events, the prothrombin time was beyond the desired range for the therapeutic ratio of between 1.8 and 2.6 to 1. Unlike several other series, this large study demonstrated no higher bleeding propensity with advancing age.

Although reports of higher rates of bleeding complications are common,[14,15] several factors are identifiable in the literature as likely to contribute to a lower rate of major problems. Careful followup in specialized clinics appears to result in complication rates of 4 percent or lower.[16,17] At least for some indications for anticoagulation, a reduction in the therapeutic ratio results in fewer complications at no appreciable cost in treatment failures. Thus, Hull and coworkers[18] found no increase in recurrence of deep venous thrombosis but did note a significant decrease in bleeding complications when the mean prothrombin time was decreased from 19.4 to 15 seconds. Similarly, Hughes and coworkers[19] documented a significant decrease in bleeding when the therapeutic aim was a ratio of between 1.4 and 1.6 to 1 as compared with a goal between 1.5 and 2.0 to 1. At least for a group of patients whose indication for anticoagulation was either a cerebrovascular accident or a transient ischemic attack, there was no difference between the two groups in the incidence of therapeutic failures. At the other end of the spectrum, even in those studies that report relatively high overall complication rates, a high proportion of severe problems has been encountered in patients whose prothrombin time was excessively prolonged.[13,14] Many studies cite advancing age as one of the risk factors for complications during long-term anticoagulation,[17,19–21] and though other series show no such predilection, patients over 65 years of age clearly deserve closer observation.

In summary, available information bears out the view that, whereas bleeding complications are an inevitable result of long-term anticoagulation, the risk of severe hemorrhage can be sharply limited by careful followup and assiduous attention to maintenance of the prothrombin time in the target range. In any event, the persistence of fatal or near-fatal complications in all series mandates careful consideration of appropriate indications for anticoagulation.

Recommendations

Though the statistics as to both the benefits of anticoagulation in rheumatic heart disease and the risks of long-term anticoagulation in general are less than ideal, some patterns seem so clear that it is unlikely we will ever see a rigorously conducted prospective study in this area. Accordingly, future practice will have to be based largely on the information already available.

Long-term anticoagulation with warfarin is indicated in patients with rheumatic mitral valve disease (either stenosis or regurgitation) of any severity in the presence of atrial fibrillation. Although advancing age may be a relevant consideration, there are no data that would make age an absolute contraindication in this highest-risk category. Even though the risk of embolization appears to be greatest in the year following onset of atrial fibrillation in patients with mitral valve disease,[6,22] we generally continue therapy indefinitely in this subgroup.

Both pharmacologic[23] and electrical[24,25] cardioversion from atrial fibrillation to sinus rhythm carry an appreciable risk of systemic embolization. The effectiveness of prior anticoagulation as a means of diminishing embolization at the time of cardioversion has not been conclusively demonstrated, but there are strong suggestions that such pretreatment is beneficial.[25] No information is available to determine the optimal period of anticoagulation prior to attempting cardioversion. On empirical grounds, however, when cardioversion is elective, we anticoagulate with warfarin for 2 to 3 weeks before attempting cardioversion.

A first embolus is a marker for high risk of recurrent embolization with high mortality and morbidity.[6,22] Therefore, we chronically administer anticoagulants to patients with rheumatic heart disease who have arterial emboli (except in the setting of infective endocarditis), without regard to severity of the valvular disease or the presence of rhythm disturbance.

Significant enlargement of the left atrial appendage has been cited as a risk factor for systemic embolization in patients with mitral valve disease,[26] but this finding has not been confirmed by other large-scale studies.[5,7] Accordingly, we do not routinely give anticoagulants to patients with valvular disease solely on the basis of an echocardiographic demonstration of left atrial enlargement. The coexistence of heart failure presents a more complex problem that is treated separately below.

Although these recommendations deal entirely with long-term warfarin therapy, recent work indicates that, at least for some patients with rheumatic heart disease and shortened platelet survival, platelet-active agents such as sulfinpyrazone may be of benefit.[9–11] Inasmuch as the risks of such therapy are likely to be smaller than those associated with warfarin treatment, those patients who are not at high enough risk of embolization to warrant the risks of warfarin may eventually be treated with platelet suppression. At present, however, assessment of platelet survival is not easily available, and further studies with large numbers of patients will be necessary before platelet suppression can be routinely recommended. Currently, we reserve antiplatelet agents as an alternative for patients for whom long-term anticoagulation with warfarin presents an unacceptable risk owing to poor compliance or a high risk for bleeding complications resulting from other conditions.

Other Problems in Nonoperative Valvular Disease

A number of special situations merit separate analysis regarding the advisability of anticoagulation.

Right Heart Failure

Unoperated valvular disease may lead to chronic elevation of right atrial pressure with or without left-sided abnormalities. Particularly in conjunction with forced inactivity, such right-sided heart failure may predispose to venous stasis, thrombosis, and pulmonary thromboembolism. Elderly patients in this group with right heart failure appear to be at increased risk for cerebral venous thrombosis.[27]

Though an early controlled study involving hospitalized patients showed a dramatic decrease in the incidence of thromboembolism with anticoagulation,[28] there have been no investigations of the risk-benefit ratio of such treatment on a chronic outpatient basis. After careful exclusion for the presence of risk factors for hemorrhage, we consider patients with severe right-sided heart failure candidates for chronic warfarin treatment. Inasmuch as recent information indicates that, at least for the prevention of deep venous thrombosis, a lower prothrombin ratio may result in fewer complications without increasing treatment failures,[18] consideration should be given to defining a lower prothrombin ratio as the goal in this group of patients.

Left Heart Failure

In their late stages, some unoperated valvular lesions, such as mitral or aortic regurgitation, may result in a dilated, myopathic left ventricle with severe global depression of left ventricular function and in left atrial hypertension. Studies of patients with other forms of dilated cardiomyopathy have demonstrated a consistently high frequency of systemic embolization and mural thrombus formation.[29–32] There have been, to our knowledge, no systematic studies evaluating the effect of anticoagulation on the embolization rate in any of the dilated cardiomyopathies, though embolization in the presence of adequate warfarin treatment is reported as rare in primary dilated cardiomyopathy.[33] As with right-sided heart failure, our practice is to screen patients carefully for contraindications to anticoagulation and to treat patients with left-sided heart failure with warfarin if there is no evident increased hemorrhagic risk.

Mitral Valve Prolapse

Mitral valve prolapse (MVP), a lesion that has come to be recognized as one of the most prevalent cardiac abnormalities, is regarded as having a generally benign prognosis.[34] Recently, however, Barnett and coworkers,[35] in followup of their earlier report,[36] have suggested an association between MVP and cerebral ischemic events, at least in younger patients. They found that, of 60 patients less than 45 years old with a history of transient ischemic attacks or partial strokes, 40 percent (24) had MVP as compared with 6.8 percent (5) of age-matched controls. In only 6 of the 24 patients was another potential cause for cerebral ischemia identified. There was no correlation between cerebral ischemia and MVP in patients older than 45 years. These findings are especially fascinating in view of previous reports of shortened platelet survival in a group of patients with MVP and a history of thromboembolism.[37]

Variations in echocardiographic techniques and criteria as well as the high prevalence of both MVP and cerebral ischemic events suggest the need for caution in interpreting these data. Certainly, no case has been established for routine prophylactic antiplatelet treatment of patients with MVP. Nevertheless, if the results of these studies are confirmed, young patients with MVP and otherwise unexplained episodes of cerebral ischemia will be candidates for assessment of platelet survival and treatment with platelet-suppressant agents, at least when platelet longevity is found to be impaired.

Calcified Mitral Annulus

Mitral annular calcification has been reported to be the most common cardiac abnormality in autopsy series of elderly persons who had had systolic murmurs,[38] and this disorder is especially common in patients with significant calcific aortic valvular stenosis.[39] In a series of 14 patients with "massive calcification of the mitral annulus," four were found at autopsy to have arterial emboli that were significant enough to be listed as the cause of death.[40] Other reports of series of patients with cerebral or retinal ischemic events[41] and of patients with roentgenographically demonstrated calcification of the mitral annulus[42] have confirmed the impression that arterial embolization is an important complication of this common syndrome. Though some of the emboli are calcific, many are not and may originate instead from platelet-fibrin depositions on the irregular, calcified annular surface.

There is no evidence to suggest that routine prophylaxis with either warfarin or antiplatelet agents is beneficial in this large group of predominantly elderly patients. Paroxysmal or chronic atrial fibrillation has been reported in as many as 29 percent of patients with calcified mitral annulus,[42] but the available literature does not reveal whether this subgroup is particularly susceptible to embolization. Nonetheless, in view of evidence that atrial fibrillation per se may predispose to arterial embolization,[43] patients with echocardiographically proven mitral annular calcification and atrial fibrillation should, in the absence of contraindications, be considered for treatment with warfarin or antiplatelet agents.

Calcific Aortic Valvular Stenosis

Calcification of the aortic valve has not been notably associated with clinically recognized systemic embolization. Autopsy reports, however, have demonstrated a surprisingly high incidence of calcific emboli.[44] Because of the content of the embolic material and the absence of clinical sequelae, we do not recommend prophylactic anticoagulant treatment in patients with calcific aortic stenosis.

AFTER VALVE SURGERY

Mitral Commissurotomy

Early reports of the long-term followup of patients who had undergone closed mitral commissurotomy indicated a persistently high rate of embolization, most notably in those patients whose rhythm was atrial fibrillation.[45] However, as experience accumulated with both valve reconstructive surgery[46] and open radical mitral commissurotomy,[47] the postoperative incidence of emboli has been significantly reduced.

We treat all patients with warfarin for 2 to 3 months following commissurotomy to allow time for tissue healing and stabilization of heart rhythm. We recommend chronic treatment with warfarin postoperatively in those with chronic atrial fibrillation, with left atrial thrombus found at surgery, or with a prior postoperative embolic episode.

Valve Replacement

The surgical literature may be most conveniently categorized according to valve type and location. Because of improvements in surgical technique, patient selection, and timing of surgery, the date of insertion has proven to be an important variable in assessment of thrombotic and embolic risks postoperatively. Though reporting of complications is highly variable, we will attempt a comparative review of the complication rates of the most commonly used prostheses in the aortic and mitral positions, and we will make recommendations as to appropriate use of anticoagulants in each group.

Mechanical Aortic Valve Prostheses

STARR-EDWARDS. The Starr-Edwards ball-valve prosthesis has undergone a series of design changes over the past two and a half decades aimed both at improved hemodynamics and decreased risk of thrombosis and embolization. Prior to 1966, the pre-1000 and 1000 series aortic prostheses were in use. Despite long-term anticoagulation in most patients, only 66 percent of patients with pre-1000 and 76 percent with 1000 series prostheses remained free of systemic emboli 5 years after implantation.[48]

The 1200 series introduced cloth covering for portions of the metal seat, and this modification appeared to result in a modest long-term decrease in embolic complications. That improved tehniques and careful patient selection also may have played a significant role is suggested by the series of Macmanus and associates, who found a 77 percent 5-year embolus-free rate for the 1200 series among patients who had their valves replaced between 1965 and 1972 compared with an 87 percent embolus-free rate at 5 years for patients who had prostheses of the same series implanted between 1973 and 1979.[49] The most recent long-term comparison between 1000 and 1200 series showed no statistically significant long-term difference in rates of embolization.[50]

The fully cloth-covered 2300 series, introduced in 1968, was designed to encourage endothelialization of the entire seat and sewing ring. Despite early hopes that the need for anticoagulation would be obviated by this modification, it became quickly apparent that the embolic rate without permanent anticoagulation following use of this prosthesis was unacceptably high.[51,52] To eliminate the problem of strut cloth wear, the Model 2400 composite strut ("track") valve was introduced in 1972, with a metal track on the inner aspect of each strut. In the absence of anticoagulation, these valves proved to have a dramatically high incidence of restenosis owing to pannus and thrombus formation in the inflow orifice.[53] However, anticoagulation appears effective in eliminating this complication.[54]

Because of the aforementioned risks of long-term anticoagulation with warfarin, a few prospective studies have attempted to ascertain the adequacy of treatment with only platelet-active agents, but they have concluded that aspirin alone[55] or aspirin in combination with dipyridamole[56] provided insufficient protection against systemic embolization, even with the cloth-covered series.

Anticoagulation with warfarin for the cloth-covered 2300 series has been demonstrated to lower significantly the incidence of embolic complications. Starr and coworkers[57] found that, at 5 years after valve replacement, 92 percent of their patients were free of embolic events, and other authors have cited similar or more impressive figures for anticoagulant-treated patients.[52,58]

Although the need for indefinite therapy with warfarin for patients with Starr-Edwards aortic prostheses can no longer be doubted, most major series, as noted above, confirm that thromboembolic complications are not completely eliminated even with assiduous long-term warfarin treatment. Reports that adequacy of anticoagulation may not correlate with embolic risk,[50] coupled with preliminary evidence that emboli from aortic prostheses may consist primarily of platelets,[59] raise the possibility that platelet inhibition may eventually play a particularly important role in patients with mechanical aortic prostheses. Steele and coworkers[60] found that significantly shortened platelet survival occurred after aortic valve replacement with any of the Starr-Edwards series. The most significant diminution in platelet survival was in patients with the 1000 series prosthesis and in those who had a history of thromboembolism. In the only completed prospective, randomized, double-blind comparison of warfarin and 400 mg/day of dipyridamole versus warfarin and placebo, Sullivan and associates[61] reported a statistically significant reduction of embolic events after 1-year followup from 14.3 percent for the placebo group to 1.3 percent for the patients taking dipyridamole, without a significant increase in the rate of bleeding complications.

Treatment with aspirin in addition to warfarin has been compared with treatment with warfarin alone in two prospective studies. Using 500 mg of aspirin/day, Altman and colleagues[62] were able to show a significant decrease at 2 years in the incidence of thromboembolic events in the aspirin-treated group, with no appreciable increase in bleeding complications. Dale and coworkers,[63] adding 1000 mg/day of aspirin to warfarin, also found a significant reduction in thromboembolic risk in patients with series 1200 and 2300 Starr-Edwards aortic prostheses. Unlike the results at lower doses of aspirin, however, this benefit was obtained at the cost of a significant increase in bleeding complications, with the difference being entirely attributable to an increase in gastrointestinal hemorrhage in the group of patients who received aspirin and warfarin together. A preliminary report of another large-scale prospective study indicated a trend toward diminished thromboembolic risk with the addition of dipyridamole to warfarin, without an increased risk of bleeding complications, but these investigators found an unacceptably high bleeding rate when aspirin was added to warfarin.[64]

Although some authorities now routinely treat their patients with mechanical prosthetic valves with a combination of warfarin and platelet-active agents,[65] we believe there is, as yet, insufficient information as to the long-term risks and benefits of such multi-agent therapy. Accordingly, we reserve the addition of a platelet-active agent for those patients who have evidence of embolization while receiving adequate anticoagulant therapy, and for patients with selected prostheses, such as the pre-1000 and 1000 series, that appear to be associated with the highest thromboembolic risk. The results of ongoing studies may warrant changes in these recommendations.

BJÖRK-SHILEY. The Björk-Shiley tilting-disk aortic prosthesis, designed to diminish the gradient across the prosthetic valve, has been in use since approximately 1969. With continuous warfarin anticoagulation, these valves have had an embolic rate somewhat lower than the Starr-Edwards prostheses as a whole and approximately equal to the rates reported for the cloth-covered Starr-Edwards series.[66–68] Attempts at limiting anticoagulant complications by treating with the combination of dipyridamole and aspirin instead of warfarin resulted, in one study, in thromboembolic episodes in 11 of 64 patients during a mean followup period of only 9 months.[69] In another series of patients with aortic, mitral, or combined valve replacements, treatment with dipyridamole alone resulted in a marked increase of thromboembolic complications, when compared with warfarin treatment, regardless of valve location, with 50 percent of the late deaths attributed to thromboembolism.[70]

In addition to systemic embolism, thrombotic partial obstruction or outright occlusion of the prosthesis itself is a major threat in patients with Björk-Shiley prostheses. Although this complication is more common with mitral prostheses, reported rates for aortic implants have ranged from 0.7 to 5 percent.[71,72] Even though the majority of the reports are of patients who were not given anticoagulants,[73] whose anticoagulation was not in the desired range,[71] or who were receiving only platelet-active agents,[74] it is, nevertheless, clear that thrombosis may occur even in the face of adequate anticoagulation with warfarin.[72]

Based on the aforementioned information, we recommend continuous anticoagulation with warfarin for all patients with Björk-Shiley aortic prostheses. In view of the potentially disastrous complication of thrombosis of the prosthesis, scrupulous attention to the adequacy of anticoagulation is of utmost importance. As with Starr-Edwards prostheses, we do not believe there is yet sufficient information to mandate addition of platelet-active medications in all cases, though patients who have suffered thromboembolic complications despite warfarin treatment certainly merit combination therapy.

OTHER MECHANICAL AORTIC VALVE PROSTHESES. The Lillehei-Kaster aortic pivoting disk prosthesis has a thromboembolic rate similar to that of the Björk-Shiley and Starr-Edwards cloth-covered prostheses in anticoagulant-treated patients, and there have been reports of thrombosis of the prosthesis.[68,75] Patients with this prosthesis who are not given anticoagulants suffer an unacceptably high rate of thromboembolic complications.[76] Though one reported series comparing aspirin with warfarin treatment found warfarin only slightly preferable, we recommend an approach identical with that for the Björk-Shiley prosthesis.

The St. Jude Medical mechanical bileaflet valve has been in use since the late 1970s in patients with a small aortic root. Early followup reports indicate a high risk of thromboembolic problems among patients who are not given anticoagulants, and there have been occasional cases of prosthetic thrombosis.[77] In the presence of adequate anticoagulation with warfarin, this valve appears to present among the lowest thromboembolic risks of the mechanical prostheses.[78-80] In the absence of information as to the efficacy of other regimens, full anticoagulation with warfarin is indicated.

The recently introduced Björk-Shiley convex prosthesis and the Hall-Kaster tilting-disk prosthesis may diminish the incidence of prosthetic thrombosis. Though data have not yet been published, embolic complications are expected to be about as frequent with these newer prostheses as with the older disk valves,[81] and continuous warfarin anticoagulation is recommended.

Mechanical Mitral Valve Prostheses

STARR-EDWARDS. The development of the Starr-Edwards mitral ball-valve prosthesis paralelled the changes in the aortic prosthesis. The earliest model, the 6000, featuring a cloth sewing ring with exposed metal inflow and outflow faces, was in general use between 1960 and 1965. Despite universal therapy with warfarin, the embolus-free rate 10 years after valve replacement is generally reported to be approximately 50 percent,[50] but in one series, as low as 19 percent.[82]

The introduction of cloth covering of the valve seat in the model 6120 resulted in little diminution in the thromboembolic rate, with Starr and coworkers reporting a 66 percent embolus-free rate at 5 years and 51 percent embolus-free rate at 10 years after valve replacement.[83] It is worth noting that, as was the case with aortic valve replacement, patients who had a non-cloth-covered mitral prosthesis implanted during the early years had a far higher thromboembolic rate than did patients undergoing mitral valve replacement with the same model prosthesis in later years.[49]

The Starr-Edwards 6300 series, with cloth covering for the entire seat and cage, provided a significant decrease in the risk of thromboembolism, with an 85 percent embolus-free rate at 6 years[83] and 70 percent at 10 years.[50] The model 6400, which is designed to diminish cloth wear by the addition of metal tracks on the inner aspects of the valve struts, is expected to have thromboembolic rates no higher than those of the 6300 series.

Factors that predispose to thromboembolism vary among reported series. Barnhorst and colleagues[84] found a large left atrium, the presence of left atrial thrombus at the time of surgery, and inadequacy of anticoagulation to be important predictors. Fuster and coworkers,[50] however, found no correlation with either heart size or left atrial thrombus at the time of operation, but agreed that inadequate anticoagulation was a risk factor. The presence of atrial fibrillation in a large percentage of patients in all of the mitral series undoubtedly represents an important explanation for the persistently high embolic rate.

Additional predisposing factors may include significantly diminished platelet survival after mitral valve replacement, with the shortest survivals in patients with emboli and in those who have received a series 6000, non-cloth-covered Starr-Edwards prosthesis.[85] Autopsy studies have raised the possibility that postoperative mural thrombosis of the left atrium may result from trauma during the operative procedure and may present a postoperative risk factor for systemic embolization.[86]

Despite the possibility that lower- and higher-risk subgroups of patients after ball-valve mitral valve replacement may be identifiable, we recommend treating all patients with warfarin indefinitely. As with aortic valve replacement, currently ongoing studies may demonstrate that addition of platelet-inhibiting agents to warfarin may yield additional benefits, but, in our opinion, that approach is not yet warranted on the basis of available data. We currently reserve addition of platelet-active agents for patients who have suffered systemic emboli despite adequate anticoagulation with warfarin.

BJÖRK-SHILEY. The thromboembolic rate of Björk-Shiley mitral prostheses in anticoagulant-treated patients is similar to rates reported for the Starr-Edwards cloth-covered 6300 series and still significantly higher than for Björk-Shiley aortic prostheses, with an incidence of embolism at 5 years after valve replacement of 19 percent.[87] The incidence of thrombosis of these prostheses is generally reported as approximately 4 percent.[72] The primary predisposing factor appears to be unreliability of anticoagulation. Faced with the incidence of thrombosis as high as 8 percent, some groups have stopped using this prosthesis in the mitral position unless adequate followup for anticoagulation is a certainty.[88] Because of the very significant risk of thrombosis, patients who have had this prosthesis implanted in the mitral position require the closest possible attention to their anticoagulant status, regardless of the presence of other predisposing features.

OTHER MECHANICAL MITRAL PROSTHESES. The Lillehei-Kaster tilting-disk mitral prosthesis has thromboembolic rates of the same order as the Björk-Shiley mitral valve.[89] Because of a significant incidence of tissue ingrowth, some centers have abandoned the use of this valve in the mitral position.[90] Certainly, patients who have had the valve implanted in the mitral position require careful followup of their warfarin anticoagulation as well as attention to the possibility of development of prosthetic obstruction by either thrombus or tissue ingrowth.

The St. Jude mechanical bileaflet prosthesis in the mitral position has been reported to have approximately five times the thromboembolic risk of the same valve in the aortic position. Nevertheless, with a thromboembolism-free rate of better than 95 percent at 3 years following valve replacement, this prosthesis appears to have perhaps the lowest thromboembolic rate of any of the mechanical mitral prostheses. All patients receiving this prosthesis are routinely given anticoagulant therapy with warfarin.

The Smeloff-Cutter ball valve with open cage has approximately the same thromboembolic rate as that generally reported for the non-cloth-covered Starr-Edwards 6100 series and requires continuous warfarin treatment.[91]

As in the case of their aortic counterparts, little information is as yet available about the recently introduced Björk-Shiley convex or the Hall-Kaster mitral prostheses. It is likely, however, that their major advantage over older models will be a diminished incidence of valve thrombosis, with no major change in embolization rate. In any case, both these and all other currently available mechanical prostheses in the mitral position continue to require indefinite warfarin anticoagulation.

Aortic Valve Bioprostheses

The continuing need for anticoagulation in all patients with mechanical aortic valve prostheses provided a major impetus for the introduction of glutaraldehyde-treated porcine bioprostheses in 1970. The results, in terms of reduction of thromboembolic risk, have been as dramatic as anticipated, in particular for aortic bioprostheses.

Cohn and coworkers,[92] reporting a 5- to 8-year followup of 43 patients who had had aortic valve replacements with Hancock porcine bioprostheses, found that only two had suffered embolic episodes despite the fact that nearly all did not receive anticoagulants. They projected an embolus-free rate at 8 years after surgery of 97 percent without routine warfarin treatment. These excellent results have been repeatedly confirmed in other series.[93,94]

The thromboembolic rate of the Carpentier-Edwards porcine aortic bioprosthesis has been at least as low as that reported for the Hancock valve. Geha and colleagues[95] reported that, at a mean followup period of more than 2 years, they had found no emboli in 134 patients who had had aortic valve replacement with the Carpentier-Edwards prosthesis, despite a policy of not anticoagulating routinely. Though other series report less perfect results, the embolic rate remains very low even without routine anticoagulation, with atrial fibrillation presenting the major risk factor.[96]

The less frequently used Ionescu-Shiley bovine pericardial bioprosthesis matches the porcine prostheses in limiting sharply the risk of thromboembolism when implanted in the aortic position. Becker and associates[97] reported a thromboembolism-free rate at 3 to 4 years of 94 percent with no anticoagulation.

Tissue degeneration and valve dysfunction have been increasingly recognized as important potential threats with the porcine bioprostheses, particularly in children and young adults.[98,99] There is, at present, no reliable evidence to support the hypothesis that anticoagulation delays or eliminates degeneration of these prostheses. Scanning electron microscopic examination of degenerated valves has been reported to demonstrate exposed collagen fibers with adhering activated platelets, providing at least a theoretical basis for the use by some groups of platelet-active agents in many patients who are not treated with warfarin following valve replacement with a porcine bioprosthesis.[98]

Our recommendation for patients who undergo aortic valve replacement with a bioprosthesis is warfarin for a period of 3 months to allow endothelialization. We then discontinue anticoagulation in all patients who are in sinus rhythm and who do not have residual marked depression of ventricular function. Although treatment with platelet suppressants appears to present a low risk, evidence for the efficacy of such intervention is lacking, and we do not routinely undertake it prophylactically.

Mitral Valve Bioprostheses

Mitral valve replacement with a bioprosthesis has been less successful than aortic valve replacement in limiting the thromboembolic risk despite early reports indicating an incidence of embolism of 1 to 2 percent at 2 years after surgery in the absence of anticoagulation.[100,101] When longer and more detailed followup became available, it became clear that there were subgroups of patients at particularly high risk for embolization. Hannah and Reis[102] reported an overall embolus-free rate at 5 years of 93 percent, but they found that all of the recognized embolic episodes had occurred in patients with low postoperative cardiac index. Edmiston and his group[103] found emboli in 5 of 22 anticoagulated patients followed for a mean period of only 16 months after Hancock mitral valve replacement. All of the patients who suffered emboli had atrial fibrillation as their predominant rhythm, and three of the five had had emboli before the valve replacement. Cohn and associates[92] projected an 8-year embolus-free rate of 82 percent for their series of patients with Hancock mitral bioprostheses, and they found that atrial fibrillation was the most important risk factor for embolism. A past history of emboli and the presence of left atrial throbus at the time of valve replacement are other factors that have been thought to increase the risk of embolism.[104]

In a series of 108 patients with Carpentier-Edwards and 17 with Hancock mitral prostheses, 34 patients in sinus rhythm were placed on antiplatelet agents and suffered no emboli at a mean followup of nearly 26 months.[95] Of 14 patients in sinus rhythm who were not on platelet-active agents, 2 had emboli. There were no emboli among 61 patients whose rhythm was atrial fibrillation but who were treated with warfarin, whereas 4 of 16 patients with atrial fibrillation who were on platelet-suppressant treatment had emboli.

Reports of results with the Ionescu-Shiley bovine pericardial mitral prosthesis are in conflict. Becker and coworkers[97] found a 3- to 4-year thromboembolism-free rate of only 71 percent. None of the patients suffering emboli was anticoagulated, and 80 percent were in atrial fibrillation. The much larger series of Ionescu and his group[105] had an 11-year embolus-free rate of 96.4 percent despite the fact that 75 percent of the patients were in atrial fibrillation and no patient received anticoagulants for longer than 6 weeks following surgery.

In addition to the disagreements in the literature about the frequency of thromboembolism after bioprosthetic mitral valve replacement, the efficacy of warfarin in diminishing the embolic rate has been questioned. A large-scale comparative study concluded that warfarin was not more effective at reducing the embolic rate than aspirin alone, while there were significantly fewer bleeding complications in the aspirin group.[106] Another recently reported retrospective analysis of 124 patients who had undergone isolated mitral valve replacement with a Hancock prosthesis found no difference in embolic rates between groups of patients treated with warfarin alone, warfarin and aspirin, aspirin alone, or neither agent. There was, however, a significantly increased bleeding risk among patients receiving warfarin therapy.[107] Because of the relatively small numbers of patients in each group and the retrospective nature of the study, the authors rightly conclude that further investigation is necessary before firm conclusions can be drawn from their work.

The risk of tissue degeneration and valve failure is at least as great with the mitral bioprostheses as with those in the aortic position. We know of no convincing evidence that warfarin treatment diminishes the rate of degeneration.

As is evident from this discussion, the analysis of the risks and benefits of anticoagulation is least straightforward in the group of patients with a bioprosthesis in the mitral position. Despite some evidence to the contrary, we believe the literature does generally indicate that the thromboembolic rate of those subgroups who are at highest risk is diminished by warfarin therapy. Careful followup in a specialized anticoagulation clinic should limit the risk of bleeding complications sufficiently to allow chronic anticoagulation therapy for patients most vulnerable to thromboembolic events. We, therefore, recommend indefinite warfarin treatment after bioprosthetic mitral valve replacement for patients who are in atrial fibrillation, have significantly impaired postoperative ventricular function, or remain in a low-output state. In addition, in the absence of strong contraindication, a history of preoperative arterial embolization or a finding of left atrial thrombus at the time of surgery, leads us to advise chronic warfarin treatment. When none of these risk factors is present, we discontinue warfarin 3 months after surgery. The decision to administer platelet-active agents to patients who are not treated with warfarin must be made on a case-by-case basis in the absence of scientific evidence of the value of treatment.

SPECIAL PROBLEMS OF PATIENTS ON ANTICOAGULANTS

The need for chronic warfarin anticoagulation, in addition to its general risks, presents difficulties in a number of special circumstances. We will briefly review the most commonly encountered problems and delineate our approach.

Infective Endocarditis

Patients with damaged native heart valves or prosthetic valves are at significantly increased risk for development of infective endocarditis. Infection with organisms such as fungi, slowly growing gram-negative bacilli, and nutritionally variant Streptococcus viridans produce large valvular vegetations and result in the highest frequency of embolic complications.[108] In a well-documented study, Pruitt and coworkers[109] reported clinically recognized embolic cerebral infarctions in 17 percent of their 218 patients with native valve endocarditis. Though the majority of embolic episodes occurred while blood cultures were still positive, one third of the strokes were recognized later, with one episode reported 2 years after completion of antibiotic treatment. Five patients with cerebral emboli had been on anticoagulants prior to the embolus and an additional two were given anticoagulants within the following 24 hours. Three of these seven patients on anticoagulants suffered major hemorrhage at the site of the embolic infarction. It is noteworthy that although 10 of the remaining 211 patients not receiving anticoagulants also developed intracranial hemorrhage, 23 percent of the hemorrhagic events occurred in the 3 percent of patients who received anticoagulants. In a smaller unpublished series, Karchmer and Dismukes[110] found central nervous system complications in 32 percent of 43 patients with prosthetic valve endocarditis. All but one of their patients had been given anticoagulants prior to the appearance of infection, and half of the patients on anticoagulants with neurologic complications were found to have intracerebral hemorrhage or hemorrhagic infarction. In addition to hemorrhage into the area of a recent embolic infarction, the possibility of bleeding from rupture of a mycotic aneurysm presents a substantial threat to anticoagulant-treated patients with infective endocarditis.[109,111]

The risk of hemorrhagic complications has led some authorities to favor routine discontinuation of anticoagulation upon recognition of infective endocarditis,[112] though others have suggested treatment may be carefully continued.[113] Hall and colleagues,[114] in a retrospective study of 52 patients with prosthetic valve endocarditis, found an increase in mortality and central nervous system complications among patients whose anticoagulation had been discontinued when compared with patients who were maintained on warfarin. Though the results of this investigation are of major importance, the limited numbers involved do not permit generalization with confidence.

Assuming the indication for initial anticoagulation was appropriate, we believe routine cessation of warfarin therapy for patients with either native or prosthetic valve infective endocarditis is not justified. When the infection is caused by a fungus or one of the other organisms particularly prone to formation of large vegetations or when such vegetations are actually documented by echocardiography, consideration should be given to suspension of anticoagulation in all but the highest-risk patients, such as those with non-cloth-covered ball valves or standard tilting-disk mitral prostheses. When an anticoagulant-treated patient with infective endocarditis suffers an apparent embolic event, we recommend discontinuing anticoagulation for an arbitrarily selected period of 72 hours in the hope of diminishing the risk of complicating a bland infarction with hemorrhage. Because of the absence of dependable data, these recommendations are intended to represent only flexible general guidelines that should be varied in accordance with the assessment of individual risks and benefits.

Pregnancy

The management of anticoagulation in young women who expect to become or are pregnant presents another difficult issue in the treatment of patients who have undergone valve replacement or who have native valvular disease that puts them at high risk for thromboembolic complications. With the advent of bioprostheses, it was hoped the need for continued anticoagulation would be eliminated for women of childbearing age. However, the apparently heightened likelihood of early tissue degeneration in young adults, noted above, has resulted in diminished enthusiasm for implanting bioprostheses in young women.

Warfarin freely crosses the placental barrier and has been implicated as the etiologic agent in a distinctive embryopathy when administered during the first trimester of pregnancy, a variety of fetal central nervous system abnormalities regardless of the trimester of exposure, and a high rate of fetal wastage.[114] Because heparin does not cross the placental barrier, a variety of combinations of heparin and warfarin have been proposed.[115] The most commonly recommended approach calls for discontinuation of warfarin during the first trimester, substituting subcutaneous heparin in doses of 7,000 to 10,000 units every 12 hours. Between 12 and 37 weeks of gestation, warfarin is resumed and at 37 weeks, subcutaneous heparin is once again substituted.[116] Although we believe these recommendations are appropriate, we note that at least one retrospective analysis of pregnancies in which heparin was the primary anticoagulant has failed to demonstrate significantly improved outcome for the fetus when compared with warfarin treatment, but the study did document greater maternal morbidity owing to hemorrhagic complications in the heparin-treated group.[114] Successful completion of pregnancy has been reported in patients with ball-valve prostheses treated with dipyridamole alone,[117] but this approach has been followed in too few patients to allow its recommendation as an alternative to warfarin and heparin. In view of the substantial risk to the fetus, and to a lesser extent to the mother, imposed by continuation of anticoagulation during pregnancy, careful and detailed counseling is an essential feature of the treatment of all women of childbearing age who must receive chronic anticoagulant therapy.

Subsequent Noncardiac Surgery

The necessity for changes in anticoagulation in patients with prosthetic heart valves who require other surgery will, in general, present major problems only in those patients at highest thromboembolic risk. Dental extractions can be done in the face of prothrombin times that are from 1½ to 2½ times control, with no major increase in postoperative hemorrhage.[118] We generally allow the prothrombin time to drift down to about 1½ times control on the day of the extraction. For more invasive procedures, prior to which anticoagulation must be completely stopped, discontinuing warfarin 2 to 3 days prior to surgery and reinstituting it 2 to 3 days following the operation are thought to be safe for most patients.[119] Patients at highest risk for thromboembolic complications, however, appear to benefit from continuation of anticoagulation to within 12 to 24 hours of their surgery.[120] In these patients, we generally switch to heparin therapy 2 to 3 days preoperatively, stop the heparin 8 to 12 hours before surgery, and restart it postoperatively as soon as possible from a surgical standpoint. This approach permits maximal anticoagulant protection with good hemostasis during surgery while avoiding the small but worrisome risk of hepatitis associated with the administration of fresh-frozen plasma for preoperative correction of a prolonged prothrombin time. Heparin is continued until the resumption of warfarin therapy has resulted in the return of the prothrombin ratio to the desired range.

SUMMARY

We have reviewed the risks and benefits of anticoagulation for cardiac valve disease before and after valve surgery. Though the absence of standardized reporting of complications and the paucity of well-designed comparative studies mandate careful consideration of the variables of individual cases, we have made the following general recommendations:

(1) Unoperated patients with rheumatic mital valvular disease and atrial fibrillation should be chronically treated with warfarin, regardless of the hemodynamic severity of their valvular lesion.

(2) The presence of right- or left-sided heart failure is an indication for warfarin treatment, in the absence of significant contraindications.

(3) There is emerging evidence that platelet-suppressant therapy may be of benefit in diminishing the thromboembolic risk of at least a subset of patients with rheumatic valvular disease and decreased platelet survival. Until platelet-survival studies are more readily available and larger-scale studies can be performed, however, we do not recommend routine treatment with platelet-active agents.

(4) We recommend chronic warfarin anticoagulation in all patients with mechanical prostheses in either the aortic or mitral position, regardless of cardiac rhythm or prosthesis model. We do not routinely add platelet-active agents except in the case of embolism despite adequate anticoagulation with warfarin.

(5) Patients with aortic bioprostheses generally do not require warfarin treatment for more than 3 months following valve replacement. The presence of atrial fibrillation and marked depression of postoperative ventricular function are indications for chronic anticoagulation.

(6) In the case of mitral bioprostheses, we recommend indefinite warfarin treatment for patients with atrial fibrillation, depressed ventricular function, or low cardiac output. We consider a preoperative history of embolism or an operative finding of left atrial thrombus to be an additional indication for anticoagulation, in the absence of significant contraindications.

(7) Patients on anticoagulant therapy should be followed closely—when possible in specialized anticoagulation clinics—to minimize the risks of treatment.

(8) Specific recommendations are made for management of anticoagulation during infective endocarditis, pregnancy, and noncardiac surgery.

REFERENCES

1. Wood, P: *An appreciation of mitral stenosis: Part I. Clinical features.* Br Med J 1:1054, 1954.
2. Casella, L, Abelman, WH, and Ellis, LB: *Patients with mitral stenosis and systemic emboli: Hemodynamic and clinical observations.* Arch Intern Med 114:773, 1964.
3. Selzer, A and Cohn, KE: *Natural history of mitral stenosis: A review.* Circulation 45:878, 1972.
4. Mahapatra, RH, Agarwal, JB, and Chopra, P: *Systemic thromboembolism in rheumatic heart disease.* Jpn Heart J 21:773, 1980.
5. Coulshed, N, Epstein, EJ, McKendrick, CS, et al: *Systemic embolism in mitral valve disease.* Br Heart J 32:26, 1970.
6. Szekely, P: *Systemic embolism and anticoagulant prophylaxis in rheumatic heart disease.* Br Med J 1:1209, 1964.
7. Fleming, HA and Bailey, SM: *Mitral valve disease, systemic embolism and anticoagulants.* Postgrad Med J 47:599, 1971.
8. Adams, GF, Merrett, JF, Hutchinson, WM, et al: *Cerebral embolism and mitral stenosis: Survival with and without anticoagulants.* J Neurol Neurosurg Psychol 37:378, 1974.
9. Steele, PP, Weily, HS, Davies, H, et al: *Platelet survival in patients with rheumatic heart disease.* N Engl J Med 290:537, 1974.
10. Ludlam, CA, Allan, N, Blandford, RB, et al: *Platelet and coagulation function in patients with abnormal cardiac valves treated with sulphinpyrazone.* Thromb Haemost 46:743, 1981.
11. Steele, P and Rainwater, J: *Favorable effect of sulfinpyrazone on thromboembolism in patients with rheumatic heart disease.* Circulation 62:462, 1980.
12. Goodnight, SH: *Editorial: Antiplatelet therapy for mitral stenosis?* Circulation 62:466, 1980.
13. Forfar, JC: *A 7-year analysis of haemorrhage in patients on long-term anticoagulant treatment.* Br Heart J 42:128, 1979.
14. Pollard, JW, Hamilton, HJ, Christensen, NA, et al: *Problems associated with long-term anticoagulant therapy.* Circulation 25:311, 1962.
15. Husted, S and Andreasen, F: *Problems encountered in long-term treatment with anticoagulants.* Acta Med Scand 200:379, 1976.
16. Davis, FB, Estruch, MT, Samson-Corvera, EB, et al: *Management of anticoagulation in outpatients.* Arch Intern Med 137:197, 1977.
17. Roos, J and Van Joost, HE: *The cause of bleeding during anticoagulant treatment.* Acta Med Scand 178:129, 1965.
18. Hull, R, Hirsh, J, Jay, R, et al: *Different intenstities of oral anticoagulant therapy in the treatment of proximal vein thrombosis.* N Engl J Med 307:1677, 1982.
19. Hughes, RA, Steinberg, EP, Barnett, GO, et al: *Analysis of 1315 courses of oral anticoagulant therapy.* (submitted for publication, 1983).
20. Coon, WW and Willis, PW: *Hemorrhagic complications of anticoagulant therapy.* Arch Intern Med 133:386, 1974.
21. Husted, S and Andreasen, F: *The influence of age on the response to anticoagulants.* Br J Clin Pharmacol 4:559, 1977.
22. Abernathy, WS and Willis, PW: *Thromboembolic complications of rheumatic heart disease.* Cardiovasc Clin 5(2):131, 1973.

23. Askey, JM: *Embolism and atrial fibrillation: The effect of restoration to normal heart rhythm with quinidine.* Am J Cardiol 9:491, 1962.

24. Turner, JR and Towers, JR: *Complications of cardioversion.* Lancet 2:612, 1965.

25. Bjerkelund, C and Orning, OM: *The efficacy of anticoagulant therapy in preventing embolism related to DC electrical cardioversion of atrial fibrillation.* Am J Cardiol 23:208, 1969.

26. Sommerville, W and Chambers, RJ: *Systemic embolism in mitral stenosis: Relation to the size of the left atrial appendix.* Br Med J 2:1167, 1964.

27. Towbin, A: *The syndrome of latent cerebral venous thrombosis: Its frequency and relation to age and congestive heart failure.* Stroke 4:419, 1973.

28. Griffith, GC, Strognell, R, Levinson, DC, et al: *A study of the beneficial effects of anticoagulant therapy in congestive heart failure.* Ann Intern Med 37:867, 1952.

29. Wexler, LF, Boucher, CA, Dinsmore, RE, et al: *Primary cardiomyopathy and cardiomyopathy syndrome due to coronary artery disease: A comparison of natural history.* Circulation 54(Suppl II):II-79, 1976.

30. Harvey, WP, Segal, JP, and Gurel, T: *The clinical spectrum of primary myocardial disease.* Prog Cardiovasc Dis 7:17, 1964.

31. Demakis, JG, Shahbudin, HR, Sutton, GC, et al: *Natural course of peripartum cardiomyopathy.* Circulation 44:1053, 1971.

32. Demakis, JG, Proskey, A, Rahimtoola, SH, et al: *The natural course of alcoholic cardiomyopathy.* Ann Intern Med 80:293, 1974.

33. Massumi, RA, Rios, JAC, Gooch, AS, et al: *Primary myocardial disease.* Circulation 31:19, 1965.

34. Devereux, RB, Perloff, JK, Reichek, N, et al: *Mitral valve prolapse.* Circulation 54:3, 1976.

35. Barnett, HJM, Boughner, DR, Taylor, DW, et al: *Further evidence relating mitral valve prolapse to cerebral ischemic events.* N Engl J Med 302:139, 1980.

36. Barnett, HJM, Jones, MW, Boughner, DR, et al: *Cerebral ischemic events associated with prolapsing mitral valve.* Arch Neurol 33:777, 1976.

37. Steele, P, Weily, H, Rainwater, J, et al : *Platelet survival time and thromboembolism in patients with mitral valve prolapse.* Circulation 60:43, 1979.

38. Pomerance, A: *Cardiac pathology and systolic murmurs in the elderly.* Br Heart J 30:687, 1968.

39. Roberts, WC, Perloff, JK, and Costantino, J: *Severe valvular aortic stenosis in patients over 65 years of age.* Am J Cardiol 37:497, 1971.

40. Korn, D, DeSanctis, RW, and Sell, S: *Massive calcification of the mitral annulus.* N Engl J Med 267:900, 1962.

41. de Bono, DP and Warlow, CP: *Mitral-annulus calcification and cerebral or retinal ischemia.* Lancet 2:383, 1979.

42. Fulkerson, PK, Beaver, BM, Auseon, JC, et al: *Calcification of the mitral annulus. Etiology, clinical associations, complications and therapy.* Am J Med 66:967, 1979.

43. Hinton, RC, Kistler, JP, Fallon, JT, et al: *Influence of etiology of atrial fibrillation on incidence of systemic embolism.* Am J Cardiol 40:509, 1977.

44. Holley, KE, Bahn, RC, McGoon, DC, et al: *Spontaneous calcific embolization associated with calcific aortic stenosis.* Circulation 27:197, 1963.

45. Kellogg, F, Liu, CK, Fishman, IW, et al: *Systemic and pulmonary emboli before and after mitral commissurotomy.* Circulation 24:263, 1961.

46. Carpentier, A, Chauvaud, S, Fabiani, JN, et al: *Reconstructive surgery of mitral valve incompetence: Ten-year appraisal.* J Thorac Cardiovasc Surg 79:338, 1980.

47. Laschinger, JC, Cunningham, JN, Baumann, FG, et al: *Early open radical commissurotomy: Surgical treatment of choice for mitral stenosis.* Ann Thorac Surg 34:287, 1982.

48. Barnhorst, DA, Oxman, HA, Conolly, DC, et al: *Isolated replacement of the aortic valve with the Starr-Edwards prosthesis: A 9 year review.* J Thorac Cardiovasc Surg 71:230, 1976.

49. MacManus, Q, Grunkemeier, GL, Lambert, LE, et al: *Year of operation as a risk factor in the late results of valve replacement.* J Thorac Cardiovasc Surg 80:843, 1980.

50. Fuster, V, Pumphrey, CW, McGown, MD, et al: *Systemic thromboembolism in mitral and aortic Starr-Edwards prostheses: A 10-19 year follow-up.* Circulation 66(Suppl I):I-157, 1982.

51. Larsen, GL, Alexander, JA, and Stanford, W: *Thromboembolic phenomena in patients with prosthetic aortic valves who did not receive anticoagulants.* Ann Thorac Surg 23:323, 1977.

52. Limet, R, Lepage, G, and Grondin, CM: *Thromboembolic complications with the cloth-covered Starr-Edwards aortic prosthesis in patients not receiving anticoagulants.* Ann Thorac Surg 23:529, 1977.

53. Stein, DW, Rahimtoola, SH, Kloster, FE, et al: *Thrombotic complications with nonanticoagulated, composite-strut aortic prostheses.* J Thorac Cardiovasc Surg 71:680, 1976.

54. Smithwick, W, Kouchoukos, NT, Karp, RB, et al: *Late stenosis of Starr-Edwards cloth-covered prostheses.* Ann Thorac Surg 20:249, 1975.

55. Dale, J and Myhre, E: *Can acetylsalicylic acid alone prevent arterial thromboembolism? A pilot study in patients with aortic ball valve prostheses.* Acta Med Scand (Suppl) 645:73, 1981.

56. Brott, WH, Zajtchuk, R, Bowen, TE, et al: *Dipyridamole–aspirin as thromboembolic prophylaxis in patients with aortic valve prosthesis. A prospective study with the Model 2320 Starr-Edwards prosthesis.* J Thorac Cardiovasc Surg 81:632, 1981.

57. Starr, A, Grunkemeier, GL, Lambert, LE, et al: *Aortic valve replacement: A ten-year follow-up of non-cloth-covered vs cloth-covered caged-ball prostheses.* Circulation 56(Suppl II):II-133, 1977.

58. Isom, OW, Williams, CD, Falk, EA, et al: *Evaluation of anticoagulant therapy in cloth-covered prosthetic valves.* Circulation 48(Suppl III):III-48, 1973.

59. Fuster, V and Chesebro, JH: *I. Current concepts of thrombogenesis: Role of platelets.* Mayo Clin Proc 56:102, 1981.

60. Steele, P, Weily, H, Davies, H, et al: *Platelet survival time following aortic valve replacement.* Circulation 51:358, 1975.

61. Sullivan, JM, Harken, DE, and Gorlin, R: *Pharmacologic control of thromboembolic complications of cardiac valve replacement.* N Engl J Med 284:1391, 1971.

62. Altman, R, Boullon, F, Rouvier J, et al: *Aspirin and prophylaxis of thromboembolic complications in patients with substitue heart valves.* J Thorac Cardiovasc Surg 72:127, 1976.

63. Dale, J, Myhre, E, and Loew, D: *Bleeding during acetylsalicylic acid and anticoagulant therapy in patients with reduced platelet activity after aortic valve replacement.* Am Heart J 99:746, 1980.

64. Chesebro, JH, Fuster, V, Pumphrey, CW, et al: *Combined warfarin-platelet inhibitor antithrombotic therapy in prosthetic heart valve replacement.* Circulation 64(Suppl IV):IV-76, 1981.

65. Fuster, V and Chesebro, JH: *III. Management of arterial thromboembolic and atherosclerotic disease.* Mayo Clin Proc 56:265, 1981.

66. Björk, VO and Henze, A: *Results five to seven years after aortic valve replacement with the original Delrin disc model Björk-Shiley prosthesis.* Scand J Thorac Cardiovasc Surg 11:177, 1977.

67. Cheung, D, Flemma, RJ, Mullen, DC, et al: *Ten-year follow-up in aortic valve replacement using the Björk-Shiley prosthesis.* Ann Thorac Surg 32:138, 1981.

68. Dale, J: *Arterial thromboembolic complications in patients with Björk-Shiley and Lillehei-Kaster aortic disc valve prostheses.* Am Heart J 93:715, 1977.

69. Björk, VO and Henze, A: *Management of thrombo-embolism after aortic valve replacement with the Björk-Shiley tilting disc valve. Medicamental prevention with dicumarol in comparison with dipyridamole-acetylsalicylic acid. Surgical treatment of prosthetic thrombosis.* Scand J Thorac Cardiovasc Surg 9:183, 1975.

70. Sutton, MG, Miller, GA, Oldershaw, PJ, et al: *Anticoagulants and the Björk-Shiley prosthesis. Experience of 390 patients.* Br Heart J 40:558, 1978.

71. Martinell, J, Salas, J, de Vega, NG, et al: *Thrombotic obstruction of the Björk-Shiley aortic valve prosthesis. Report of four cases.* Scand J Thorac Cardiovasc Surg 13:255, 1979.

72. Wright, JO, Hiratzka, LF, Brandt, B, et al: *Thrombosis of the Björk-Shiley prosthesis: Illustrative cases and review of the literature.* J Thorac Cardiovasc Surg 84:138, 1982.

73. de la Rocha, AG, Plume, SK, and Baird, RJ: *Thrombosis of Björk-Shiley aortic prosthesis: Report of three cases.* Canad Med Assoc J 116:1158, 1977.

74. Moreno-Cabral, RJ, McNamara, JJ, Mamiya, RT, et al: *Acute thrombotic obstruction with Björk-Shiley valves: Diagnostic and surgical considerations.* J Thorac Cardiovasc Surg 75:321, 1978.

75. Thevenet, A: *Lillehei-Kaster prosthesis in the aortic position with and without anticoagulants.* J Cardiovasc Surg (Torino) 21:669, 1980.

76. Thomsen, PB and Alstrup, P: *Thromboembolism in patients without anticoagulants after aortic valve replacement with the Lillehei-Kaster disc valve.* Thorac Cardiovasc Surg 27:313, 1979.

77. Moulton, AL, Singleton, RT, Oster, WF, et al: *Fatal thrombosis of an aortic St. Jude Medical valve despite "adequate" anticoagulation: Anatomic and technical considerations.* J Thorac Cardiovasc Surg 83:472, 1982.

78. Hunt, D, Sloman, G, and Sutton, L: *The St. Jude Medical valve—the Australian experience.* Med J Aust 2:276, 1981.

79. NICOLOFF, DM, EMERY, RW, AROM, KV, ET AL: *Clinical and hemodynamic results with the St. Jude Medical cardiac valve prosthesis. A three year experience.* J Thorac Cardiovasc Surg 82:674, 1981.

80. GILL, CC, KING, HC, LYTLE, BW, ET AL: *Early clinical evaluation after aortic valve replacement with the St. Jude Medical valve in patients with a small aortic root.* Circulation 66(Suppl I):I-147, 1982.

81. EDMUNDS, LH: *Thromboembolic complications of current cardiac valvular prostheses.* Ann Thorac Surg 34:96, 1982.

82. MACMANUS, Q, GRUNKEMEIER, G, THOMAS, D, ET AL: *The Starr-Edwards Model 6000 valve: A fifteen year follow-up of the first successful mitral prosthesis.* Circulation 56:623, 1977.

83. STARR, A, GRUNKEMEIER, G, LAMBERT, L, ET AL: *Mitral valve replacement: A 10-year follow-up of non-cloth-covered vs cloth covered caged-ball prostheses.* Circulation 54(Suppl III):III-47, 1976.

84. BARHNORST, DA, OXMAN, HA, CONOLLY, DC, ET AL: *Long-term follow-up of isolated replacement of the aortic or mitral valve with the Starr-Edwards prosthesis.* Am J Cardiol 35:228, 1975.

85. WEILY, HS, STEELE, PP, DAVIES, H, ET AL: *Platelet survival in patients with substitute heart valves.* N Engl J Med 290:534, 1974.

86. SHACHAR, GB, VLODAVER, Z, JOYCE, LD, ET AL: *Mural thrombosis of the left atrium following replacement of the mitral valve.* J Thorac Cardiovasc Surg 82:595, 1981.

87. BJÖRK, VO AND HENZE, A: *Ten years' experience with the Björk-Shiley tilting disc valve.* J Thorac Cardiovasc Surg 78:331, 1979.

88. COPANS, H, LAKIER, JB, KINSLEY, RH, ET AL: *Thrombosed Björk-Shiley mitral prostheses.* Circulation 61:169, 1980.

89. ZWART, HHJ, HICKS, G, SCHUSTER, B, ET AL: *Clinical experience with the Lillehei-Kaster valve prosthesis.* Ann Thorac Surg 28:158, 1979.

90. MARVASTI, MA, MARKOWITZ, RH, EICH, FB, ET AL: *Late results of Lillehei-Kaster valve.* Circulation 62(Suppl III):III-238, 1980.

91. OXMAN, HA, CONOLLY, DC, AND ELLIS, FM: *Mitral valve replacement with the Smeloff-Cutter prosthesis.* J Thorac Cardiovasc Surg 69:247, 1975.

92. COHN, LH, MUDGE, GH, PRATTER, F, ET AL: *Five to eight year follow-up of patients undergoing porcine heart valve replacements.* N Engl J Med 304:259, 1981.

93. GALLO, JI, RUIZ, B, CARRION, MF, ET AL: *Heart valve replacement with the Hancock bioprosthesis: A 6-year review.* Ann Thorac Surg 31:444, 1981.

94. OYER, PE, STINSON, EB, REITZ, BA, ET AL: *Long-term evaluation of porcine xenograft bioprostheses.* J Thorac Cardiovasc Surg 78:343, 1979.

95. GEHA, AS, HOLTER, AR, LANGOU, RA, ET AL: *Dysfunction and thromboembolism associated with cardiac valve xenografts in adults.* Circulation 64(Suppl II):II-172, 1981.

96. JAMIESON, WR, JANUSZ, MT, MIYAGISHIMA, RT, ET AL: *Embolic complications of porcine heterograft valves.* J Thorac Cardiovasc Surg 81:626, 1981.

97. BECKER, RM, SANDOR, L, TINDEL, M, ET AL: *Medium-term follow-up of the Ionescu-Shiley heterograft valve.* Ann Thorac Surg 32:120, 1981.

98. GEHA, AS, HAMMOND, GL, LAKS, H, ET AL: *Factors affecting performance and thromboembolism after porcine xenograft cardiac valve replacement.* J Thorac Cardiovasc Surg 83:377, 1982.

99. PLATT, MR, MILLS, LJ, ESTRERA, AS, ET AL: *Marked thrombosis and calcification of porcine heterograft valves.* Circulation 62:862, 1980.

100. STINSON, EB, GRIEPP, RB, AND SHUMWAY, NE: *Clinical experience with a porcine aortic valve xenograft for mitral valve replacement.* Ann Thorac Surg 18:391, 1974.

101. MCINTOSH, CL, MICHAELIS, LL, MORROW, AG, ET AL: *Atrioventricular valve replacement with the Hancock porcine xenograft: A five year clinical experience.* Surgery 78:768, 1975.

102. HANNAH, H AND REIS, RL: *Current status of porcine heterograft prostheses: A five year appraisal.* Circulation 54(Suppl III):III-27, 1975.

103. EDMISTON, WA, HARRISON, EC, DUICK, GF, ET AL: *Thromboembolism in mitral porcine valve recipients.* Am J Cardiol 41:508, 1978.

104. HETZER, R, HILL, JD, KERTH, WJ, ET AL: *Thromboembolic complications after mitral valve replacement with Hancock xenograft.* J Thorac Cardiovasc Surg 75:651, 1978.

105. IONESCU, MI, SMITH, DR, HASAN, SS, ET AL: *Clinical durability of the pericardial xenograft valve: Ten years' experience with mitral valve replacement.* Ann Thorac Surg 34:265, 1982.

106. NUNEZ, L, AGUADO, MG, CELEMIN, D, ET AL: *Aspirin or coumadin as the drug of choice for valve replacement with porcine bioprosthesis.* Ann Thorac Surg 33:354, 1982.

107. Hill, JD, LaFollette, L, Szarnicki, RJ, et al: *Risk-benefit analysis of warfarin therapy in Hancock mitral valve replacement.* J Thorac Cardiovasc Surg 83:718, 1982.

108. Wilson, WR, Giuliani, ER, Danielson, GK, et al: *Management of complications of infective endocarditis.* Mayo Clin Proc 57:162, 1982.

109. Pruitt, AA, Rubin, RH, Karchmer, AW, et al: *Neurologic complications of bacterial endocarditis.* Medicine 57:329, 1978.

110. Karchmer, AW and Dismukes, W: Unpublished data.

111. Lieberman, A, Hass, WK, Pinto, R, et al: *Intracranial hemorrhage and infarction in anticoagulated patients with prosthetic heart valves.* Stroke 9:18, 1978.

112. Kanis, JA: *The use of anticoagulants in bacterial endocarditis.* Postgrad Med J 50:312, 1974.

113. Lerner, PI and Weinstein, L: *Infective endocarditis in the antibiotic era.* N Engl J Med 274:323, 388, 1976.

114. Hall, JG, Pauli, RM, and Wilson, KM: *Maternal and fetal sequelae of anticoagulation during pregnancy.* Am J Med 68:122, 1980.

115. Tejani, N: *Anticoagulant therapy with cardiac valve prosthesis during pregnancy.* Obstet Gynecol 42:785, 1973.

116. Editorial: *Anticoagulants and heart valve replacement in pregnancy.* Br Med J 1:1047, 1977.

117. Biale, Y, Cantor, A, Lewenthal, H, et al: *The course of pregnancy in patients with artificial heart valves treated with dipyridamole.* Int J Gynaecol Obstet 18:128, 1980.

118. McIntyre, H: *Management during dental surgery of patients on anticoagulants.* Lancet 2:99, 1966.

119. Tinker, JH and Tarhan, S: *Discontinuing anticoagulant therapy in surgical patients with cardiac valve prostheses. Observations in 180 operations.* JAMA 239:738, 1978.

120. Katholi, RE, Nolan, SP, and McGuire, LB: *The management of anticoagulation during noncardiac operations in patients with prosthetic heart valves.* Am Heart J 96:163, 1978.

Drug Therapy for Hyperlipidemia

Frank A. Franklin, Jr., M.D., Ph.D.,
and Simeon Margolis, M.D., Ph.D.

The purpose of this chapter is to provide physicians and surgeons interested in cardiovascular disorders with a practical approach to the use of drugs in the treatment of adult patients with hyperlipidemia. Drug therapy cannot be approached reasonably without first considering the rationale for treatment, diagnosis, and dietary management, the first step in the treatment of hyperlipidemia. More extensive recent reviews of the structure and metabolism of lipoproteins,[1–3] genetics of hyperlipidemia,[3–6] and the diagnosis and treatment[3,7,8] of hyperlipidemia are available.

Hyperlipidemia is defined as an elevation in the concentration of cholesterol and/or triglycerides in the plasma of individuals after a 12-hour fast. These lipids are transported in association with apoproteins in macromolecular complexes called lipoproteins. Characterizing the hyperlipidemias by determining which lipoprotein(s) carries the excess lipid is useful in understanding the pathogenesis and treatment of these disorders (see below). After an overnight fast, the plasma lipids are carried normally on three classes of lipoproteins that differ in density and composition (Table 1). The very low-density lipoproteins (VLDL) are rich in triglycerides (about 50 percent by weight) and transport triglycerides from liver to peripheral tissues. Cholesterol and cholesterol esters comprise approximately 50 percent of the weight of low-density lipoproteins (LDL). LDL are formed in the plasma after the removal of most of the triglyceride from VLDL by the enzyme lipoprotein lipase. The major apoprotein of both of these lipoproteins is apoprotein B. A separate family of lipoproteins is the high-density lipoproteins (HDL), which are rich in protein (about 50 percent by weight), particularly apoprotein A-1. Following a fat-containing meal, absorbed triglycerides are transported from the intestine by a fourth type of lipoprotein, chylomicrons (CM). The degradation of these chylomicrons occurs in two phases. Initially, the triglycerides are hydrolyzed, as with VLDL, by lipoprotein lipase. This produces a cholesterol-enriched chylomicron remnant with the density of VLDL but with beta migration on electrophoresis (β-VLDL). The chylomicron remnant acquires apoprotein E, which serves as the signal for the rapid uptake of the lipoprotein by the liver.[9] Because they are rapidly cleared from the blood stream, chylomicrons and their remnants are never present in the fasting plasma of normal subjects.

Elevations in cholesterol and/or triglycerides can be related to increased concentrations of the various lipoproteins based on their composition (see Table 1). It is evident that hypertriglyceridemia can result from an increased concentration of VLDL or chymicrons or both. Inasmuch as each of these lipoproteins also carries some cholesterol, a severe elevation in plasma triglycerides is often associated with some increase in cholesterol levels. Hypercholesterolemia with normal or modestly elevated triglycerides is usually caused by increased levels of LDL. Occasionally, an isolated increase in cholesterol results from high levels of HDL.

Table 1. Plasma lipoproteins

Lipoprotein	*Abbreviation*	*Electrophoretic Migration*	*Major Components*		*Major Apoproteins*
Chylomicron	CM	Origin	Triglycerides	(90%)	Apo B, apo C
Chylomicron remnant	β-VLDL	Beta	Triglycerides	(35%)	Apo B, apo E
			Cholesterol	(35%)	
Very low-density	VLDL	Prebeta	Triglycerides	(60%)	Apo B, apo C
Low-density	LDL	Beta	Cholesterol	(50%)	Apo B
High-density	HDL	Alpha	Protein	(50%)	Apo A

Significant elevations of both cholesterol and triglycerides may be produced by an increase in both VLDL and LDL or an isolated increase in β-VLDL.

RATIONALE FOR TREATMENT

The major aims in the treatment of hyperlipidemia are the prevention of premature atherosclerosis and acute pancreatitis. Because our focus in this chapter is on the prevention of atherosclerosis and its cardiovascular manifestations, we will only briefly mention the prevention of pancreatitis. Severe hypertriglyceridemia, usually greater than 2000 mg/dl, can provoke attacks of acute pancreatitis, and control of severe hypertriglyceridemia does prevent such attacks.[10]

LDL is considered an atherogenic lipoprotein[11] because epidemiologic studies clearly demonstrate that increased levels of LDL are associated with an enhanced risk of premature coronary artery disease (CAD). Epidemiologic data also show that levels of HDL are inversely related to the incidence of CAD; HDL is therefore viewed as antiatherogenic.[12] The atherogenic potential is often assessed by the ratio of LDL (or total cholesterol) to HDL. Presently, there is no evidence that high levels of tryglycerides, on either VLDL or chylomicrons, pose an independent risk for premature CAD.[13] However, hypertriglyceridemia may serve as a risk factor indirectly because high levels of VLDL or chylomicrons are almost invariably associated with low values of HDL.[13] In contrast to the lack of direct risk from increased levels of normal VLDL, β-VLDL is a potent atherogenic lipoprotein.[9]

There is still no conclusive proof that lowering the concentrations of the atherogenic lipoproteins, LDL and β-VLDL, or raising levels of the protective HDL will delay or prevent the development of premature vascular disease. Results will be available in 1984 from a major clinical trial of the effectiveness of lowering LDL by drug therapy in preventing myocardial infarction.[14] Meanwhile, the high rates and serious consequences of vascular disease, the strong data from epidemiologic studies, and the findings in many animal experiments all justify our efforts to control elevated levels of the atherogenic lipoproteins. Our therapeutic goals are to lower plasma LDL and β-VLDL, using measures that raise or maintain HDL levels.

DIAGNOSIS OF HYPERLIPIDEMIA

Early identification and treatment of patients with elevated LDL levels are essential. Severe primary hypercholesterolemia is often expressed during childhood. For these reasons, it is advisable to perform at least one screening lipid examination in all children or young adults. However, abnormalities of plasma triglycerides may not develop until later, after sexual maturation or excess weight gain.

A screening lipid examination is indicated particularly in patients with a family history of either hyperlipidemia or premature vascular disease; in individuals with major risk factors such as hypertension, cigarette smoking, diabetes mellitus, or extreme obesity; and in those

Table 2. Cutoff points for cholesterol and triglycerides in fasting white subjects

	Age (yr)	Cholesterol (mg/dl)			Triglycerides (mg/dl)*
		Total*	LDL*	HDL†	
Males					
	10–14	202	132	37	125
	15–19	197	130	30	148
	20–24	218	147	30	201
	25–29	244	165	31	249
	30–34	254	185	28	266
	35–39	270	189	29	321
	40–44	268	186	27	320
	45–49	276	202	30	327
	50–54	277	197	28	320
	55–59	276	203	28	286
	60–64	276	210	30	291
Females					
	10–14	201	136	37	131
	15–19	200	135	35	124
	20–24	216	136	37	131
	25–29	222	151	37	145
	30–34	231	150	38	151
	35–39	242	172	34	176
	40–44	252	174	33	191
	45–49	265	187	33	214
	50–54	285	215	37	233
	55–59	300	213	36	262
	60–64	297	234	36	239

*95th percentile.
†5th percentile.

settings known to produce secondary hyperlipidemia. Lipid screening is also worthwhile when patients first develop clinical manifestations of atherosclerotic vascular disease. The patient should not be screened until 3 months after a myocardial infarction, which may lower cholesterol levels transiently.[15] Inasmuch as many primary hyperlipidemias are familial (genetic and environmental), all household members and first-degree relatives of affected individuals should also be screened.

The screening lipid examination should be done after a 12-hour fast and include determinations of plasma total cholesterol, triglycerides, and HDL-cholesterol. The results should be compared with values obtained from population studies for subjects of the same age and sex. Many laboratories still base their upper limit of normal for total cholesterol on some rather arbitrary value (such as 250 mg/dl) or use outdated normal ranges derived from a small group of subjects.[16] Up-to-date diagnostic decisions require the utilization of data (shown in Table 2) obtained in a more recent large population study.[17] These values were determined on plasma samples, which are generally 3 percent less than in serum. The new upper limits of normal are generally lower for plasma cholesterol and considerably higher, especially in men, for plasma triglycerides. These normal ranges are based on the values found in the reference population of white subjects and are necessarily statistical (i.e., between the 5th and 95th percentiles). For the dietary therapy for hyperlipidemia, some authorities have chosen the 90th percentile as the cutoff point for the normal range.[18] Because our focus is on drug therapy, we have chosen the 95th percentile. This cutoff point should be viewed as flexible and considered in relation to the patient's other risk factors and family history for premature atherosclerotic vascular disease (see below). A normal range ("ideal range") based on values that minimize cardiovascular risk awaits the results from intervention trials that lower plasma cholesterol levels.

Sole reliance on plasma total cholesterol levels may be misleading. Some patients with elevated levels of LDL or depressed levels of HDL may present with values for total cholesterol that are well within the normal range. Conversely, in rare individuals, a high total cholesterol may be due to increased HDL concentrations. Levels of LDL-cholesterol (LDL_{ch}) can be estimated, using the lipid values described above, as follows:

$$LDL_{ch} = \text{total plasma cholesterol} - HDL_{ch} - \frac{\text{plasma TG}}{5}$$

This formula is applicable whenever the plasma triglycerides do not exceed 400 mg/dl and dysbetalipoproteinemia (type III) is not present.[19]

When plasma triglyceride values exceed the upper limits of normal, it is important to be certain the subject was fasting for an adequate time. Next, it is generally useful to determine which lipoprotein is responsible for the hypertriglyceridemia. This distinction can usually be made by examining a sample of turbid plasma that has stood overnight in the refrigerator. Chylomicrons will form a cream layer on top of the plasma, whereas VLDL remain evenly distributed through the plasma. Lipoprotein electrophoresis is not helpful in the diagnosis of hyperlipidemia except to identify β-VLDL after isolation of VLDL in those uncommon patients with dysbetalipoproteinemia (see below).

A generally accepted and useful classification of the hyperlipidemias originally developed at the National Institutes of Health (NIH) is based on the lipoprotein(s) responsible for the elevated plasma lipids. These types represent phenotypes inasmuch as a patient may vary between types during treatment. Also patients within the same family may have different types. Types I and IV have high levels of triglycerides owing to increased chylomicrons and VLDL, respectively. Type II, characterized by elevated concentrations of LDL (and therefore by hypercholesterolemia), is subdivided into types IIa and IIb. In the former type, only LDL levels are increased; patients with type IIb have high levels of both LDL and VLDL and thus present with the combination of hypercholesterolemia and hypertriglyceridemia. Elevations of both chylomicrons and VLDL are found in type V, which usually produces severe hypertriglyceridemia. Defective catabolism of chylomicrons produces an accumulation of abnormal VLDL (β-VLDL) that are unusually rich in cholesterol compared with the composition of normal VLDL. Individuals with this disorder are defined as having dysbetalipoproteinemia, broad-beta disease, or type III hyperlipoproteinemia. Dysbetalipoproteinemia should be suspected when both cholesterol and triglycerides are increased to similar degrees or when characteristic planar xanthomas are present in the palmar creases. A definitive diagnosis of dysbetalipoproteinemia, however, requires special laboratory procedures to isolate VLDL in an ultracentrifuge and to demonstrate that the ratio of VLDL cholesterol to plasma triglycerides exceeds 0.3.[19]

Although laboratory determinations are required to diagnose hyperlipidemia, its presence is strongly suggested by certain skin lesions. Eruptive xanthomas are characteristic of severe hypertriglyceridemia with chylomicronemia and rapidly clear with correction of the hypertriglyceridemia. Eruptive xanthomas appear as erythematous papules, 1 to 5 mm in diameter, with a central yellow nodule, and they are distributed over the buttocks and proximal portion of the extremities. Xanthelasmas are often present in patients with hypercholesterolemia, but plasma cholesterol levels are normal in about half the individuals with xanthelasma. Xanthomas in extensor or Achilles tendons are almost always due to elevated LDL levels. Premature arcus senilis, particularly in whites, may suggest hypercholesterolemia. Yellowish planar lesions in the palmar creases (palmar xanthomas) may be seen in patients with elevated β-VLDL.

GENERAL PRINCIPLES OF MANAGEMENT

General principles for the management of hyperlipidemia are outlined in Table 3. No treatment of hyperlipidemia should be initiated before obtaining adequate baseline values of serum lipids and lipoproteins. Generally, three determinations, spaced at least a week apart, are adequate. These samples should be obtained while patients are on their regular diet, at a stable weight, on no lipid-lowering agents, not pregnant, and without intercurrent infection. Adequate baseline values from a reliable laboratory assure that long-term therapy is justified and allow evaluation of the efficacy of treatment. Care must be taken to identify and treat any underlying disorders known to cause secondary hyperlipidemia. These include hypothyroidism, diabetes mellitus, chronic renal failure, nephrotic syndrome, obstructive liver disease, dysgammaglobulinemia, and the administration of sex steroids or glucocorticoids. For the management of patients with hypertriglyceridemia, it is important to discontinue medications containing estrogen and to tightly regulate diabetes mellitus.

Dietary treatment is the initial step in the management of all types of hyperlipidemia. Dietary modifications should also be recommended for hypertensive patients, cigarette smokers, and patients with diabetes, if their LDL levels are in the high-normal range, or if HDL is low. Some experts recommend a modified diet for all individuals with LDL levels in the high-normal range. In fact, the American Heart Association has chosen the 90th percentile of cholesterol or triglycerides for its definition of hyperlipidemia.[18] All patients with hyperlipidemia should be counseled to quit smoking, should be treated for hypertension or hyperglycemia, and should be encouraged to exercise. Drugs should be started only after dietary management of patients with hyperlipidemia has failed to lower plasma lipids sufficiently or when the patient does not comply with the diet. Hyperlipidemia can usually be controlled by a combination of diet and medication, even when there is an underlying genetic predisposition.

Drug treatment is recommended for all individuals whose levels of LDL fail to decrease to below the 95th percentile with diet, with the possible exception of patients older than 65, particularly those with a history of myocardial infarction. It seems reasonable to use lipid-lowering drugs in patients with hyperlipidemia after bypass surgery of coronary or other vessels because control of LDL levels may slow the development of atherosclerosis in the newly anastomosed vessles. Because of the atherogenicity of β-VLDL, drug therapy should be used in any patient with dysbetalipoproteinemia whose β-VLDL level persists with diet.

To prevent attacks of acute pancreatitis, treatment is essential in individuals whose triglycerides exceed 1000 mg/dl. The fastest method of decreasing plasma triglycerides in an acute situation is to prescribe a fat-free, hypocaloric diet. Drug therapy is required if a longer-term trial of dietary treatment (weight loss and restricted fat) fails to maintain the plasma triglycerides below 1000 mg/dl, and drugs should be strongly considered if triglyceride levels still exceed 600 mg/dl. Patients with triglycerides between 600 and 1000 mg/dl should be treated with drugs if there is a history of pancreatitis or premature vascular disease in the patient or family, or if HDL levels are low or other cardiovascular risk factors (smoking, hypertension, diabetes) are present. Some patients who initially present with hypertriglycer-

Table 3. General principles in the management of hyperlipidemia

1. Obtain two or three baseline values of plasma cholesterol, triglycerides, and HDL-cholesterol before initiating treatment.
2. Identify and treat secondary causes of hyperlipidemia.
3. Screen family members for hyperlipidemia.
4. Dietary measures are the keystone of management; drugs are used only if dietary treatment is unsuccessful.
5. Start with low dose of drugs, then increase slowly.
6. During therapy, monitor plasma lipids, lipoproteins, and adverse effects. The goal of treatment is to lower LDL and/or VLDL while raising, or at least not reducing, HDL levels.

idemia develop abnormal levels of LDL during diet or drug therapy. These patients should then be treated with a medication which can lower both triglycerides and LDL.

During the course of treatment, the lipid examination should be repeated on several occasions. Usually the effectiveness of diet or drug is apparent within 6 weeks of full compliance. Repeat lipid testing at that time will demonstrate the effects of diet or drugs on LDL and triglycerides. It also permits us to assess possible changes in HDL levels to be sure that a beneficial effect on the atherogenic lipoproteins is not counterbalanced by an unwanted fall in HDL.

PRINCIPLES OF DIET THERAPY

Although reviewed here only briefly, dietary management is the first line of therapy in hyperlipidemia. No drug should be started prior to the initiation of a proper diet and evaluation of the response of the plasma lipids and lipoproteins.

Four dietary measures have proven successful in lowering plasma lipid and lipoprotein levels (Table 4): reduced intake of saturated fat, increased intake of polyunsaturated fat, decreased dietary cholesterol, and weight loss.[20] Inasmuch as the usual American diet contains about 40 percent fat with a ratio of polyunsaturated to saturated fats (P/S ratio) of approximately 0.4, the first two dietary measures can be achieved by reducing the total intake of fat while partially substituting foods containing polyunsaturated fats for those rich in saturated fats. These dietary modifications will raise the P/S ratio. A small further reduction in plasma cholesterol is achieved by restricting dietary cholesterol to less than 300 mg/day. These changes in the type of fat and the amount of dietary cholesterol may lower total cholesterol and LDL by 5 to 15 percent, depending on the extent of change from the patients's previous diet.

Dietary modifications, particularly weight reduction in overweight patients, usually are more effective in lowering triglyceride-rich lipoproteins (CM, VLDL, β-VLDL) than cholesterol-rich lipoproteins (LDL). Alcohol must also be restricted in diets aimed at reducing VLDL or β-VLDL. Fasting chylomicronemia (types I and V) can be controlled by more severe restriction of dietary fat. Such fat-restricted diets may be made more palatable by supplementation with medium-chain triglycerides.

Based on these principles, two forms of diet instruction have been prepared for patients with hyperlipidemia. In general, both forms agree on the major elements already described for the control of hyperlipidemia. The first, developed initially at the NIH, specifies a different diet for each type of hyperlipidemia. Our recommendations (Table 5) differ in several respects from these diets and are similar to the Phase I diet of the American Heart Association (see below). For example, to lower plasma cholesterol and LDL the NIH diet increased the polyunsaturated fats to achieve a P/S ratio > 2. More recent diets aim for a P/S = 1 because

Table 4. Dietary measures to reduce plasma levels of LDL, VLDL, or chylomicrons and raise levels of HDL

Plasma Lipoprotein	*Dietary Measures*
LDL	Reduction in total dietary fat
	Replace saturated fat with polyunsaturated fat
	Restrict dietary cholesterol
VLDL and β-VLDL	Weight reduction
	Alcohol restriction
Chylomicrons	Severe reduction in total dietary fat
	Weight reduction
HDL	Weight reduction
	Moderate alcohol intake

Table 5. Management of hyperlipidemia

Type	*Elevated Lipoprotein**	*Diet†*	*Drug*	
			1st Line	*2nd Line*
I	CM	Fat intake < 15% of calories	None	
IIa	LDL	Total fat intake < 35% of calories P/S = 1	Bile acid sequestrants +/−	
IIb	LDL VLDL	Cholesterol < 300 mg Weight reduction	Nicotinic acid	Probucol D-Thyroxine
III	β-VLDL	Weight reduction Total fat intake < 35% of calories	Clofibrate	
IV	VLDL	P/S = 1 Cholesterol < 300 mg Replace simple sugars with complex carbohydrates Limit alcohol	Clofibrate Gemfibrozil Nicotinic acid	
V	CM VLDL	Weight reduction Total fat intake < 25% of calories Replace simple sugars with complex carbohydrates Limit alcohol	Clofibrate Nicotinic acid	Medroxyprogesterone acetate (women) Oxandrolone (men)

*HDL levels are decreased in all types except IIA.
†Dietary measures are listed in order of efficacy.

high levels of polyunsaturated fats reduce both LDL and HDL.[21] The NIH triglyceride-lowering diet reduced the intake of all carbohydrates. Although the intake of simple sugars is still limited, complex carbohydrates are no longer restricted for several reasons. The restriction of total carbohydrate intake necessarily raises the fat content of the diet. In addition, the fiber components of complex carbohydrates may lower LDL-cholesterol.[20]

The second approach (the unified diet) was developed by the American Heart Association (AHA). The AHA suggests a progressive, three-phase reduction in the intake of total fat and cholesterol for patients with either hypercholesterolemia or hypertriglyceridemia. In Phase I, 30 to 35 percent of calories are derived from fat, and cholesterol is limited to 300 mg/day. In Phase II, the fat intake is essentially the same, but cholesterol is further restricted to 100 to 250 mg per day. In Phase III, total fat is reduced to 20 to 25 percent of calories and cholesterol is restricted to 100 mg per day. In all three phases, less than 10 percent of the calories are saturated fat and approximately 10 percent are polyunsaturated fat. Another principle of the diet is to lower energy intake to achieve an ideal weight. When patients with hypertriglyceridemia do not respond to these measures, the diet is supplemented with polyunsaturated fat. An even further reduction in fat intake is recommended for patients with chylomicronemia. In Phase II and Phase III of the AHA diet, the reduction in fat and cholesterol may lower both LDL and HDL,[22] and adherence may be difficult for many patients. Booklets that describe this approach to the dietary management of hyperlipidemia are available from the American Heart Association.

The problem of achieving patient compliance with diet is complex, but several general principles are helpful. The dietary instruction should be performed by someone experienced in nutrition counseling, for example, a registered dietitian, and periodically reviewed and reinforced by the physician. The dietary plan must be adjusted to the patient's life style as well as to any requirements imposed by other medical conditions (e.g., sodium restriction and weight reduction for hypertension). Several months may be required to teach the diet to the patient and to the person who prepares the meals. Maintenance of consistently good dietary adherence usually requires continued followup by the dietitian and physician. To make appropriate food choices, the patient should understand the recommended nutrient changes and have reliable and readily available sources of information on the dietary modifications and the nutrient content of foods. All family members may safely eat the same meals that are low in saturated fat and cholesterol. This approach makes food preparation easier and may benefit other family members inasmuch as hyperlipidemia is frequently familial.

GENERAL PRINCIPLES OF DRUG THERAPY

Although dietary modifications are generally considered to be associated with minimal risk, their effectiveness is limited. As a result, many patients, particularly those with significantly elevated LDL levels, become candidates for drug treatment. Because their use is often long-term, drugs should not only be safe and effective but also be well tolerated in order to maintain the patient's cooperation. Unfortunately, none of the lipid-lowering agents meets all of these criteria. Thus, the physician must assess the risk versus the benefit for each patient.

Before prescribing any medication, the physician must consider its efficacy and potential side effects and determine its suitability for a given patient. For example, nicotinic acid should be used with caution in patients with glucose intolerance, gout, or liver disease because this agent can produce hyperglycemia, hyperuricemia, and alterations of liver function. Some lipid-lowering medications, for example, the bile acid sequestrants and clofibrate, alter the absorption or metabolism of certain other drugs. Thus, it is important to review the patient's other medications before starting a lipid-lowering regimen and during followup visits.

Cooperation by the patient requires an understanding of the rationale for the medication, the need to take the drug as prescribed, and the type of followup. Long-term compliance is improved when the patient has few negative experiences with a medication. Inasmuch as the treatment of hyperlipidemia is an emergency only in cases of massive hypertriglyceridemia, the physician can minimize side effects by slowly increasing the dose of a bile acid–binding resin or nicotinic acid until the fully effective dose is achieved.

Lipid determinations should be repeated in about 6 weeks to assess the efficacy of the medication because most lipid-lowering drugs exert their full effects within a few weeks. If the drug is partially or completely ineffective, it may be necessary to change to or add another medication. Drugs lower the levels of plasma lipoproteins either by decreasing their synthesis or by increasing their catabolism. Thus, when drug combinations are required, the use of one drug that reduces lipoprotein synthesis and another that enhances lipoprotein catabolism may have complementary or even synergistic effects on lipoprotein levels. If the patient loses weight, significantly improves other aspects of dietary compliance, or improves diabetic control, he or she can be given a trial off the medication, particularly in the treatment of hypertriglyceridemia. If there is no major rebound, the patient may be continued without drug treatment. After lipoprotein levels are controlled on an established dose of medication, the patient is encouraged to maintain this pattern and is seen approximately three to four times a year. Dietary compliance is emphasized at each return visit inasmuch as there is a natural tendency for patients to slip away from their diets once they believe their lipid problem is successfully managed with drugs.

INDIVIDUAL DRUGS

Because the goal of this review is to be practical rather than all-inclusive, we will discuss individually only the first- and second-line drugs. The major indications, efficacy, dosage, and

Table 6. Drugs for treatment of hyperlipidemia

Drug	*Indications: Elevated Lipoproteins*	*Dose*	*Efficacy**	*Cost†‡ ($/year)*		*Common Short-Term Adverse Effects*
Bile acid sequestrants	LDL	2–3 packs bid	TG ↑ LDL ↓↓↓ HDL →	935 460	(Questran) (Colestid)	Constipation and hemorrhoids Heartburn, bloating Impaired absorption of vitamins and drugs
Nicotinic acid	VLDL LDL	1.5–3.0 gm bid	TG ↓↓↓ in IIb, IV LDL ↓↓ HDL ↑	305 208	(Nicobid) (Nicolar)	Cutaneous flushing and pruritus Gastric distress and peptic ulceration Increased blood glucose, transaminases, and uric acid
Probucol	LDL	500 mg bid	LDL ↓↓ HDL ↓	265		Diarrhea, eosinophilia
D-Thyroxine	LDL	4–8 mg qd	LDL ↓↓↓ HDL ↓↓	182		Arrhythmias, angina, thyrotoxicosis
Clofibrate	CM VLDL β-VLDL	1gm bid	TG ↓↓↓ β-VLDL ↓↓↓ LDL ↓ (II) ↑ (IV) HDL ↑	130		Myositis Decreased libido Potentiate warfarin anticoagulants Gallstones
Gemfibrozil	VLDL	600 mg bid	TG ↓↓ HDL ↑↑	275		Similar to clofibrate
Medroxyprogesterone acetate	CM VLDL	5–10 mg qd	TG ↓↓↓ HDL →	128		Fluid retention Thrombosis
Oxandrolone	CM VLDL	2.5 mg tid	TG ↓↓↓ LDL ↑↑ HDL ↓↓↓	145		Masculinization of women Fluid retention and edema

*→ = unchanged; ↑ = <10% change; ↑↑ = 10–20% change; ↑↑↑ = >20% change.
†Wholesale price, June 1982.[71]
‡Cost based on lower of specified doses.

adverse effects of these drugs are shown in Table 6. Third-line agents like neomycin and phytosterols are rarely used in the treatment of hyperlipidemia.

Agents to Lower Total Cholesterol, Particularly LDL-Cholesterol

Bile Acid Sequestrants (Cholestyramine and Colestipol)

Although they are different resins, cholestyramine (Questran) and colestipol (Colestid) are discussed together because they are virtually identical in their mechanism of action, dosage schedule, and side effects. Bile acid sequestrants have been used for about two decades and are the drugs of choice for patients with increased LDL levels. Both compounds are nonabsorbable anion exchange resins that bind bile acids and prevent their reabsorption from the small intestine. The increased fecal loss of bile acids stimulates their synthesis from cholesterol in the liver. Because LDL-cholesterol is used for bile acid synthesis, intestinal binding of bile acids leads to an increased uptake of plasma LDL by the liver.[4,23]

Bile acid sequestrants are available as granular powders provided in packets (cholestyramine 4 gm per packet, colestipol 5 gm per packet) or in cans with a scoop that measures the equivalent of one packet. The full dosage is six packets per day, but the most common dose is four packets per day. At full dosage, the resins produce a 25 to 35 percent lowering of LDL and no change in HDL-cholesterol. In severe hypercholesterolemia, the resins may be combined with nicotinic acid (see below) to lower LDL by 50 percent.[24] Triglyceride levels are increased occasionally during resin therapy.[26] The increase is transient and generally not significant in patients with normal baseline triglyceride values. However, the increase may be persistent and severe in patients whose triglycerides are elevated before therapy. Thus, the use of the resins alone should be reserved primarily for patients with an isolated increase in LDL (type IIa).

The medications are usually taken 10 to 15 minutes after suspension in cold water or fruit juices to assure proper hydration of the powder. The patient should be started on one or at most two packets per day. Over a period of several months, the dose is gradually increased to four to six packets per day as necessary to achieve the desired lowering of LDL. For full efficacy, the medication is taken twice daily within 30 minutes of a meal. Other drugs should be taken 1 hour before the resins to minimize the potential for their binding to the resin and subsequent malabsorption.

Cholestyramine and colestipol produce few systemic side effects inasmuch as they are not absorbed. However, they may interfere with absorption of vitamins and drugs, and they often cause unpleasant effects within the intestine. These agents can interfere with the absorption of folic acid and iron and, at high doses, fat-soluble vitamins.[7] Although significant problems rarely result from vitamin malabsorption, administration of a multiple vitamin with folic acid and iron provides an added margin of safety. Binding to resins of anionic drugs, for example, digitalis glycosides, warfarin derivatives, salicylates, thiazides, and thyroxine, may decrease their absorption. When patients are treated with both digitalis and resins, digitalis levels and cardiac status should be monitored carefully until a consistent medication regimen is established. Significant problems may be avoided by adjusting dosage schedules so that the resins and other drugs are not simultaneously present in the gut. Alternatively, the dosage of the other drugs that may be bound during their enterohepatic recirculation may be appropriately increased. The resins may exacerbate the symptoms of gastroesophageal reflux and cause a feeling of epigastric bloating. Binding of bile acids may reduce the movement of water into the colon and produce constipation and hemorrhoids. The addition of bran to the diet and the use of a stool softener, such as docusate sodium (Colace), frequently relieve these symptoms. It is helpful for the patient to initiate these anticonstipation measures prophylactically. The bile acid–binding resins should be introduced cautiously in patients with a significant history of gastrointestinal symptoms.

Poor compliance and expense are the major limitations of the bile acid–binding resins. Both children and adults often take less than 40 percent of their prescribed dose because of constipation and the unpleasant taste and texture of the medication. Additionally, many patients have problems mixing the medication in the required fluid volume in social settings. Many of these problems that limit compliance can be overcome by careful and consistent guidance by the physician. The use of a new preparation of microcrystalline cholestyramine, as yet unavailable in the United States, may increase efficacy, eliminate this problem of mixing, and minimize constipation.

Nicotinic Acid

Nicotinic acid, also called niacin (Nicobid or Nicolar), has been used for more than two decades for the treatment of hypercholesterolemia and hypertriglyceridemia. Nicotinic acid is the drug of choice for the treatment of hypercholesterolemia in patients who cannot tolerate or do not respond adequately to the bile acid sequestrants. Nicotinic acid, in full doses of 3 to 6 gm/day, significantly lowers VLDL and LDL and raises HDL levels.[27] The major action of nicotinic acid is to decrease indirectly the secretion of VLDL from the liver.[28] Nicotinic acid reduces the release of fatty acids from adipose tissue[29]; the resultant decrease in the availability of fatty acids for liver uptake lowers the synthetic rate of VLDL lipid and apo B.[28] The decline in VLDL synthesis leads to a fall in plasma LDL, the major product of VLDL catabolism.[30] The increase in HDL results from a decrease in the fractional catabolic rate of HDL.[31] The combination of nicotinic acid with a bile acid–binding resin has an additive effect and may lower the very elevated LDL levels of patients with familial hypercholesterolemia into the normal range.[24] This combination is recommended for patients who develop significant hypertriglyceridemia or who fail to achieve normal LDL levels on the bile acid sequestrants.

Patients may experience cutaneous flushing, pruritus, urticaria, and gastric distress within ½ to 1 hour following each dose when they first take nicotinic acid. Gradual introduction of the medication and taking it with meals three times a day can diminish these adverse effects. The patient should begin with 100 mg/day and increase the dosage over a period of several months at the rate of 2.5 gm/month to reach a full therapeutic dose. This gradual increase in dose generally prevents most of the flushing. If therapy is interrupted, tachyphylaxis is rapidly lost and a gradual increase of dosage is again necessary. In patients whose flushing episodes persist, administration of 300 mg aspirin 30 minutes prior to the nicotinic acid is suggested since the flushing appears to be mediated by prostaglandins.[24] Nicotinic acid therapy may also activate peptic ulcer disease. Thus, patients with symptoms of active peptic ulcer should not be started on nicotinic acid. In patients with a prior history of peptic ulcer disease, nicotinic acid may be used cautiously with monitoring of symptoms, signs, and laboratory evidence of intestinal bleeding. The vasodilating effects of ganglionic blocking agents may be potentiated by nicotinic acid, and orthostatic hypotension may develop. For this reason, ganglionic blocking agents, if used to treat hypertension, should be administered with significant caution.

Nicotinic acid may impair glucose tolerance in some nondiabetic patients and make some diabetic patients more difficult to regulate. During glucose tolerance tests in the Coronary Drug Project, fasting and 1-hour post-challenge blood glucose levels were 3 and 10 mg/dl higher, respectively, in patients receiving nicotinic acid compared with placebo.[32] Nicotinic acid is often well tolerated by patients with mild adult-onset diabetes whose disease is controlled by diet alone. Blood glucose should be monitored frequently in such patients and the medication stopped if a significant decrease in glucose tolerance develops. Glucose tolerance returns to pretreatment levels with discontinuance of the nicotinic acid. Nicotinic acid probably should not be used in patients with insulin-dependent diabetes.

Elevations of SGOT and SGPT are common, and the drug should not be started in patients with abnormal liver function test results. Increases in transaminase levels are more frequently encountered with higher doses (greater than 3 gm/day) and with the longer-acting, time-release preparations.[33] These changes, usually mild and transient, diminish once the patient is stabilized at a particular dose. During therapy, liver function tests should be routinely monitored; the drug dose is reduced or discontinued if significant abnormalities persist.

Uric acid levels should be monitored during treatment with nicotinic acid, which frequently causes hyperuricemia.[34] The incidence of acute gouty arthritis was also increased in patients on nicotinic acid during the Coronary Drug Project.[32] Nicotinic acid may decrease the renal clearance of uric acid, possibly by competing for the organic acid secretory mechanism. Nicotinic acid may act synergistically with thiazide diuretics to increase plasma uric acid levels. If hyperuricemia persists during therapy, simultaneous administration of allopurinol should be considered.

Nicotinic acid must be used with caution in patients with mild glucose intolerance or gout, and probably not at all in patients with insulin-dependent diabetes, active peptic ulcer, or liver disease. There is a frequent association of hypertriglyceridemia with elevated blood glucose[35] and uric acid or abnormal liver function tests. In patients with this syndrome, it may be preferable to treat the hypertriglyceridemia with clofibrate (see below).

D-Thyroxine

D-Thyroxine (Choloxin), the D-isomer of thyroid hormone, is an effective agent to lower plasma cholesterol, but its use is limited by its side effects and propensity to lower HDL-cholesterol as well as LDL levels. Treatment is started with 2 mg daily, and the drug dose is raised over a period of several months to 4 to 8 mg a day. D-Thyroxine lowers cholesterol levels by increasing the conversion of cholesterol to bile acids and possibly by stimulating the uptake and catabolism of LDL-cholesterol in the liver.[36]

D-Thyroxine is well tolerated by most young individuals. An occasional patient may experience symptoms of thyrotoxicosis, and the severity of diabetes may be aggravated. D-Thyroxine also potentiates the action of warfarin anticoagulants. Because D-thyroxine may precipitate serious arrhythmias and anginal episodes in patients with coronary artery disease and previous myocardial infarction,[37] the drug is contraindicated in such individuals as well as in those with congestive heart failure, other causes of arrhythmias, significant hypertension, and advanced renal or liver disease. D-Thyroxine may be useful in young adults who have elevated LDL levels without clinically manifest heart disease and cannot tolerate the bile acid sequestrants or nicotinic acid.

Probucol

Probucol (Lorelco), 4,4′-(isopropylidenedithio)bis(2,6-di-t-butyl phenol), a new agent with no structural similarities to other lipid-lowering drugs, is effective in reducing plasma cholesterol. In its usual dose of 500 mg bid, probucol lowers plasma cholesterol by 10 to 15 percent with little change in plasma triglycerides.[38] Both the cholesterol and apoproteins of LDL and HDL are lowered by probucol. In fact, the percent lowering of HDL cholesterol may exceed that for LDL-cholesterol.[39] Thus, the LDL/HDL ratio frequently increases during probucol therapy. Therefore, the major indication for probucol is in patients with elevated LDL levels who cannot tolerate the bile acid–binding resins, nicotinic acid, or D-thyroxine.

Probucol is lipophilic and is concentrated in adipose tissue. As a result, plasma levels increase gradually during chronic administration and reach a steady state after 3 to 4 months. The peak effect of probucol occurs after about 3 to 7 weeks of administration, and some effect persists for several weeks after discontinuing treatment. The mechanism of action for probucol has not been clearly defined, but the fecal loss of bile acids doubled and the fractional catabolic rate of LDL increased in patients taking probucol.[40] In another study, the decrease in LDL appeared to be due to decreased synthesis.[41] However, both studies agree that the decrease in HDL reflects reduced apo A-1 synthesis.[41,42] The change in HDL apoprotein synthesis may be related to altered transport of cholesterol in the intestinal mucosa.

The advantage of probucol is that it is well tolerated and leads to good patient compliance. The most common short-term side effect is diarrhea, which was reported in approximately 10 percent of patients. Flatulence, abdominal pain, nausea, and vomiting have occasionally occurred. A mild, transient eosinophilia was noted in 10 to 32 percent of patients. Four of eight monkeys fed a high-fat, high-cholesterol diet died suddenly after several weeks of probucol therapy. Their blood levels of the drug were comparable to those encountered in humans, and ECG changes were noted.[43] The drug also appears to sensitize the myocardium of dogs to epinephrine-induced ventricular fibrillation.[44] Although arrhythmias have not been reported yet during probucol treatment in humans, the drug must be used with caution in patients with arrythmias. The long-term side effects of probucol are not known, and too few patients have been treated to identify infrequent adverse effects. Additional investigation is needed to determine whether the long half-life and the accumulation of probucol in adipose tissue produce late adverse effects.

The simultaneous reduction in LDL and HDL by probucol has diminished the enthusiasm for its use among many physicians who specialize in the treatment of lipid disorders. However, several preliminary reports suggest that the combination of probucol with a bile acid–binding resin produced a greater regression of atherosclerosis in monkeys than either agent alone.[45] Others showed that probucol decreased xanthomas in patients with homozygous familial hypercholesterolemia.[45] In an uncontrolled 5-year study, probucol decreased the incidence of sudden death and myocardial infarction.[46] If confirmed, these preliminary reports would suggest that probucol either alone or in combination with a bile acid sequestrant may decrease tissue concentrations of cholesterol. More complete studies in humans on the protective role of HDL in atherosclerosis are needed before it is known whether the proportionately greater decrease in HDL will cancel out any benefit derived from lowering LDL with probucol.

Agents to Lower Plasma Triglycerides

Clofibrate

Clofibrate (Atromid-S), chlorophenoxyisobutyric acid ethyl ester, is the first-line agent to lower plasma triglyceride levels or β-VLDL. After absorption, the ester group is hydrolyzed and the free acid circulates largely bound to albumin. The drug is excreted in the urine, and its clearance is decreased in patients with chronic renal failure. The usual dose is 1 gm bid.

Clofibrate is particularly effective in the treatment of dysbetalipoproteinemia (type III) in which even small doses may normalize cholesterol and triglyceride levels although some β-VLDL persists in the plasma. Clofibrate also reduces triglyceride and VLDL levels by 15 to 50 percent in patients with type IV and may lower plasma triglycerides in type V hyperlipidemia by as much as 60 percent.[48] During clofibrate treatment of patients with hypertriglyceridemia, both HDL and LDL concentrations tend to rise.[49] Clofibrate produces a reduction in LDL of 5 to 10 percent in some patients with type II hyperlipidemia but is not recommended as the drug of choice for such individuals because of concerns regarding its long-term side effects.

Multiple actions of clofibrate have been described, but its most important effects on VLDL probably reflect enhanced clearance of triglyceride-rich lipoproteins by increasing lipoprotein lipase activity.[50] Clofibrate also decreases hepatic VLDL synthesis and raises the excretion of cholesterol in the bile and feces.[51] The latter action reduces the total body pool of cholesterol in most patients with hypercholesterolemia but also increases the lithogenicity of the bile and the incidence of gallstones during treatment.[52]

Most patients tolerate clofibrate quite well. The most common side effect is gastrointestinal discomfort, particularly nausea, which occurs in 5 to 10 percent of patients. In the Coronary Drug Project, approximately 14 percent of male patients receiving clofibrate reported decreased libido compared with 10 percent in those receiving placebo.[32] These differences were significant statistically and support a trial period off clofibrate in patients with this complaint. Clofibrate may stimulate appetite and produce slight to moderate weight gain. Liver enlargement may also occur, and serum transaminases are sometimes elevated. These hepatic changes are reversible and clinical signs of hepatotoxicity are unusual.

Clofibrate displaces acidic drugs such as warfarin anticoagulants, phenytoin, and tolbutamide from binding sites on plasma proteins. Inasmuch as clofibrate potentiates warfarin anticoagulants and may decrease platelet stickiness,[53] careful attention to prothrombin time and clotting parameters is necessary when clofibrate is used in conjunction with warfarin-type anticoagulants. The dosage of anticoagulant should be reduced by one third to one half in patients started on clofibrate. General malaise and myalgia are also common. An occasional patient develops a severe reversible myositis with elevated serum levels of creatine phosphokinase during clifibrate treatment. This problem is especially common in patients with the nephrotic syndrome, presumably because the low plasma albumin levels increase the proportion of unbound drug, and in chronic renal failure.[54] The half-life of clofibrate is greatly prolonged in renal failure because the drug is eliminated predominantly by urinary excretion as a glucuronide. If used at all in such patients, the medication dose must be drastically reduced, at times to as little as 0.5 gm twice weekly.

A multicenter trial of the benefits of clofibrate in the treatment of hypercholesterolemia showed that the drug did reduce the incidence of nonfatal myocardial infarction.[52,55] However, there was a 25 percent increase in overall mortality, mainly from disorders of the liver, gallbladder, pancreas, and intestine, in the clofibrate-treated group when compared with placebo-treated controls.[52,55] Because of these findings, and the increase in cholelithiasis, clofibrate should be used to treat hypertriglyceridemia only when significantly elevated triglyceride concentrations persist despite maximal efforts at dietary management and the patient has a significant risk of pancreatitis or atherosclerosis and cannot tolerate nicotinic acid.

Nicotinic Acid

Nicotinic acid is a useful agent for the treatment of hypercholesterolemia and hypertriglyceridemia. The pharmacology of nicotinic acid was described in the previous section. The choice between nicotinic acid and clofibrate for the treatment of hypertriglyceridemia is still unresolved. Several points should be emphasized. Most patients with hypertriglyceridemia can be controlled with diet, discontinuation of estrogens, and tight regulation of diabetes mellitus. No drug is effective in the very rare patient with primary type I hyperlipidemia. Clofibrate is the drug of choice for type III hyperlipidemia. In patients with persistent hypertriglyceridemia refractive to diet and without diabetes mellitus, liver disease, or peptic ulcer, nicotinic acid is preferred. In hypertriglyceridemic patients with glucose intolerance or hyperuricemia, clofibrate may be used, or nicotinic acid may be administered cautiously. If the patient cannot tolerate nicotinic acid, clofibrate may be substituted. If diet adherence improves and there is significant weight loss, medications can be discontinued and the lipid values followed.

Gemfibrozil

Gemfibrozil (Lopid), which is related chemically to clofibrate, is the most recent drug approved for the treatment of hyperlipidemia. The usual dose is 600 mg bid. Reduction of VLDL levels in the treatment of type IV and possibly IIb hyperlipidemia is the major indication for the use of gemfibrozil. Reports have shown a 40 to 50 percent reduction of serum triglycerides in patients with type IV hyperlipidemia.[56] The medication reduces LDL levels by only about 5 to 10 percent in subjects with hypercholesterolemia and, like clofibrate, may raise LDL levels in those with type IV hyperlipidemia. The drug increases HDL levels by about 20 percent in patients with both type IIa and type IV hyperlipidemia.[57] As a consequence, the ratio of LDL (or total cholesterol) to HDL is favorably modified (decreased) in both types of patients. The major mechanism for the lipid-lowering effect of gemfibrozil is uncertain. However, the agent does inhibit the release of fatty acids from adipose tissue, and this action should reduce VLDL synthesis in the liver.[58]

Gemfibrozil is generally well tolerated. The most common adverse effects are gastrointestinal symptoms. Other side effects include skin rash, anemia, leukopenia, myositis, and blurred vision. Gemfibrozil potentiates the action of warfarin anticoagulants. Because of the limited clinical experience with the drug, and especially the lack of long-term studies, the full range of adverse effects from gemfibrozil is not known. Since gemfibrozil resembles clofibrate chemically, it is quite likely that the two drugs will demonstrate similar adverse effects. For example, both drugs are largely excreted through the kidneys, primarily as glucuronides, but it is not yet clear whether patients with chronic renal failure are as prone to the development of myositis during gemfibrozil treatment as they are with clofibrate. Gemfibrozil does increase the lithogenicity of the bile by the same mechanism but perhaps not to the same extent as clofibrate.[59] Studies completed to date have not determined whether gemfibrozil has the same tendency to increase cholelithiasis. Finally, there has been no long-term comparison of gemfibrozil with placebo treatment to determine whether this new agent has a beneficial effect on the frequency of myocardial infarctions or possibly shares with clofibrate an increased overall mortality when treated patients are compared with a control group. At present, there is little objective evidence to recommend the use of gemfibrozil over clofibrate.

Progestational Agents and Anabolic Steroids

Progestational agents, such as medroxyprogesterone acetate (Provera) and norethindrone acetate (Norlutate), and the androgenic steroid oxandrolone (Anavar) may be useful as adjunctive drugs in the treatment of adults with type V hyperlipidemia when dietary measures and other triglyceride-lowering medications (clofibrate or nicotinic acid) fail to maintain plasma triglyceride levels below 1000 mg/dl. The progestational agents or oxandrolone may be used in combination with clofibrate or nicotinic acid. Progestational agents are effective in females; oxandrolone should be used in males. Oxandrolone has also been used to treat patients with type IV hyperlipidemia. The mechanism of action of these hormones is uncertain, but both progestational agents and oxandrolone increase lipoprotein lipase.[60,61]

The recommended dose of medroxyprogesterone acetate is 5 to 10 mg daily. The response to the drug is variable, but in many women triglyceride levels may fall by 50 percent or more. This hormone has no significant effect on HDL levels. Because they may cause congenital anomalies in the fetus, progestational agents should not be used in the first 4 months of pregnancy. The drug is also contraindicated in women with a history of thrombophlebitis, thromboembolic disorders, and known or suspected malignancy of the breasts or uterus. Fluid retention is common. Occasional patients may exhibit cholestatic jaundice, anorexia, or mental depression.

The usual dose of oxandrolone is 2.5 mg three times per day. This drug may lower plasma triglycerides by as much as 50 percent in responsive patients and has produced normal lipid levels in some. Although this agent is usually well tolerated, occasional side effects include sodium retention, edema, leukopenia, and abnormal liver function tests. Oxandrolone should be used with caution in men with cardiac, renal, or hepatic disease and should not be used concomitantly with adrenal corticosteroids or ACTH. Women may show signs of virilization. Caution is warranted in the long-term use of oxandrolone because it causes profound reductions of HDL levels, often by more than 30 percent.[62]

SURGICAL TREATMENT OF HYPERCHOLESTEROLEMIA

Partial Ileal Bypass

The problems of adverse effects, long-term compliance, and cost of drugs have stimulated an interest in surgical treatment of hypercholesterolemia. Partial ileal bypass is currently used in some centers for the treatment of patients with severely elevated LDL levels. The small intestine is transected 200 cm from the ileocecal valve, or between the proximal two thirds and distal one third, depending on which procedure bypasses the greater segment.[63] The bypassed segment is considerably shorter than in the jejunoileal bypass procedure used for the treatment of massive obesity. Partial ileal bypass is associated with about a 40 percent lowering of total cholesterol and LDL.[64] Essentially, no changes occur in HDL or triglycerides. Qualitatively, the mechanism for cholesterol reduction in these patients appears similar to that for the bile acid sequestrants. The distal ileum is the major site for bile acid reabsorption, and bypassing this segment induces an approximately fivefold increase in the fecal loss of bile acids. This loss triggers a compensatory increase in the hepatic uptake of LDL and conversion of its cholesterol to bile acids. The decrease in bile acids also may decrease cholesterol absorption.

The major side effect of partial ileal bypass is an increase in stool frequency to more than five times per day in the majority of patients. This reflects an exaggeration of the cathartic action of bile acids to stimulate water secretion by the colonic mucosa. The increased stool frequency has been treated with bile acid–binding resins and antidiarrheal medications; however, we are aware of no report demonstrating the efficacy of cholestyramine in the treatment of the diarrhea in these patients. Diarrhea has been severe enough for an occasional patient to request restoration of the normal anatomy. The small, but clinically insignificant, increase in fecal fat may cause the weight loss of about 6 percent observed within a year after surgery.[65] The operation decreases calcium absorption and increases oxalate absorption and excretion in the urine. However, these effects have not been associated with the clinically important problems of osteoporosis or oxalate kidney stones. Malabsorption of vitamin B_{12} occurs after partial ileal bypass, and it is routine to inject vitamin B_{12} every 3 months after surgery. The incidence of cholelithiasis is not increased in the operated patients.

The place for partial ileal bypass in the treatment of hyperlipidemia is not well established. We would consider the operation for well-motivated adult patients without advanced atherosclerosis, who are at high risk because of a very high LDL/HDL ratio and cannot tolerate a bile acid sequestrant, nicotinic acid, or D-thyroxine, and in addition are cigarette smokers or hypertensive. Partial ileal bypass is generally not effective in the patient with homozygous familial hypercholesterolemia. These patients are rare, one in a million in the general population, usually with xanthomas before the age of 10 and have total cholesterol in the range of 600 to 1000 mg/dl. They develop clinical atherosclerosis in the second decade, and about 20 percent die before age 20.[4] For these patients, biweekly plasmapheresis is currently the treatment of choice for lowering the plasma cholesterol.[66]

FUTURE DEVELOPMENTS

Recent results from several trials of intervention for multiple risk factors suggest that lowering cholesterol by diet, discontinuing smoking, and treatment of hypertension may decrease the rate of fatal and nonfatal myocardial infarction in middle-aged men.[67] In early 1984, the results of the Coronary Primary Prevention Trial of the Lipid Research Clinics will be presented.[14] In this double-blind trial, men with elevated LDL were randomized to cholestyramine or a placebo and followed for at least 7 years. Demonstration of a significant benefit in the prevention of myocardial infarction by pharmacologic lowering of plasma cholesterol in this trial would provide a considerably greater impetus to identify and manage patients with hypercholesterolemia. Newer methods also are being applied for the diagnosis of patients with lipoprotein disorders. Apoprotein B of LDL, apoprotein A-1 of HDL, and apoprotein E of β-VLDL can now be measured in whole plasma by immunochemical methods. These methods may simplify and improve our ability to identify patients at a high risk for atherosclerosis because of high LDL or β-VLDL and low HDL.

The interest in identification and treatment of lipid disorders has stimulated pharmaceutical companies to improve the formulations of currently available products and to develop new drugs. Two new types of agents with particular promise are in early phases of clinical testing. One is sucrose polyester, a nonabsorbable artificial fat.[68] Substitution of sucrose polyester for regular fats in food preparation decreases energy intake and may assist patients to lose weight. Within the lumen of the small intestine, cholesterol, whether derived from the diet or from biliary secretion, is dissolved in the nonabsorbable sucrose polyester and excreted in the feces. This agent may act synergistically to lower plasma cholesterol with drugs like clofibrate that stimulate the biliary secretion of cholesterol. Another promising family of compounds are fungal derivatives that inhibit the rate-limiting enzyme of cholesterol synthesis.[69] These agents (compactin and mevinolin) stimulate the liver to take up LDL-cholesterol to meet its needs for cholesterol.[70] They also diminish the hepatic secretion of lipoproteins by limiting the amount of cholesterol available for lipoprotein synthesis. These agents act synergistically with the bile acid sequestrants to stimulate the catabolism of LDL in the liver. The advent of improved methods for the screening, diagnosis, and management of hyperlipidemia should aid the ongoing efforts of physicians and surgeons to prevent premature atherosclerosis.

ACKNOWEDGMENTS

This work was supported by NHLBI contract 1-HV-1-2158L. We express our appreciation to Dr. Peter O. Kwiterovich, Jr. for critical review of the manuscript and to Ms. Carol McGeeney for assistance in preparation of the manuscript.

REFERENCES

1. Miller, JP and Gotto, AM Jr: *The plasma lipoproteins, their formation and metabolism.* In Neuberger, A and Van Deenen, LLM (eds): *Comprehensive Biochemistry,* Vol 19b, Part II. Elsevier Scientific, Amsterdam, 1982.
2. Kane, JP: *Plasma lipoproteins: Structure and metabolism.* In Snyder, F (ed): *Lipid Metabolism in Mammals.* Plenum, New York, 1977.
3. Havel, RJ, Goldstein, JL, and Brown, MS: *Lipoproteins and lipid transport.* In Bondy, PK and Rosenberg, LE (eds): *Metabolic Control and Disease,* ed 8. WB Saunders, Philadelphia, 1980.
4. Goldstein, JL and Brown, MS: *Familial hypercholesterolemia.* In Stanbury, JB, Wyngaarden, JB, Fredrickson, DS, et al (eds): *The Metabolic Basis of Inherited Disease,* ed 5. McGraw-Hill, New York, 1982.
5. Nikkila, EA: *Familial lipoprotein lipase deficiency and related disorders of chylomicron metabolism.* In Stanbury, JB, Wyngaarden, JB, Fredrickson, DS, et al (eds): *The Metabolic Basis of Inherited Disease,* ed 5. McGraw-Hill, New York, 1982.
6. Brown, MS, Goldstein, JL, and Fredrickson, DS: *Familial type 3 hyperlipoproteinemia (dysbetalipoproteinemia).* In Stanbury, JB, Wyngaarden, JB, Fredrickson, DS, et al (eds): *The Metabolic Basis of Inherited Disease,* ed 5. McGraw-Hill, New York, 1982.
7. Hunninghake, DB and Probstfield, JL: *Drug treatment of hyperlipidemia.* In Rifkind, BM and Levy, RI (eds): *Hyperlipidemia, Diagnosis and Therapy.* Grune & Stratton, New York, 1977.
8. Lewis, B: *The Hyperlipidemias, Clinical and Laboratory Practice.* Blackwell Scientific, Oxford, 1976.
9. Mahley, RW: *Atherogenic hyperlipoproteinemia: The cellular and molecular biology of plasma lipoproteins altered by dietary fat and cholesterol.* Med Clin North Am 66:375, 1982.
10. Brunzell, JD and Bierman, EL: *Chylomicronemia syndrome: Interaction of genetic and acquired hypertriglyceridemia.* Med Clin North Am 66:455, 1982.
11. Kannel, WB, Castelli, WP, Gordon, T, et al: *Serum cholesterol, lipoproteins and the risk of coronary heart disease: The Framingham study.* Ann Intern Med 74:1, 1971.

12. Castelli, WP, Doyle, JT, Gordon, T, et al: *HDL cholesterol and other lipids in coronary heart disease. The cooperative lipoprotein phenotyping study.* Circulation 55:767, 1977.

13. Hulley, SB, Rosenman, RH, Bawol, RD, et al: *Epidemiology as a guide to clinical decisions. The association between triglyceride and coronary heart disease.* N Engl J Med 302:1383, 1980.

14. The Lipid Research Clinics Program: *The Coronary Primary Prevention Trial: Design and implementation.* J Chronic Dis 32:609, 1979.

15. Ballantyne, FC, Melville, DA, McKenna, JP, et al: *Response of plasma lipoproteins and acute phase proteins to myocardial infarction.* Clin Chim Acta 99:85, 1979.

16. Fredrickson, DS, Levy, RI, and Lees, RS: *Fat transport in lipoproteins—an integrated approach to mechanisms and disorders.* N Engl J Med 276:32, 94, 148, 215, 273, 1967.

17. *The Lipid Research Clinics. Population Studies Data Book,* Vol 1. U.S. Department of Health and Human Services, Public Health Service, National Institutes of Health, Lipid Metabolism Branch, NHLBI, Bethesda, NIH Publication No 80-1527, 1980.

18. *Recommendations for the Unified Diet Approach to the Treatment of Hyperlipidemia, Statement for Physicians.* American Heart Association, Dallas (in press, 1982).

19. Lipid Research Clinics Program: *Manual of Laboratory Operations, Vol 1. Lipid and Lipoprotein Analysis.* DHEW Publication No. (NIH) 75-628, Government Printing Office, Washington, DC, 1974.

20. Connor, WE and Connor, SL: *The dietary treatment of hyperlipidemia, rationale, technique and efficacy.* Med Clin North Am 66:485, 1982.

21. Ernst, N, Fisher, M, Bowen, P, et al: *Changes in plasma lipids and lipoproteins after a modified fat diet.* Lancet 2:111, 1980.

22. Gonen, B, Patsch, W, Kuisk, I, et al: *The effect of short-term feeding of a high carbohydrate diet on HDL subclasses in normal subjects.* Metabolism 30:1125, 1981.

23. Grundy, SM, Ahrens, EH Jr, and Salen, G: *Interruption of the enterohepatic circulation of bile acids in man: Comparative effects of cholestyramine and ileal exclusion on cholesterol metabolism.* J Lab Clin Med 78:94, 1971.

24. Kane, JP, Malloy, MJ, Tun, P, et al: *Normalization of LDL levels in heterozygous familial hypercholesterolemia with a combined drug regimen.* N Engl J Med 304:251, 1981.

25. Glueck, CJ, Ford, S Jr, Scheel, D, et al: *Colestipol and cholestyramine resin: Comparative effects in familial type II hyperlipoproteinemia.* JAMA 222:676, 1972.

26. Lees, AM, McCluskey, MA, and Lees, RS: *Results of colestipol therapy in type II hyperlipoproteinemia.* Atherosclerosis 24:129, 1976.

27. Carlson, LA, Olsson, A, and Ballantyne, D: *On the rise in low density and high density lipoproteins in response to the treatment of hypertriglyceridemia in type IV and type V hyperlipoproteinemias.* Atherosclerosis 26:603, 1977.

28. Carlson, LA, Oro, L, and Ostman, J: *Effect of nicotinic acid on plasma lipids in patients with hyperlipoproteinemia during the first week of treatment.* J Atheroscler Res 18:667, 1968.

29. Butcher, RW, Baird, CE, and Sutherland, EW: *Effects of lipolytic and antilipolytic substances on adenosine 3′,5′-monophosphate levels in isolated fat cells.* J Biol Chem 243:1705, 1968.

30. Eisenberg, S and Levy, RI: *Lipoprotein metabolism.* Adv Lipid Res 13:1, 1975.

31. Shepherd, J, Packard, CJ, Patch, JR, et al: *Effects of nicotinic acid therapy on plasma high density lipoprotein subfraction distribution and composition and on apolipoprotein A metabolism.* J Clin Invest 63:858, 1979.

32. Coronary Drug Project: *Clofibrate and niacin in coronary heart disease.* JAMA 231:360, 1975.

33. Christensen, NA, Achor, RWP, Berge, KG, et al: *Nicotinic acid treatment of hypercholesterolemia: Comparison of plain and sustained-action preparations and report of two cases of jaundice.* JAMA 177:546, 1961.

34. Berge, KG, Achor, RWP, Christensen, NA, et al: *Hypercholesterolemia and nicotinic acid: A long-term study.* Am J Med 31:24, 1961.

35. Glueck, CJ, Levy, RI, and Fredrickson, DS: *Immunoreactive insulin, glucose tolerance and carbohydrate inducibility in types II, III, IV and V hyperlipoproteinemia.* Diabetes 18:739, 1969.

36. Miettinen, TA: *Mechanism of serum cholesterol reduction by thyroid hormones in hypothyroidism.* J Lab Clin Med 71:537, 1968.

37. The Coronary Drug Project: *Findings leading to further modifications of its protocol with respect to dextrothyroxine, the Coronary Drug Project Research Group.* JAMA 220:996, 1972.

38. Le Lorier, J, DuBreuil-Quidoz, S, Lussier-Cacan, S, et al: *Diet and probucol in lowering cholesterol concentrations: Additive effects on plasma cholesterol concentrations in patients with familial type II hyperlipoproteinemia.* Arch Intern Med 137:1429, 1977.

39. Mellies, MJ, Gartside, PS, Glatfelter, L, et al: *Effects of probucol on plasma cholesterol, high and low density lipoprotein cholesterol, and apolipoproteins A1 and A2 in adults with primary familial hypercholesterolemia.* Metabolism 29:956, 1980.
40. Nestel, PJ and Billington, T: *Effects of probucol on low density lipoprotein removal and high density lipoprotein synthesis.* Atherosclerosis 38:203, 1981.
41. Nestel, PJ: *Effects of probucol on lipoprotein protein kinetics.* Artery 10:95, 1982.
42. Magill, P, Whitting, C, Hammett, F, et al: *Probucol: Effects on the metabolism of low density and high density lipoproteins in moderate hypercholesterolemia.* Artery 10:88, 1982.
43. Marshall, FN: *Pharmacology and toxicology of probucol.* Artery 10:7, 1982.
44. Marshall, FN and Lewis, JE: *Sensitization to epinephrine-induced ventricular fibrillation produced by probucol in dogs.* Toxicol Appl Pharmacol 24:594, 1973.
45. *Medical news: Regression of atherosclerosis: Preliminary but encouraging news.* JAMA 246:2309, 1981.
46. *Medical news: Is it harmful to lower HDL levels?* JAMA 246:2311, 1981.
47. Miettinen, TA, Huttunen, JK, Kuusi, T, et al: *Clinical experience with probucol with special emphasis on mode of action and long-term treatment.* Artery 10:35, 1982.
48. Lees, AM and Lees, RS: *Agents used to treat hyperlipidemia and atherosclerosis.* In Miller, RR and Greenblatt, DJ (eds): *Handbook of Drug Therapy.* Elsevier, New York, 1979.
49. Wilson, DE and Lees, RS: *Metabolic relationships among the plasma lipoproteins.* J Clin Invest 51:1051, 1972.
50. Boberg, J, Boberg, M, Gross, R, et al: *The effect of treatment with clofibrate on hepatic triglyceride and lipoprotein lipase activities of post-heparin plasma in male patients with hyperlipidemia.* Atherosclerosis 27:499, 1977.
51. Grundy, SM, Ahrens, EH Jr, Salen, G, et al: *Mechanisms of action of clofibrate on cholesterol metabolism in patients with hyperlipidemia.* J Lipid Res 13:531, 1972.
52. Committee of Principal Investigators: *A cooperative trial in the primary prevention of ischemic heart disease using clofibrate.* Br Heart J 40:1069, 1978.
53. Carvalho, AC, Colman, RW, and Lees, RS: *Clofibrate reversal of hypersensitivity in hyperbetalipoproteinemia.* Circulation 56:114, 1977.
54. Bridgeman, JF, Rosen, SM, and Thorp, JM: *Complications during clofibrate treatment of nephrotic-syndrome hyperlipoproteinemia.* Lancet 2:506, 1972.
55. World Health Organization (WHO): *Cooperative trial on primary prevention of ischemic heart disease using clofibrate to lower serum cholesterol.* Lancet 2:379, 1980.
56. Kaukola, S, Manninen, V, Malkonen, M, et al: *Gemfibrozil in the treatment of dyslipidaemias in middle-aged male survivors of myocardial infarction.* Acta Med Scand 209:69, 1981.
57. Peabody, HM Jr: *Clinical investigation of gemfibrozil: The treatment of primary hyperlipoproteinemia.* Cardiovascular Reviews and Reports 3:1195, 1982.
58. Carlson, LA: *Effect of gemfibrozil in vitro on fat-mobilizing lipolysis in human adipose tissue.* Proc R Soc Med 69(Suppl 2):101, 1976.
59. Hall, MJ, Nelson, LM, Russell, RI, et al: *Gemfibrozil—The effect on biliary cholesterol saturation of a new lipid-lowering agent and its comparison with clofibrate.* Atherosclerosis 39:511, 1981.
60. Ehnholm, C, Huttunen, JK, Kinnunen, PJ, et al: *Effect of oxandrolone treatment on the activity of lipoprotein lipase, hepatic lipase and phospholipase A_1 of human post-heparin plasma.* N Engl J Med 292:1314, 1975.
61. Glueck, CJ, Levy, RI, and Fredrickson, DS: *Norethindrone acetate, post-heparin lipolytic activity and plasma triglycerides in familial types I, III, IV, and V hyperlipoproteinemia.* Ann Intern Med 75:345, 1971.
62. Tamai, T, Nakai, T, Yamada, S, et al: *Effects of oxandrolone on plasma lipoproteins in patients with type IIa, IIb, and IV hyperlipoproteinemia: Occurrence of hypo-high density lipoproteinemia.* Artery 5:125, 1979.
63. Buchwald, H, Moore, RB, and Varco, RL: *Surgical treatment of hyperlipidemia.* Circulation 49(Suppl 1):1, 1974.
64. Moore, RB, Buchwald, H, Varco, RL, et al: *The effect of partial ileal bypass on plasma lipoproteins.* Circulation 62:469, 1980.
65. Faergeman, O, Meinertz, H, Hylander, E, et al: *Effects and side-effects of partial ileal by-pass surgery for familial hypercholesterolemia.* Gut 23:558, 1982.
66. Thompson, GR: *Management of familial hypercholesterolemia and new approaches to the treatment of atherosclerosis.* In Paoletti, R and Gotto, AM (eds): *Atherosclerosis Reviews,* Vol 5. Raven Press, New York, 1979.
67. Editorial: *Trials of coronary heart disease prevention.* Lancet 2:803, 1982.

68. GLUECK, CJ, MATTSON, FH, AND JANDACEK, RJ: *The lowering of plasma cholesterol by sucrose polyester in subjects consuming diets with 800, 300 or less than 50 mg of cholesterol per day.* Am J Clin Nutr 32:1636, 1979.

69. MABUCHI, H, HABA, T, TATAMI, R, ET AL: *Effects of an inhibitor of 3-hydroxy-3-methylglutaryl coenzyme A reductase on serum lipoproteins and ubiquinone—10 levels in patients with familial hypercholesterolemia.* N Engl J Med 305:478, 1981.

70. BROWN, MS AND GOLDSTEIN, JL: *Lowering plasma cholesterol by raising LDL receptors.* N Engl J Med 305:515, 1981.

71. *American Druggist Blue Book.* Hearst Corp, New York, 1981.

The Therapy for Infective Endocarditis

Reuben Ramphal, M.D., and Joseph W. Shands, Jr., M.D.

Infective endocarditis, whether caused by a virulent pathogen or by a relatively avirulent commensal organism, is a lethal disease when untreated. Even when treated appropriately, the morbidity and mortality can be substantial. Not only is the risk of physical disability great, the economic impact can be devastating. Four to 6 weeks of hospitalization coupled with loss of income for a similar period can be a serious economic setback. Furthermore, therapeutic failure that necessitates an even lengthier course of therapy, with or without cardiac surgery, may easily push the dollar cost of illness as high as $30,000. For these reasons, the treatment of infective endocarditis is a very serious matter.

APPROACH TO THE PATIENT WITH SUSPECTED ENDOCARDITIS

Diagnosis

Because of the wide variety of bacteria that may cause endocarditis and because of their varying susceptibilities to antibiotics, it is obviously of extreme importance to isolate the causative organism. This information is needed for diagnosis and for appropriate therapy. In fact, the definitive diagnosis of endocarditis depends on data from blood cultures, because the clinical features of infective endocarditis are nonspecific and may be mimicked by other disorders.[1]

A continuous bacteremia is characteristic of bacterial endocarditis. When the result of one blood culture is positive, usually all subsequent culture results are positive.[2] For diagnostic purposes, a number of blood cultures sufficient to document continuous bacteremia should be taken in the first few hours. In our opinion, a sufficient number is three. Because the bacteremia is continuous, one need not synchronize the cultures with fever spikes, but each culture should come from a separate venipuncture to avoid the risk of uniform contamination.

Blood culture results in bacterial endocarditis are usually positive in more than 90 percent of the cases.[3,4] Occasionally, microbial growth will be delayed or inhibited by prior antibiotic therapy or delayed by the fastidious nature of the infecting microorganism.[5] When the initial cultures are negative after 24 hours of incubation, another set of three cultures should be taken to help establish the diagnosis. Rarely will more than six cultures be required from the symptomatic, febrile patient. If, however, the patient has received antibiotics and has become asymptomatic, one may have to wait for the recrudescence of symptoms to obtain positive culture results.

In some cases of infective endocarditis, culture results are uniformly negative. These include infections by Coxiella burnetii, which cannot be cultured on artificial media; by Histoplasma capsulatum[6]; and by molds, such as Aspergillus,[7] in which the intertwining of the hyphae with the fibrin clot probably prevents the loss of small fragments that ordinarily would pass through the capillary circulation to be picked up by venipuncture.

Use of the Microbiologic Data Base

The identification of the infecting microorganism and the determination of its sensitivity to antibiotics are data that are essential for rational medical management. Every attempt must be made to isolate the causative organism and identify the genus and species. The reported isolation of "staphylococci" or "streptococci" is not sufficient information for the clinician to define optimal therapy. Moreover, the organism that has been isolated must be retained by the laboratory for a period of 2 to 3 months, to be used to monitor the therapy or to re-evaluate therapy if there is a relapse. Facilities for identification and sensitivity testing are available in any accredited microbiology laboratory. Additional data, however, may or may not be available, depending on the sophistication of the laboratory or the interest of the infectious disease consultant.

Minimal inhibitory concentrations of antibiotics (MICs) for the infecting microorganism are available in most but not all laboratories. The determination of minimal bactericidal concentrations of antibiotics (MBCs) are somewhat less available, as are the determination of the bacteriostatic and bactericidal power of serum and the testing of antibiotic synergy. In some institutions, all of these tests are performed routinely for management of endocarditis, and modulations of therapy are based on the results.[8] This laudable scientific approach to antibiotic therapy may optimize therapeutic benefits. We offer the caveat, however, that none of these tests singly or collectively is a "gold standard" and that "optimizing" therapy according to these tests is no guarantee of success. We assume that the use of these tests increases the chance of successful therapy. However, there are currently no compelling data indicating that this assumption is correct.

Empiric antibiotic regimens have been established for the major causes of infective endocarditis. The choice of the appropriate regimen depends on the identification of the causative organism and the pattern of antibiotic sensitivity and resistance. Resistance to antibiotics detectable by routine sensitivity tests usually is mediated by one of several possible mechanisms, that is, enzymes that inactivate the antibiotic, alterations in permeability to the antibiotic, or a mutation in the binding site of the antibiotic.[9] These mechanisms produce high-level resistance and necessitate the choice of alternative therapy.

A more subtle form of antibiotic resistance has been described in recent years and has been termed "tolerance." The growth of bacteria that exhibit "tolerance" is readily inhibited by an antibiotic, but the bacteria are less readily killed.[10] Tolerance cannot be detected by MICs alone, because the phenomenon is defined by a difference between the minimal inhibitory concentration of the antibiotic (MIC) and the minimal bactericidal concentration of the antibiotic (MBC). Although various values of the MBC/MIC ratio have been used to define tolerance, the minimum value used has been 8.[11] The phenomenon of tolerance can be determined in the clinical laboratory by comparing the MIC and the MBC of antibiotics for the causative organism. By testing a variety of antibiotics, one can usually find an antibiotic to which the organism is not tolerant. Alternatively, one can assess the bacteriostatic and bactericidal power of the patient's serum against the causative organism after the institution of therapy. This approach will detect tolerance and also will provide some quantitation of the adequacy of the antibiotic in the blood. The influence of the phenomenon of tolerance on the therapeutic response to antibiotics has not been clarified. There are reports suggesting that tolerance results in a higher incidence of therapeutic failure.[11,12] Conversely, other investigators have questioned the influence of the phenomenon on the effectiveness of therapy.[13] In any event, when tolerant bacteria are encountered, one can usually select an alternative antibiotic to which the bacterium is not tolerant, or one can add an additional antibiotic to the regimen to boost the bactericidal titer of the serum.

In general, one tends to be reassured that antibiotic therapy for infective endocarditis is adequate if the bactericidal titer of the serum is 1:8 or greater—a value that has usually been associated with successful therapy.[14] If the titer is less than 1:8, one either increases the amount of antibiotic administered or adds an additional antibiotic. The bactericidal power of the serum is then retested to determine "adequacy." Because there are uncertainties in the interpretation of the bactericidal power of blood, the results of the test should be used only as one of many pieces of data to judge the "adequacy" of therapy. There are known instances in which bacteria can be cultured from blood in the presence of a bactericidal titer of 1:8.[15] Conversely, it is quite possible that therapy may be effective even at titers less than 1:8.

In vitro antibiotic synergy studies are expensive, time consuming, usually unavailable, and rarely needed, even in enterococcal endocarditis in which combination antimicrobial therapy is always used. The potential synergy of streptomycin (but not necessarily all aminoglycosides) with penicillin can be predicted by the sensitivity of the bacterium to the aminoglycoside alone. Synergy with streptomycin occurs when the sensitivity is $<2000\ \mu g/ml$.[16]

Monitoring Therapy

Clinical and Bacteriologic Response. Once the antimicrobial therapy is "optimized" in accord with the microbiologic data base, the patient with endocarditis must be followed carefully to determine that the regimen is indeed effective. The rates of "normalization" of signs of inflammation will vary among individuals with the same infecting organism and will differ with different causative agents. For instance, the fever associated with endocarditis caused by Streptococcus viridans may subside within a day or two of the institution of therapy, whereas that associated with endocarditis due to Staphylococcus may require a week to normalize.[17] Therefore, it is important to determine early that sterilization of the blood is actually accomplished by the antibiotics. During the first week of therapy, several blood cultures should be taken. With some exceptions, persistently positive culture results suggest either inappropriate therapy, inadequate therapy, or a complication such as abscess formation in a valve ring. Negative blood culture results, decreasing fever and malaise, and with time a lowering of the blood sedimentation rate and the level of rheumatoid factor, if present, indicate that microbial growth and bacteremia have been suppressed. One should keep in mind, however, that suppression of bacteremia and symptoms does not mean that a cure necessarily follows.

If potentially toxic antibiotics are used, for instance, gentamicin, blood levels should be monitored periodically to ensure that excessive levels are not achieved. Because there may be changing renal function during endocarditis and its therapy, these levels should be obtained soon after beginning therapy and every fourth day thereafter.

Watching for Complications. Valvular destruction, myocardial abscesses, and embolism are the major complications that lead to morbidity and death in patients with infective endocarditis. Patients should be watched closely for signs of valvular destruction, arrhythmias, pericarditis, and congestive heart failure. The development of congestive heart failure that is not easily controlled medically is a major indication for surgical intervention. Similarly, the development of arrhythmias or pericarditis, particularly in association with an infected aortic valve, suggests the occurrence of myocardial abscess or a ring abscess that may require surgical intervention.[18]

The Role of Surgery in Endocarditis

Without question, cardiac surgery plays a prominent role in the management of infective endocarditis. A cardiovascular surgeon should at least be made aware of the cases undergoing

Table 1. Major criteria for early surgery in infective endocarditis

1. Progressive heart failure
2. Heart failure that fails to resolve on medical therapy
3. Multiple emboli
4. Uncontrolled bacteremia
5. Fungal infection
6. Development of conduction defects or pericarditis
7. Prosthetic valve dehiscence or obstruction
8. Relapse after "adequate" antibiotic therapy

medical management, and optimally should be part of the team caring for such patients. There are accepted general guidelines that govern surgical intervention in infective endocarditis. These guidelines have been established in institutions where there is ample expertise in cardiovascular surgery and where the results of such surgery have been good. Obviously, one needs to compare medical versus surgical risk in one's own setting. The latter may vary considerably from hospital to hospital, and this fact should temper the aggressiveness with which valve replacement is approached. Unfortunately, an assessment of surgical risk is sometimes difficult to obtain.

An excellent review of the role of surgery in infective endocarditis has been provided by Dinubile.[19] He has suggested major and minor criteria for early surgery in infective endocarditis. The criteria outlined in Tables 1 and 2 are among those listed by Dinubile.[19] He has suggested that the presence of one major criterion mandates surgical intervention. The presence of two or three of the minor criteria necessitates serious consideration of surgical intervention.

The Test of Cure

The gold standard of microbiologic cure of the patient with infective endocarditis is the demonstration of the absence of signs and symptoms and the lack of positive blood cultures after the cessation of antibiotic therapy. When therapy fails, symptoms may return and blood cultures may become positive within a day or two, or relapse may occur after several weeks but usually before 2 months.[20] Generally, patients should be observed in the hospital for 2 days after the cessation of therapy, and blood cultures obtained each week for 2 months. These cultures should be obtained even if the patient remains asymptomatic. Patients should also be advised to record their afternoon temperature daily during this interval, and they should report any febrile episodes or symptoms.

Prevention of Recurrence

Inadequate attention often is given to the prevention of recurrent endocarditis. Patients with endocarditis due to viridans streptococci should have a dental evaluation while on ther-

Table 2. Minor criteria for early surgery in infective endocarditis

1. Heart failure that resolves on medical therapy
2. Single embolus
3. Vegetation demonstrated by M-mode echocardiography
4. Early mitral valve closure or flail leaflets
5. Early prosthetic endocarditis caused by organisms insensitive to penicillin
6. Persistent symptoms without other identifiable cause
7. Resistance to or inability to use bactericidal antibiotics

Table 3. Procedures requiring antibiotic prophylaxis

Oral Cavity
1. Any dental manipulation, including dental prophylaxis
2. Endoscopy with rigid instruments
3. Surgery of the upper respiratory tract

Genitourinary
1. Urethral instrumentation or catheterization
2. Prostatectomy
3. Gynecologic instrumentation or surgery

Gastrointestinal
1. Surgery or instrumentation with biopsy

Skin
1. Incision and drainage of abscesses

apy, and if dental procedures are needed, these should be done prior to the cessation of therapy. Similarly, patients should be educated concerning antibiotic prophylaxis for endocarditis. They should have an understanding of the sorts of procedures that require prophylaxis and should be advised to inform dentists and other medical professionals they visit about their potential needs for prophylaxis.

Procedures that are very likely to result in bacteremia and therefore increase the risk of infective endocarditis are those that traumatize mucosal surfaces laden with the indigenous microflora. The sorts of procedures that should require prophylaxis are listed in Table 3. Although other procedures also increase the risk of bacteremia, for example, sigmoidoscopy, colonoscopy, and barium enema, there are currently no data associating these procedures with endocarditis.

Although the effectiveness of antibiotic prophylaxis for endocarditis is unknown, very specific suggestions have been made. The data to show adequacy or inadequacy of the current regimens are now being collected. The current recommendations of the American Heart Association[21] are listed in Tables 4 and 5.

Table 4. Prophylaxis of infective endocarditis for dental procedures or surgery of the upper respiratory tract

Regimens for adults without prosthetic valves:

I. *Without Penicillin Allergy*

Aqueous crystalline penicillin G 1,000,000 units plus 600,000 units procaine penicillin I.M. 30 to 60 min prior to procedure followed by penicillin V 500 mg po q 6 h for 8 doses

or

Penicillin V 2.0 gm po 30 to 60 min prior to procedure followed by 500 mg penicillin V po q 6 h for 8 doses

II. *Penicillin Allergy*

Vancomycin 1 gm I.V. 30 to 60 min prior to procedure followed by erythromycin 500 mg po q 6 h for 8 doses

or

Erythromycin 1.0 gm orally 90 to 120 min prior to procedure followed by 500 mg po q 6 h for 8 doses

Regimens for adults with prosthetic valves:

I. *Without Penicillin Allergy*

Aqueous crystalline penicillin G 1,000,000 units plus 600,000 units procaine penicillin I.M.

PLUS

Streptomycin 1 gm I.M. 30 to 60 min prior to procedure followed by erythromycin 500 mg po q 6 h for 8 doses

II. *Penicillin Allergy*

Vancomycin 1 gm I.V. 30 to 60 min prior to procedure followed by erythromycin 500 mg po q 6 h for 8 doses

Table 5. Prophylaxis of infective endocarditis for gastrointestinal and genitourinary procedures

Regimens for Adults:

I. *Without Penicillin Allergy*

Aqueous crystalline penicillin G 2,000,000 units I.M. or I.V. 30 to 60 min prior to procedure

or

Ampicillin 1.0 gm I.M. or I.V.

PLUS

Gentamicin 1.5 mg/kg I.M. or I.V.

or

Streptomycin 1.0 gm I.M.

II. *Penicillin Allergy*

Vancomycin 1.0 gm I.V.

PLUS

Streptomycin 1.0 gm I.M. 30 to 60 min prior to procedure

SPECIFIC THERAPY

Rationale for Bactericidal Antibiotics and Prolonged Therapy

The inability of the "normal" host to eradicate an intravascular focus of infection, even when caused by relatively avirulent microorganisms, is well known and suggests that such foci occupy an immunologically privileged site. Examination of valves infected experimentally in animal models of endocarditis and even "naturally" infected valves removed from humans may show few inflammatory cells in the vegetation per se.[22,23] The reasons for the latter are not established. It has been assumed that the fibrin-platelet meshwork harboring the infecting microorganisms provides some sort of barrier against inflammatory cells.[24] However, it is more likely that circulatory dynamics in the heart or in larger vessels prevent the establishment of chemotactic gradients that are essential for the attraction of inflammatory cells.

Regardless of reasons behind the failure of host defenses in endocarditis, the practical conclusion to be gained from this failure is that successful therapy depends on the use of appropriate *bactericidal* antibiotics. In fact, therapeutic trials with bacteriostatic agents in the past have shown them to be relatively ineffective.[25] Bacteriostatic antibiotics should never be used in endocarditis except in those cases caused by organisms such as Coxiella that are not susceptible to bactericidal antibiotics.

Clinical experience has shown that successful therapy for infective endocarditis depends on prolonged antibiotic therapy, and in some instances the duration of therapy appears to be more important than the dosage of antibiotic.[20] The experimental models of infective endocarditis provide a possible explanation for this observation. They have shown that within a relatively brief time after the induction of endocarditis, the concentration of microbes in the vegetation reaches a maximum.[26] At this point, it appears that most of the microbes deep within the vegetation are in the stationary phase of growth and are therefore insusceptible to antibiotics that inhibit cell-wall biosynthesis.[27] As a result, one would expect that brief treatment with antibiotics would leave a nidus of resting but viable organisms that could lead to relapse.

Streptococcal Endocarditis

The rational approach to the treatment of endocarditis due to streptococci requires a basic understanding of the classification of the streptococci. This is an area of considerable taxonomic confusion. Hence, a simplified version is presented for the clinician (Table 6). The main

Table 6. Classification of streptococci

Penicillin-Sensitive	*Relatively Pencillin-Resistant*	*Penicillin-Resistant*
α-Streptococci (S. viridans)	α-Streptococci isolated from patients on rheumatic fever prophylaxis	Enterococci
β-Streptococci (A, B, C, E, F, etc.)		
Non-enterococcal Group D streptococci	Some strains of S. bovis and S. mitior	

point of distinction is the division between penicillin-sensitive and penicillin-resistant organisms. The names used do not necessarily correspond to well-defined species but to the names commonly used in descriptions of this group of bacteria.

Penicillin-Sensitive Streptocci (Viridans, Non-Group D, β-Hemolytic, and Non-Enterococcal Group D Streptococci)

The streptococci commonly called "viridans" or α-hemolytic streptococci are responsible for the majority of cases of infective endocarditis in a nonaddict population. A vast amount of experience has been acquired in the treatment of this type of endocarditis. The first reports of successful therapy with penicillin appeared in 1944.[28] It became very clear in the early trials that moderate doses of penicillin for a moderate length of time were required for cure.[20] The exceptional patient was cured with low doses given for a short time.[20] The next improvement in the management of this type of endocarditis occurred after the demonstration of in vitro synergy with penicillin and streptomycin.[29] Clinical trials in the early 1950s quickly confirmed the efficacy of this combination in vivo.[30,31]

Today, there are three acceptable regimens for treating endocarditis due to penicillin-sensitive streptococci (Table 7). Controlled trials comparing these regimens have not been done and are hardly necessary, because all three are recognized as effective by the majority of authorities in this field. With any of these regimens, the bacteriologic cure rate is usually in excess of 90 percent.[32] The advantages of the 2-week regimen are clearly economic and psychologic. This regimen is likely to gain more favor in view of the tenuous economic situation of the health-care system. The American Heart Association does not recommend 2-week therapy for patients with complications, for example, shock, extracardiac foci of infection, and prosthetic valve infection, or for those infected with unusual, nutritionally deficient variants of viridans streptococci.[32] It must be kept in mind that in patients with some degree of renal dysfunction, streptomycin may be ototoxic unless the dose is altered.

For patients with a major allergy to penicillin (anaphylaxis, wheezing), vancomycin 10 mg/kg (maximum 500 mg) I.V. every 6 hours for 4 weeks may be used instead of penicillin. In cases of minor allergy, a first-generation cephalosporin such as cefazolin or cephalothin may be used for 4 weeks. There is no extensive experience with the use of cephalosporins and streptomycin in 2-week regimens. During therapy it is imperative that microbial sensitivity to these alternate drugs or the serum bactericidal titer with these agents be ascertained, as in all forms of therapy for endocarditis.

Table 7. Antibiotic regimens for penicillin-sensitive streptococci[32]

Regimen I:	Penicillin G 10–20 × 10^6 units I.V. a day for 4 weeks
Regimen II:	Penicillin G* 10–20 × 10^6 units a day I.V. for 4 weeks; streptomycin 10 mg/kg I.M. (maximum 500 mg) every 12 hours for 2 weeks
Regimen III:	Penicillin G* 10–20 × 10^6 units I.V. a day for 2 weeks; streptomycin 10 mg/kg I.M. (maximum 500 mg) every 12 hours for 2 weeks

*Procaine penicillin 1.2 × 10^6 units I.M. every 6 hours may be used in regimens II and III in lieu of penicillin G.

Relatively Penicillin-Resistant Streptococci

These streptococci have been recognized to cause endocarditis in the setting of rheumatic fever prophylaxis[33] as well as in untreated persons. At the New York Hospital the frequency of these organisms from cases of endocarditis has been about 20 percent.[34] The most frequent isolates are strains of S. mitis and S. sanguis (oral organisms falling within the appellation of Streptococcus viridans), and some strains of S. bovis, an organism related to colonic cancer in some obscure way.[35] Although these organisms have been called relatively penicillin-resistant (i.e., MIC $> 0.1\ \mu g/ml$), the use of penicillin alone or in combination with streptomycin has resulted in microbiologic cure. The documented experience with these bacteria has not been large, but it appears that high doses of penicillin, 12 to 20 $\times 10^6$ units daily for up to 30 days, or lower doses in combination with streptomycin (10 mg/kg, maximum 500 mg I.M.) twice a day for 2 weeks have been used successfully.[36] Experience indicates that the longer-term therapy used to treat enterococcal endocarditis is not required for these bacteria, but the American Heart Association does recommend penicillin G 20 $\times 10^6$ units I.V. daily and streptomycin 10 mg/kg I.M. (maximum dose 500 mg) twice a day for 4 weeks.[32] The need for this very conservative approach has not been supported by case studies. The penicillin-allergic patient may receive vancomycin where there is a major penicillin allergy, or a first-generation cephalosporin where there is minor allergy (rash).

Penicillin-Resistant Streptococci (Enterococci)

Enterococci possess a high degree of intrinsic resistance to penicillin. Hence, the therapeutic approach to enterococcal endocarditis is quite different. Even with relatively large doses of penicillin, the treatment results were poor. There were occasional cures, but most patients relapsed after penicillin therapy.[37] Although ampicillin has greater activity against enterococci than does penicillin, both cures and failures occurred when ampicillin was used in this condition.[38] Thus, neither penicillin nor ampicillin is recommended as sole therapy for enterococcal endocarditis.

The regimen associated with the highest success rates was first used in 1947 by Hunter.[39] Subsequently, many other investigators have confirmed that penicillin combined with streptomycin results in a cure rate of about 85 percent.[40] Some controversy exists as to whether this combination is feasible when there is high-level resistance to streptomycin ($> 2000\ \mu g/ml$). For this reason, some advocate the use of gentamicin instead of streptomycin.[41] On theoretical grounds, gentamicin would seem to offer an advantage because these streptomycin-resistant enterococci are almost always gentamicin-sensitive (MIC $< 2000\ \mu g/ml$),[42] but it should be borne in mind that despite 25 to 50 percent streptomycin resistance among enterococci from endocarditis,[42] there are very few documented failures with streptomycin.[43] The recommended regimens are interchangeable (Table 8).

The important point in choosing any regimen is to document that the generally accepted serum bactericidal titer is attainable. Ampicillin 12 gm/day may be substituted for penicillin. Vancomycin is an acceptable replacement for penicillin where there is minor or major allergy. Cephalosporins should not be used as penicillin substitutes in enterococcal endocarditis

Table 8. Treatment regimens for enterococcal endocarditis[46]

Penicillin 20 $\times 10^6$ units I.V. daily for 6 weeks
PLUS
Streptomycin 10 mg/kg I.M. (maximum dose 500 mg) every 12 hours
or
Gentamicin 1 mg/kg I.M. or I.V. every 8 hours for 6 weeks

because of the high MICs of this group of antibiotics[44] and their documented lack of effectiveness.[45] Although 6 weeks is the commonly recommended length of therapy, some argue that 4 weeks is sufficient therapy.[46] If there are mitigating circumstances, for example, unacceptable drug toxicity or economic hardship, or if the course is uncomplicated, we see no reason why 4 weeks cannot be used.

Staphylococcal Endocarditis

Endocarditis due to Staphylococcus aureus ranks next in frequency after that due to streptococci. S. aureus has been notoriously difficult to treat and is often associated with suppurative complications.[47] It is the most common cause of endocarditis in narcotic addicts, but it is also acquired as a nosocomial infection and less commonly in the community in nonaddicts. There appears to have been an increase in the incidence of this disease in recent decades. It should be realized that this disease has a fatality rate higher than the other major forms of endocarditis. The mortality rate is between 25 and 50 percent even with "effective" therapy. This type of endocarditis is often "acute," and it is recommended that treatment be started immediately after blood cultures have been drawn. Besides the propensity to cause metastatic suppurative complications, certain other features should be appreciated: (1) patients may remain bacteremic between 3 and 5 days after the onset of therapy; (2) fever may persist for up to a week after initiation of therapy; and (3) valvular destruction may occur even with initiation of appropriate treatment.

Staphylococcal endocarditis has been treated with semisynthetic penicillins for some time, but despite the sensitivity of the organism to these drugs, the failure rate has been much higher than in other forms of endocarditis. The addition of an aminoglycoside to nafcillin in vitro[48] and in vivo in animal models[49] demonstrated more rapid and complete killing of these organisms. Hence, it was reasonable to believe that this combination might be more efficacious in the treatment of staphylococcal endocarditis. Several clinical studies have now addressed this issue.[50–52] Watanakunakorn and Baird[50] reported a retrospective study that showed that the addition of gentamicin to penicillin was no better than penicillin alone, both groups having a mortality of 40 percent. Abrams and coworkers[51] compared a β-lactam drug with the combination of a β-lactam and gentamicin in a group of addicts with staphylococcal endocarditis and showed that the outcome was equally good in both groups (zero mortality). More recently, Sande and Korzeniowski[52] reported the results of a multicenter trial that showed a similar low mortality in addicts, using either regimen, and a 22 to 30 percent mortality in nonaddicts with or without the addition of an aminoglycoside. This latter study showed that the combination chemotherapy sterilized the blood faster in right-sided endocar-

Table 9. Therapy for staphylococcal endocarditis

I. *Methicillin-sensitive*
Nafcillin 8–12 gm/day I.V. for 4 weeks
or
Oxacillin 8–12 gm/day I.V. for 4 weeks
or
Methicillin 12–16 gm/day I.V. for 4 weeks
II. *Methicillin-resistant*
Vancomycin 2 gm/day for 4 weeks
III. *Tolerant*
Semisynthetic penicillin ± vancomycin for 4–6 weeks
or
Semisynthetic penicillin + rifampin or gentamicin for 4–6 weeks
or
Vancomycin + rifampin for 4–6 weeks

ditis, and reduced the number of febrile days on therapy from 7 to 3. However, patients receiving aminoglycosides suffered more renal toxicity. Although there may have been difficulties in stratifying patients in such a multicenter trial, it may be concluded that the addition of the aminoglycoside, despite earlier sterilization of the blood, cannot be recommended as routine therapy because it adds little to the eventual outcome and is potentially nephrotoxic.

The multicenter trial also compared 4 weeks of therapy with 6 weeks of therapy and could find no difference in outcome. However, if there is a suspicion of metastatic complications, 6 weeks of treatment may be required (Table 9).

Patients with minor allergies to penicillin can receive a first-generation cephalosporin such as cephalothin 8 to 12 gm/day or cefazolin 6 to 8 gm/day. Patients with a major allergy should receive vancomycin 2 gm/day.

Staphylococcal Endocarditis due to Resistant Staphylococci

Staphylococci have proven to be extremely versatile bacteria in evolving resistance to penicillins. In addition to β-lactamase production, these organisms have evolved two other major forms of antimicrobial resistance that are of great concern in the treatment of staphylococcal endocarditis. The first form, called methicillin-type resistance, is now a serious emergent problem in this country.[53] The second form, called "tolerance," has been recently recognized,[10] but its significance is not totally clear.[13] It must be pointed out, however, that at least two studies report that patients infected with tolerant staphylococci suffer more complications[11,12] than those with nontolerant staphylococci. When there is the methicillin type of resistance, it is recommended that vancomycin be used.[54] If the staphylococcal strain is tolerant, it is prudent to achieve reasonable serum bactericidal activity by increasing the dose of the semisynthetic penicillin, or by using vancomycin instead. However, tolerance may extend across the pencillins, cephalosporins, and even to vancomycin; in such a case, one may have to resort to the addition of rifampin and/or aminoglycosides.[55] The adequacy of any combination should be verified by serum bactericidal activity.

Other Causes of Endocarditis

A whole host of other organisms cause endocarditis, but there is relatively limited clinical experience in dealing with the majority of these infections. The groups of organisms with which there is some experience are the fungi and aerobic gram-negative rods. It is noteworthy that both of these types of endocarditis occur almost solely in well-defined populations, that is, narcotic addicts or postoperatively following prosthetic valve insertion. A detailed discussion of these entities is beyond the scope of this review, but certain general statements can be made. The best results of medical therapy in gram-negative endocarditis (Pseudomonas aeruginosa, Serratia marcescens) were achieved with combination chemotherapy,[56,57] but left-sided disease appears to require adjunctive surgery in a fair percentage of cases.[57,58] Fungal endocarditis, on the other hand, almost always requires valve replacement, but even with combined medical and surgical therapy the survival rate is dismal.[7] If the diagnosis of fungal endocarditis is definite, surgery must be done urgently to reduce the risk of major embolization—a complication not uncommon in fungal endocarditis.[59] Any apparent medical cures of these two entities should be viewed with caution, and patients should be followed closely because relapse is frequent. After valve replacement, medical therapy should be continued for 6 weeks, limited only by the toxicity of the aminoglycoside in gram-negative endocarditis or amphotericin B in fungal endocarditis.

Besides these two groups of organisms, some other bacteria have been noted with increasing frequency. Several species of Haemophilus,[60] anaerobic bacteria,[61] and diphtheroids[62] have been reported in recent reviews; for completeness, the drugs of choice for these bacteria are indicated in the list in Table 10.

Table 10. Therapy for uncommon forms of endocarditis

Organism	*Regimen*
P. aeruginosa*[56]	Carbenicillin 30 gm/day plus Tobramycin or gentamicin 8 mg/kg/day
Serratia marcescens*[57]	Carbenicillin or cefoxitin or trimethoprim-sulfamethoxazole plus Gentamicin or tobramycin
Candida sp./Torulopsis[59]	Amphotericin B plus + Surgery 5-Flurocytosine
Aspergillus sp.[67,68]	Amphotericin B plus + Surgery 5-Flurocytosine or rifampin
Haemophilus sp.[69] H. aphrophilus	Penicillin + streptomycin
H. paraphrophilus H. parainfluenzae H. influenzae	Ampicillin† 8–12 gm/day
Diphtheroids[69]	Vancomycin 2 gm/day
Anaerobes[69]	High-dose penicillin (except B. fragilis) Metronidazole (B. fragilis)

*Left-sided disease will often require surgery.
†β-lactamase production by some of these strains may require change to a second- or third-generation cephalosporin.

Prosthetic Valve Endocarditis

This form of endocarditis is particularly difficult to treat for several reasons. Foreign bodies per se make eradication of infection by antimicrobial agents alone very difficult. In addition, the majority of organisms causing prosthetic valve endocarditis (PVE) are intrinsically difficult to eradicate. Therefore, the tendency has been to utilize surgery in many cases. The rationale for this approach can be appreciated by examining a recent compendium of some of the microorganisms causing early or late PVE (Table 11).[63]

In both early and late groups, there is a predominance of nonstreptococcal organisms that are notoriously difficult to treat even on native heart valves. Besides the presence of a foreign body and the microbial etiology of this condition that make treatment problematic, there is also a tendency to valve ring abscess formation between the seat of the prosthesis and the endocardium.[64] The old surgical adage that pus must be drained also applies to this situation. Most cases of PVE caused by non-enterococcal streptococci can be treated by regimens discussed earlier. The treatment of other types of PVE must be individualized. Certainly, heart failure is an accepted surgical indication, as well as major embolization and persistent infection, but the choice of surgical versus medical therapy for specific organisms remains contro-

Table 11. Etiology of prosthetic valve endocarditis[63]

Early (<60 days)		*Late (>60 days)*	
S. epidermidis	67%	S. epidermidis	24%
Diphtheroids	18%	Streptococci	21%
S. aureus	2.5%	Aerobic gram-negative rods	12%
Aerobic gram-negative rods	2.5%	S. aureus	9%
Fungi	2.5%	Diphtheroids	11%
Streptococci	2.5%	Enterococci	7.5%
		Fungi	4.5%

versial.[65] Fungal PVE is generally accepted as requiring early surgery,[59] but not all patients with staphylococcal endocarditis require surgery.[65] Early recognition of those who will require surgery should reduce the dismal prognosis of these patients. Relapse after an apparent medical cure of PVE often requires surgery.[66]

REFERENCES

1. Johnson, WD Jr: *The clinical syndrome.* In Kaye, D (ed): *Infective Endocarditis.* University Park Press, Baltimore, 1977.
2. Werner, AS, Cobbs, CG, Kaye, D, et al: *Studies on the bacteremia of bacterial endocarditis.* JAMA 202:199, 1967.
3. Belli, J and Waisbren, BA: *The number of blood cultures necessary to diagnose most cases of bacterial endocarditis.* Am J Med Sci 232:284, 1956.
4. Cannaday, PB Jr and Sanford, JP: *Negative blood cultures in infective endocarditis.* South Med J 69:1420, 1976.
5. Washington, JA II: *The role of the microbiology laboratory in the diagnosis and antimicrobial treatment of infective endocarditis.* Mayo Clin Proc 57:22, 1982.
6. Akbarian, M, Salfelder, K, and Schwarz, J: *Experimental histoplasmic endocarditis.* Arch Intern Med 114:784, 1964.
7. Rubinstein, E, Noriega, ER, Simberkoff, MD, et al: *Fungal endocarditis: Analysis of 24 cases and review of the literature.* Medicine (Baltimore) 54:331, 1975.
8. Wilson, WR, Giuliani, ER, Davidson, GK, et al: *General considerations in the diagnosis and treatment of infective endocarditis.* Mayo Clin Proc 57:81, 1982.
9. Davies, J: *General mechanisms of antimicrobial resistance.* Rev Infect Dis 1:23, 1979.
10. Sabath, LD, Wheeler, N, Laverdiere, M, et al: *A new type of penicillin resistance of Staphylococcus aureus.* Lancet 1:443, 1977.
11. Denny, AE, Peterson, LR, Gerding, DN, et al: *Serious staphylococcal infections with strains tolerant to bactericidal antibiotics.* Arch Intern Med 139:1026, 1979.
12. Rajashekaraiah, KR, Rice, T, Rao, VS, et al: *Clinical significance of tolerant strains of Staphylococcus aureus in patients with endocarditis.* Ann Intern Med 93:796, 1980.
13. Kaye, D: *The clinical significance of tolerance of Staphylococcus aureus.* Ann Intern Med 93:924, 1980.
14. Coleman, DL, Horwitz, RI, and Andriole, VT: *Association between serum inhibitory and bactericidal concentrations and therapeutic outcome in bacterial endocarditis.* Am J Med 73:260, 1982.
15. Reymann, MT, Holley, MP, and Cobbs, CG: *Persistent bacteremia in staphylococcal endocarditis.* Am J Med 65:729, 1978.
16. Moellering, RC, Korzeniowski, OM, Sande, MA, et al: *Species-specific resistance to antimicrobial synergism in Streptococcus faecium and Streptococcus faecalis.* J Infect Dis 140:203, 1979.
17. Thompson, RL: *Staphylococcal infective endocarditis.* Mayo Clin Proc 57:106, 1982.
18. Arnett, EN and Roberts, WC: *Valve ring abscess in active infective endocarditis: Frequency, location, and clues to clinical diagnosis from the study of 95 necropsy patients.* Circulation 54:140, 1976.
19. Dinubile, MJ: *Surgery in active endocarditis.* Ann Intern Med 96:650, 1982.
20. Cates, JE and Christie, RV: *Subacute bacterial endocarditis.* Q J Med 20:93, 1951.
21. American Heart Association, Committee on Rheumatic Fever and Bacterial Endocarditis: *Prevention of bacterial endocarditis.* Circulation 56:139A, 1977.
22. Spain, DM: *Endocarditis.* In Gould, SE: *Pathology of the Heart.* Charles C Thomas, Springfield, Ill, 1968.
23. Sande, MA, Bowman, CR, and Calderone, RA: *Experimental Candida albicans endocarditis: Characterization of the disease and response to therapy.* Infect Immun 17:140, 1977.
24. Friedman, M, Katz, LN, and Howell, K: *Experimental endocarditis due to Streptococcus viridans: Biologic factors in its development.* Arch Intern Med 61:95, 1938.
25. Durack, DT: *Review of early experience in treatment of bacterial endocarditis, 1940–1955.* In Bisno, HL (ed): *Treatment of Infective Endocarditis.* Grune & Stratton, New York, 1981.
26. Durack, DT and Beeson, PB: *Experimental bacterial endocarditis I. Colonization of a sterile vegetation.* Br J Exp Pathol 53:44, 1972.
27. Durack, DT and Beeson, BP: *Experimental bacterial endocarditis II. Survival of bacteria in endocardial vegetations.* Br J Exp Pathol 53:50, 1972.
28. Loewe, L, Rosenblatt, P, Greene, HJ, et al: *Combination penicillin heparin therapy of subacute bacterial endocarditis: Report of seven consecutive successfully treated patients.* JAMA 124:144, 1944.

29. Hunter, TH: *Speculations on the mechanism of cure of bacterial endocarditis.* JAMA 144:524, 1950.

30. Geraci, JE and Martin, WJ: *Antibiotic therapy of bacterial endocarditis: IV. Successful short term (2 weeks) combined penicillin-dihydrostreptomycin therapy in subacute bacterial endocarditis caused by penicillin sensitive streptococci.* Circulation 8:494, 1953.

31. Hall, B, Dowling, HF, and Kellow, W: *Successful short term therapy of streptococcal endocarditis with penicillin and streptomycin.* Am J Med Sci 230:73, 1955.

32. American Heart Association Committee Report: *Treatment of infective endocarditis due to viridans streptococci.* Circulation 63:730A, 1981.

33. Parillo, JR, Borst, GC, Mazur, MH, et al: *Endocarditis due to resistant viridans streptococci during oral penicillin chemoprophylaxis.* N Engl J Med 300:296, 1979.

34. Roberts, RB, Krieger, AG, Schiller, NL, et al: *Viridans streptococcal endocarditis: The role of various species including pyridoxal-dependent streptococci.* Rev Infect Dis 1:955, 1979.

35. Klein, RS, Catalans, MT, Edberg, SC, et al: *Streptococcus bovis septicemia and carcinoma of the colon.* Ann Intern Med 91:560, 1979.

36. Karchmer, A: *Issues in the treatment of endocarditis caused by viridans streptococci.* In Bisno, AL (ed): *Treatment of Infective Endocarditis.* Grune & Stratton, New York, 1981.

37. Loewe, L, Candel, S, and Eiber, HB: *Therapy of subacute enterococcus (Streptococcus faecalis) endocarditis.* Ann Intern Med 34:717, 1951.

38. Mandell, GL, Kaye, D, Levison, MD, et al: *Enterococcal endocarditis: An analysis of 38 patients observed at the New York Hospital-Cornell Medical Center.* Arch Intern Med 125:258, 1970.

39. Hunter, TH: *Use of streptomycin in treatment of bacterial endocarditis.* Am J Med 2:436, 1947.

40. Jawetz, E and Sonne, M: *Penicillin-streptomycin treatment of enterococcal endocarditis: A reevaluation.* N Engl J Med 274:710, 1966.

41. Watt, B: *Streptococcal endocarditis: A penicillin alone or a penicillin with an aminoglycoside.* J Antimicrob Chemother 4:107, 1978.

42. Calderwood, SA, Wennersten, C, Moellering, RC, et al: *Resistance to six aminoglycosidic aminocyclitol antibiotics among enterococci: Prevalence, evolution and relationship to synergism with penicillin.* Antimicrob Agents Chemother 12:401, 1977.

43. Tompsett, R and Berman, W: *Enterococcal endocarditis: Duration and mode of treatment.* Trans Am Clin Climatol Assoc 89:49, 1977.

44. Toala, P, McDonald, A, Wilcox, C, et al: *Susceptibility of group D streptococcus (enterococcus) to 21 antibiotics in vitro with special reference to species differences.* Am J Med Sci 258:416, 1969.

45. Rahal, JJ, Myers, PR, and Weinstein, L: *Treatment of bacterial endocarditis with cephalothin.* N Engl J Med 279:1305, 1968.

46. Kaye, D: *Treatment of enterococcal endocarditis in experimental animals and man.* In Bisno, AL (ed): *Treatment of Infective Endocarditis.* Grune & Stratton, New York, 1981.

47. Watanakunakorn, C, Tan, JS, and Phair, JP: *Some salient features of Staphylococcus aureus endocarditis.* Am J Med 54:473, 1973.

48. Watanakunakorn, C and Glotzbecker, C: *Enhancement of the effects of anti-staphylococcal antibiotics by aminoglycosides.* Antimicrob Agents Chemother 6:802, 1974.

49. Sande, M and Johnson, M: *Antimicrobial therapy of experimental endocarditis caused by Staphylococcus aureus.* J Infect Dis 131:367, 1975.

50. Watanakunakorn, C and Baird, IM: *Prognostic factors in Staphylococcus aureus endocarditis and results of therapy with a penicillin and gentamicin.* Am J Med Sci 273:133, 1977.

51. Abrams, B, Sklaver, A, Hoffman, T, et al: *Single or combination therapy of staphylococcal endocarditis in intravenous drug abusers.* Ann Intern Med 90:789, 1979.

52. Korzeniowski, O, Sande, MA, and The National Collaborative Study Group: *Combination antimicrobial therapy for Staphylococcus aureus endocarditis in patients addicted to parenteral drugs and in non addicts.* Ann Intern Med 97:496, 1982.

53. Wenzel, RP: *Editorial: The emergence of methicillin resistant Staphylococcus aureus.* Ann Intern Med 97:440, 1982.

54. Levine, DP, Cushing, RD, Jui, T, et al: *Community acquired methicillin-resistant Staphylococcus aureus endocarditis in the Detroit Medical Center.* Ann Intern Med 97:330, 1982.

55. Sande, MA and Scheld, WM: *Combination antibiotic therapy of bacterial endocarditis.* Ann Intern Med 92:390, 1980.

56. Reyes, MP, Brown, WJ, and Lerner, AM: *Treatment of patients with pseudomonas endocarditis with high dose aminoglycoside and carbenicillin therapy.* Medicine (Baltimore) 57:57, 1978.

57. Cooper, R and Mills, J: *Serratia endocarditis.* Arch Intern Med 140:199, 1980.

58. LEVITSKY, S, MAMMANA, RB, SILVERMAN, NA, ET AL: *Acute endocarditis in drug addicts: Surgical treatment for gram-negative sepsis.* Circulation 66:I-135, 1982.

59. McLEOD, R AND REMINGTON, JS: *Post operative fungal endocarditis.* In DUMA, RJ (ED): *Infections of Prosthetic Valves and Vascular Grafts.* University Park Press, Baltimore, 1977.

60. ELLNER, JJ, ROSENTHAL, MS, LERNER, PI, ET AL: *Infective endocarditis caused by slow-growing, fastidious, gram-negative bacteria.* Medicine (Baltimore) 58:145, 1979.

61. FELLNER, JM AND DOWELL, VR JR: *Anaerobic bacterial endocarditis.* N Engl J Med 283:1188, 1970.

62. GERRY, JL AND GREENOUGH, WB III: *Diphtheroid endocarditis: Report of nine cases and a review of the literature.* Johns Hopkins Med J 139:61, 1976.

63. DISMUKES, WE: *Prosthetic valve endocarditis: Factors influencing outcome and recommendations for therapy.* In BISNO, AL (ED): *Treatment of Infective Endocarditis.* Grune & Stratton, New York, 1981.

64. ARNETT, EM AND ROBERTS, WC: *Prosthetic valve endocarditis: Clinicopathologic analysis of 22 necropsy patients with comparison of observations in 74 necropsy patients with active endocarditis involving natural left sided cardiac valves.* Am J Cardiol 38:281, 1976.

65. RAPAPORT, E: *Editorial: The changing role of surgery in management of infective endocarditis.* Circulation 58:598, 1978.

66. KARCHMER, AW, DISMUKES, WE, BUCKLEY, MJ, ET AL: *Late prosthetic valve endocarditis: Clinical features influencing therapy.* Am J Med 64:199, 1978.

67. KAMMER, RB AND UTZ, JP: *Aspergillus species endocarditis.* Am J Med 56:506, 1974.

68. KITAHARA, M, SETH, VK, MEDOFF, G, ET AL: *Activity of amphotericin B, 5-flurocystosine and rifampin against six clinical isolates of aspergillus.* Antimicrob Agents Chemother 9:915, 1976.

69. WATANAKUNAKORN, C: *Antimicrobial therapy of endocarditis due to less common bacteria.* In BISNO, AL (ED): *Treatment of Infective Endocarditis.* Grune & Stratton, New York, 1981.

Index

An *italic* numeral indicates a figure. A "t" indicates a table.